MARKETING HEALTH

Marketing Health

Smoking and the Discourse of Public
Health in Britain, 1945–2000

VIRGINIA BERRIDGE

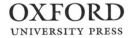

OXFORD
UNIVERSITY PRESS

OXFORD

UNIVERSITY PRESS

Great Clarendon Street, Oxford OX2 6DP

Oxford University Press is a department of the University of Oxford.
It furthers the University's objective of excellence in research, scholarship,
and education by publishing worldwide in

Oxford New York

Auckland Cape Town Dar es Salaam Hong Kong Karachi
Kuala Lumpur Madrid Melbourne Mexico City Nairobi
New Delhi Shanghai Taipei Toronto

With offices in

Argentina Austria Brazil Chile Czech Republic France Greece
Guatemala Hungary Italy Japan Poland Portugal Singapore
South Korea Switzerland Thailand Turkey Ukraine Vietnam

Oxford is a registered trade mark of Oxford University Press
in the UK and in certain other countries

Published in the United States
by Oxford University Press Inc., New York

British Library Cataloguing in Publication Data
Data available

Library of Congress Cataloging in Publication Data
Data available

Typeset by Laserwords Private Limited, Chennai, India
Printed in Great Britain
on acid-free paper by
Biddles Ltd., King's Lynn, Norfolk

ISBN 978–0–19–926030–0

1 3 5 7 9 10 8 6 4 2

For Geoff, Edward, and William

Acknowledgements

This book began life as a Wellcome Trust fellowship, awarded to me when I was a researcher on a short-term contract at the London School of Hygiene and Tropical Medicine (LSHTM) at the end of the AIDS Social History Programme, a research programme which was funded by the (then) Nuffield Provincial Hospitals Trust. Much has happened since, not least the expansion of my single temporary post into the Centre for History in Public Health at LSHTM and the development of a wide-ranging research programme. I have gained enormously from the insights of colleagues in the Centre and from the conferences and seminars organized there. In addition, my particular thanks go to Charles Webster, who has been an invaluable source of support throughout.

I would like to express my gratitude to the following people: Kelly Loughlin, who initially worked as a research assistant on HEA-funded projects and whose subsequent work on the early history of post-war public health has complemented my own interests; and Suzanne Taylor, who has helped greatly in checking and advising on all matters pertaining to technology. Penny Starns contributed through a pilot study of the Wills tobacco archive in Bristol Record Office, funded by the Wellcome Trust. My participation, as principal investigator, in the ESRC-funded study of voluntarism in the drugs field and the rise of the user group on which Alex Mold is research fellow has deepened my insights into voluntarism and its history. Ornella Moscucci made helpful suggestions for the book's title. Ingrid James has helped with the production of several versions of the book. Libraries have been of great use and here I thank the librarians of the London School of Hygiene, of the Wellcome Library for the History and Understanding of Medicine, of the British Library, and of the Royal College of Physicians.

The ASH archive, deposited in the Wellcome Library, has been invaluable, as have the National Archives and the archives of the Royal College of Physicians. The period in which the research has been undertaken has seen a greater official willingness for government papers to be made available. I thank Pauline Connor of the Department of Health records section at Nelson for her attention to my requests and for access to the papers of the Independent Scientific Committee on Smoking and Health, which fell within the then thirty-year rule.

Freedom of Information has also brought changes for contemporary historians and here I am grateful to Melody Allsebrook of the Economic and Social Research Council for her involvement in my access to the papers of the SSRC/MRC committee on smoking of the 1970s. Another change has been the accessibility of online material. Some of the US-based online tobacco industry archives have been used in the course of the study and I await the greater access to earlier (1950s–70s) UK material, which will be possible when the Guildford deposit is fully online. This offers opportunities for historians as yet unrealized.

Interviews have been an important part of the research and my thanks go to those who have endured my questioning: their insights give a dimension lacking in research which uses only published documents and archives. My location as an historian in a school of public health has greatly assisted this interaction.

Papers based on this research have been given at the University of California at San Francisco, the University of Auckland, New Zealand, the Manchester Wellcome Centre for the History of Medicine, the Wellcome Centres in London, Edinburgh, and Glasgow, the voluntary sector history society at LSE, and elsewhere. My thanks to the audiences whose comments have invariably given food for thought.

Parts of the research have been published in edited collections and in journals, *Social Science and Medicine, Twentieth Century British History, Historical Journal, Gender and History, American Journal of Public Health*, and *Bulletin of the History of Medicine*.

Finally I thank the anonymous Oxford University Press reviewers, the editors who oversaw the progress of the book, Diana LéCore who compiled the index, and my family and friends.

Virginia Berridge
LSHTM, October 2006

Contents

List of Illustrations

1. The culture of smoking. A student smokes at the laboratory bench, London School of Hygiene and Tropical Medicine, 1948. Published in *Sport and Country*.
2. Sir Austin Bradford Hill. Reproduced with permission of the London School of Hygiene and Tropical Medicine.
3. Jerry Morris. Reproduced with permission of the London School of Hygiene and Tropical Medicine.
4. *Smoking and Health*, the first Report of the Royal College of Physicians on smoking, published in 1962. Reproduced with permission of the Royal College of Physicians.
5. The Wisdom family, a Central Council of Health Education leaflet. Reproduced with permission under the terms of PSI licence C2006010511.
6. *Commonsense About Smoking* by Charles Fletcher shows the boy delinquent view of smokers in the 1960s. Reproduced with permission of Penguin books.
7. A young man smoking, with financial worries. Reproduced with Crown copyright permission and Wellcome Trust, London.
8. A young woman smoking, both by Reginald Mount for the Central Office of Information, c.196? Reproduced with Crown copyright permission and Wellcome Trust, London.
9. The naked smoking mother from the Saatchi Health Education Council campaign, 1973. Reproduced with permission under the terms of PSI licence C2006010511.
10. The Saatchi influence on health education: You can't scrub your lungs clean. Reproduced with permission under the terms of PSI licence C2006010511.
11. Women enter the picture: *The Ladykillers* by Bobbie Jacobson. Reproduced with permission of Dr Jacobson OBE.
12. The female addict: Royal College of Physicians report on *Nicotine Addiction*. Reproduced with permission of the Royal College of Physicians.

List of Abbreviations

ABPI	Association of the British Pharmaceutical Industry
ARU	Addiction Research Unit
ASH	Action on Smoking and Health
BALPA	British Airline Pilots Association
BAT	British American Tobacco
BBC	British Broadcasting Corporation
BMA	British Medical Association
BMJ	*British Medical Journal*
CCHE	Central Council for Health Education
CMO	Chief medical officer
CoI	Central Office of Information
CPAG	Child Poverty Action Group
CRIBASH	Committee for Research into the Behavioural Aspects of Smoking and Health
CSM	Committee on the Safety of Medicines
DHSS	Department of Health and Social Security
DoE	Department of Education
DoI	Department of Industry
DTI	Department of Trade and Industry
EBM	Evidence Based Medicine
EEC	European Economic Community
ESRC	Economic and Social Research Council
ETS	Environmental Tobacco Smoke
FAS	Foetal Alcohol Syndrome
FDA	Federal Drug Agency
GHS	General Household Survey
GPs	General practitioners
HEC	Health Education Council
HPRT	Health Promotion Research Trust
HSE	Health and Safety Executive

HSR	Health services research
HTC	Heat-treated cellulose
ICD	International Classification of Disease
ICI	Imperial Chemical Industries
IDL	Imperial Developments Limited
IGL	Imperial Group Limited
ISCSH	Independent Scientific Committee on Smoking and Health
ITG	Imperial Tobacco Group
IUATLD	International Union against TB and Lung Disease
LGC	Laboratory of the Government Chemist
LSHTM	London School of Hygiene and Tropical Medicine
MH	Ministry of Health
MRC	Medical Research Council
MoH	Medical Officer of Health
NACRO	National Association for the Care and Resettlement of Offenders
NAMH	National Association for Mental Health
NHS	National Health Service
NIH	National Institutes of Health
NRT	Nicotine Replacement Therapy
NSM	New Smoking Material
NSNS	National Society of Non Smokers
OPCS	Office of Population Censuses and Surveys
PQ	Parliamentary question
PR	Public Relations
RCP	Royal College of Physicians
RCT	Randomized controlled trial
RPI	Retail price index
SAC	Standing Advisory Committee
SCOTH	Scientific Committee on Tobacco and Health
SHEG	Scottish Health Education Group
SHHD	Scottish Home and Health Department
SSLC	Standing Scientific Liaison Committee
SSRC	Social Science Research Council
TAC	Tobacco Advisory Committee

TID	Tobacco Intelligence Department
TMSC	Tobacco Manufacturers' Standing Committee
TPRT	Tobacco Products Research Trust
TRC	Tobacco Research Council
TUC	Trades Union Congress
US	United States
VD	Venereal disease
VSO	Voluntary Service Overseas
WHO	World Health Organization

Introduction
Marketing Health: Smoking and the Discourse of Public Health 1945–2000

In the early 1960s Charles Rosenberg used cholera as a sampling device, a window on cultural practices and values in society.[1] This book sees smoking in a similar light. It uses the changed perception of tobacco and the ways of investigating its use in society as an emblem of public health change since the 1950s. The aim is to move from a focus on the role of professionals in public health, on public health *practice*, to a discussion of the *ideology and outlook, the discourse* of public health. Public health change can in fact be characterized in three ways, or at three levels; formal institutional change; professional change; and changes in the knowledge base and the ideology of public health. The main focus here is the third level, and how such changes in science and outlook have meshed with changes in policy.[2] The book analyses the changing ideology and compass of post-1945 public health; and uses smoking as the key 'tracer policy' which explains how public health developed, touching on other issues on the way. Smoking is the tracer policy in four broad ways. Firstly, *marketing*: the text sees the marketing of public health as defining both the beginning and the end of that fifty-year period. In the post-war years, public health adopted marketing in using the mass media to speak to and inculcate risk-avoiding behaviour in the population: it marketed the science of chronic disease epidemiology to a mass audience. By the end of the century, marketing had an added dimension as public health allied itself to treatment-focused approaches which were dependent

[1] C. Rosenberg, *The Cholera Years: The United States in 1832, 1849, and 1866* (Chicago: University of Chicago Press, 1962).
[2] See Acknowledgements at the start of this volume.

on the pharmaceutical industry. A new pharmaceutical public health promoted drug treatments as preventive strategies, as 'magic bullets' for social as well as individual behavioural problems. In the 1940s the government gave tobacco tokens as an economic supplement to old age pensions: in the late 1990s, nicotine replacement therapy was free to those in deprived areas as a remedy for inequality. The contrast in state responses shows the change which had taken place over the half-century.

Secondly, smoking symbolizes the *stages of change* of post-war public health. In the 1950s, the issue of smoking and lung cancer crystallized the post-war change of emphasis from acute infectious to chronic disease and the beginnings of a new lifestyle-oriented, activist, single-issue, public health which came to fruition in the 1970s. In the 1980s, passive smoking symbolized the reincorporation of environmentalism within public health. In the 1990s the 'discovery of addiction' for smoking also typified new developments in public health. These entwined prevention with treatment, and gave a greater role for pharmaceutical interventions and for genetics. The concept symbolized the closer relationships between substance use and public health.

Thirdly, smoking symbolizes *the tensions within public health in terms of feasible options and approaches*. The book argues for a continuing tension between 'systematic gradualism' as a public health tactic and 'coercive permissiveness'. Systematic gradualism was a strategy particularly important in the 1950s and 1960s when smoking as an activity was deeply embedded in society, in cultural and social practices. It drew on industrial alliances, which at that stage were mostly, although not exclusively, with the tobacco industry. Chemical industries were also involved, for example, in the development of New Smoking Material. But the strategy still remained in play after those decades and developed a new lease of life with the rise of pharmaceutical public health in the 1990s. Coercive permissiveness, on the other hand, was the strategy which emerged in the 1960s and 1970s and grew in importance for public health both nationally and internationally as the cultural significance of smoking began to wane. It argued for individual self-determination—but within a framework of behaviour increasingly defined by the state. Governments defined a new role for themselves in the regulation of healthy behaviour. The half-century was marked by a significant change in the attitude of governments, which took on the role, not without discussion, of advising on and regulating the individual health behaviour of the electorate.

These conceptual changes both reflected and reinforced the scientific, activist, and policy networks of post-war public health. Smoking also symbolized, as the fourth and final theme, the *post-war relationship between science and policy, between evidence, activism, and the state*. It is part of the history of evidence-based medicine. I have argued that the evidence and policy relationship has been characterized by three broad 'schools' of analysis: the rational model, which is the assumption behind present-day policy discussions; ideas of conspiracy and deliberate delay; and finally the network theories of political science studies.[3] Smoking symbolized a new public health ideology based initially on the epidemiological concept of risk, but the strategies developed around it also demonstrated a new type of 'evidence base', the rise of the social sciences as technical tools for public health. Psychology, in various forms, health economics, sociology, and the social survey were important health techniques for the observation and regulation of behaviour. And further forms of science became significant after the 1970s. The increased importance of psychopharmacology within public health reintroduced the role of 'laboratory medicine' which risk factor epidemiology had initially seemed to overthrow.

The post-war changes in the ideology of public health also elaborated a new type of science-based public health activism, whose practitioners were not those in formal public health occupations. The post-war relationship between science and the state was also played out through new types of expert committee which provided an important meeting point for science and policy. The emphasis on technical expertise typified the managerial role of post-war public health.

The overall aim is thus to deepen understanding of the scientific outlook of post-war public health and the networks which shaped it. By public health is meant the efforts of societies and individuals to prevent disease, prolong life, and promote health, a definition adapted from that used in the 1988 Acheson Report, a British policy document produced at a time when HIV/AIDS seemed to offer new possibilities for public health; these were words reiterated by the more recent (2004) Wanless Report on public health.[4] This is not what most public health history or smoking policy history is about. I have grown used to an air of

[3] V. Berridge (ed.) *Making Health Policy. Networks in Research and Policy after 1945* (Amsterdam: Rodopi, 2005).
[4] *Public Health in England: The Report of the Committee of Inquiry into the Future of the Public Health Function* (Acheson Report), (London: HMSO, 1988); D. Wanless, *Securing Good Health for the Whole Population. Final Report* (Norwich: HMSO, 2004).

puzzlement when I tell practitioners that I am studying the protagonists of public health and their changing views. It is certainly not what the history of smoking has been about. Historical research there has, in recent times, focused on the machinations of the tobacco industry.[5] And for public health history, most attention has concentrated on the nineteenth-century history and to a lesser extent, to the years up to 1945.[6] After 1945, the emphasis has been strongly on the occupational and institutional history of the public health profession.

For both areas, there are strong schools of 'practitioner history'. Public health is an historically conscious occupation and published commentary on current public health policy is far from history free. Many public health specialists present their own history of the field.[7] But some textbooks provide a survey of history which is incomprehensible in the face of historical research.[8] One tendency is to assume history is distant events—that the history is 'background' which stops some while before the present day.[9] In Petersen and Lupton's valuable book on the 'new public health' for example, the role of history is that of a bystander, the supplier of important background, but not central to their analysis of recent ideological changes.[10] Other commentary does use the history of recent events but takes it to be just the ever-changing parade of policy documents and initiatives emanating from central government.[11] Such surveys tell us what happened but they do not begin to address

[5] S. A. Glantz, J. Slade, L. A. Bero, P. Hanauer, and D. E. Barnes, *The Cigarette Papers* (Berkeley: University of California Press, 1996).

[6] C. Hamlin, *Public Health and Social Justice in the Age of Chadwick. Britain, 1800–1854* (Cambridge: Cambridge University Press, 1998); D. Porter (ed.), *The History of Public Health and the Modern State* (Amsterdam: Rodopi, 1994).

[7] J. Crown, 'The Practice of Public Health Medicine: Past, Present and Future', in S. Griffiths and D. Hunter (eds.), *Perspectives in Public Health* (Abingdon: Radcliffe Medical Press, 1999), 214–22.

[8] Naidoo and Wills, a well-known textbook in health promotion, has as its historical stages: 1800–1900, public health movement; 1900–1940, health education; 1940s to 1970s, rise of prevention; 1980s, rise of individual; 1990s, rise of market; 1997 onwards, rise of social responsibility and the new public health. None of this is referenced to the work of historians. See J. Naidoo and J. Wills, *Health Promotion. Foundations for Practice* (London: Bailliere Tindall, 1994), 138.

[9] Rob Baggott's excellent survey of recent public health policy has two chapters (2 and 3) which cover history. The book then has a number of topic-specific chapters which assume that the history has been covered in the initial contextual chapters. R. Baggott, *Public Health. Policy and Politics* (Basingstoke: Palgrave, 2000).

[10] A. R. Petersen and D. Lupton, *The New Public Health. Health and Self in the Age of Risk*, (London: Sage, 1996), 28–30.

[11] D. J. Hunter, *Public Health Policy* (Cambridge: Polity Press, 2003); D. J. Hunter, 'Public Health Policy', in J. Orme, J. Powell, P. Taylor, T. Harrison, and G. Buckingham

the important historical question of why it did—what interests, issues, activities were important. [12] In the UK, another history-using style is the role given to recent history in polemics against the emergence of the 'nanny state'. The perceived huge role of the state in health promotion is presented as historically specific to the post-war period, a dangerous intrusion of central government into the lives of individuals, supported by an increasingly dominant media.[13] For the post-war history of smoking, on the other hand, a one-dimensional 'heroes and villains' analysis has tended to dominate the post-war histories, an interpretation which stresses a gradual unveiling of scientific understanding in a manner reminiscent of the 'Whig history' which historians have long criticized.[14] The closeness of much of this work to present-day activism has meant that it is dominated by the perspectives of the present. This book aims to move away from these types of analysis. This introductory chapter therefore sets the scene both for the history of public health and for smoking prior to its career as post-war public health exemplar.[15] It then goes on to outline the history of post-war public health ideology of which smoking is part.

THE PRE-HISTORY OF POST-WAR PUBLIC HEALTH

Let us briefly survey the pre-history of this book, the nineteenth- and twentieth-century story up to mid-century. The best-known history of

(eds.), *Public Health for the 21st Century* (Maidenhead: Open University Press, 2003), 15–30.

[12] The survey of recent history in the Wanless Report (2004) is one example of the use of historical events in this way. Wanless' survey seems to be taken in part from Hunter's analysis.

[13] J. Le Fanu, *The Rise and Fall of Modern Medicine* (London: Little Brown, 1999); M. Fitzpatrick, 'Take Two Aspirins and Thank Your Caring PM', *Times Higher*, 19–26 December 2003, 28–9. See also his *The Tyranny of Health: Doctors and the Regulation of Lifestyle* (London: Routledge, 2001).

[14] P. Taylor, *Smoke Ring: The Politics of Tobacco* (London: Bodley Head, 1984); D. Pollock, *Denial and Delay. The Political History of Smoking and Health, 1951–1964: Scientists, Government and Industry as Seen in the Papers at the Public Records [sic] Office* (London: ASH, 1999).

[15] There is further discussion in V. Berridge, 'Historical and Policy Approaches', in M. Thorogood and Y. Coombes (eds.), *Evaluating Health Promotion. Practice and Methods,* 2nd edn (Oxford: Oxford University Press, 2004), 11–24, and in *eadem*, Introduction to *Medicine, the Market and the Mass Media* (London: Routledge, 2005) (with Kelly Loughlin). See also V. Berridge, D. Christie and E. M. Tansey (eds.), *Public Health in the 1980s and 90s: Decline and Rise?* (London: Wellcome Centre, 2006).

public health is that of the nineteenth century, the 'heroic' or 'golden age' often seen by present-day public health practitioners as an example to aspire to, as a model of the success of environmentalism in action. The spur to reform was epidemic disease—and especially the impact of cholera outbreaks in 1831–2, in 1848, and again in the 1860s. The 'hero' of the period (if we are writing heroic history) was Edwin Chadwick, and his famous *Report on the Sanitary Condition of the Labouring Population* (1842). Chadwick drew the link between dirt and disease, and its association with overcrowding and poor sanitation. He called for better water supplies, drainage, and sewage removal. As a follower of Jeremy Bentham's Utilitarian creed, he saw a strong role for the central state in order to achieve the greatest good for the greatest number. Chadwick's practical impact was slight. The Public Health Act of 1848 set up a Central Board of Health. But legislation was only permissive and not compulsory—and there was strong opposition to dictatorship from the centre. Chadwick was removed from his post in 1854 and the Board was abolished. In other industrializing states, however, such conflicts were avoided simply by avoiding the expansion of the central state.[16]

In Britain, it was at the local level where most was achieved. Sir John Simon, as medical officer to the Privy Council Office, helped to push through Public Health Acts in 1872 and 1875 which forced every local authority to establish a sanitary body as well as to inspect housing and monitor food supplies and 'nuisances'. His resignation in 1876 diminished central influence—but local activity still proceeded apace. The Medical Officer of Health (MoH), compulsory for the first time at the local level under the 1875 Act, could be a crucial engine of change at the local level.[17]

Looking at long-term evaluative trends, there are a number of issues to bear in mind about the nineteenth century, which are also relevant to consideration of the post-1945 story. First, the nature of the links between poverty and ill health: Chadwick was Secretary to the Poor Law Commission and his concern for health reform arose out of the concern for pauperism. Ill health caused poverty and therefore a possible reliance on the parish and poor relief. This was the 'human capital' approach to health reform, a response which has often been replicated since.

---

[16] Porter, *History of Public Health and the Modern State*.
[17] J. Eyler, *Sir Arthur Newsholme and State Medicine, 1885–1935* (Cambridge: Cambridge University Press, 1997).

The terms 'social capital' in contemporary health promotion recall this legacy. Public health reform was a surrogate and replacement in the nineteenth century for more general social reform.[18]

The question also arises of how much impact public health interventions really had? This has been a long-running debate among historical demographers which has implications for those who plan and run health services in the contemporary world. The 'McKeown thesis' view that formal medical interventions actually achieved little and rising living standards achieved more has been challenged by a view which gives a greater role for formal public health in the nineteenth century.[19]

It is important to remember, too, how the impetus behind public health was informed by fear. Fear was focused on what was seen as the growth of a 'residuum', a race of degenerates, physically stunted and morally inferior. The residuum was seen as an agent of infection—both of healthy bodies and of the body politic. Dirt was considered to be dangerous at the individual, but also at the political level. This larger ideological climate for reform was connected with the concern for environmental pollution of the late nineteenth century—the fear of contamination crossed boundaries of social and health concern. It is from this period that we derive our images of the fog-shrouded East End of London. This fear of pollution by the poor is something which we will come back to in our discussion of the 'new environmentalism' of public health in the 1980s and the rise of pharmaceutical public health directed at the poor.[20]

In the twentieth century, the ideology of public health changed and its focus narrowed. Winslow, an American public health authority, identified three phases in the development of public health: the first, from 1840 to 1890, was characterized by environmental sanitation; the second, from 1890 to 1910, by developments in bacteriology, resulting in an emphasis on isolation and disinfection; and the third, beginning

[18] Hamlin, *Public Health and Social Justice*.

[19] T. McKeown and R. G. Record, 'Reasons for the Decline of Mortality in England and Wales during the Nineteenth Century', *Population Studies*, 16 (1962), 94–122; S. Szreter, 'The Importance of Social Intervention in Britain's Mortality Decline, c.1850–1914: A Reinterpretation of the Role of Public Health', *Social History of Medicine*, 1(1) (1988), 1–37; J. Lewis, 'The Origins and Development of Public Health in the U.K.', in W. Holland et al. (eds.), *The Oxford Textbook of Public Health*, 2nd edn (Oxford: Oxford University Press, 1991), 23–33.

[20] See chapter 8 on passive smoking; also V. Berridge, 'Passive Smoking and its Pre-history in Britain: Policy Speaks to Science?', *Social Science and Medicine*, special historical issue, Science Speaks to Policy, 49(9) (1999), 1183–95.

around 1910, by an emphasis on education and personal hygiene, referred to as personal prevention. Let us take the impact of bacteriology at the end of the nineteenth century first. The discoveries of Koch and Pasteur in the late nineteenth century made public health more important as a profession—it was now possible to pinpoint specific causes of disease and bacteriology soon came to dominate the public health curriculum. But at another level, these developments moved the focus of attention away from the environment and towards the individual patient as the locus of infection. In fact, some historians have argued that these theories gained widespread acceptability quickly at the political level precisely because they provided such a circumscribed notion of appropriate intervention. Others have drawn attention to how the terminology of germs was used and only gave way to bacteria after the 1880s. Public health practice was often ahead of theory, although a linear model of innovation was presented publicly.[21] At the same time, governments took up the issue of social/welfare reform through universal education, pensions, health insurance, and school meals, and so the barriers between health and social reform became higher and more impermeable.

Some historians and sociologists argue that bacteriology had a negligible effect on the implementation of policy. Its importance lay in preparing the way for the rise of what has been called 'surveillance medicine'.[22] The new public health of the early twentieth century was indeed founded on the concept of 'personal prevention'. This was also a marriage between public health and eugenics.[23] The political imperative for reform was there, especially after the Boer War had revealed the shortcomings of British army recruits and heightened eugenic fears of 'national deterioration' and 'racial decline'. But the focus was on the individual—and especially the individual mother. The concept of 'maternal efficiency' was prevalent. Lewis has pointed to the tensions implicit in the way the infant mortality rate was conceived of as a problem of maternal ignorance.[24] The death rate was highest in poor

---

[21] M. Worboys, *Spreading Germs. Disease Theories and Medical Practice in Britain, 1865–1900* (Cambridge: Cambridge University Press, 2000).

[22] D. Armstrong, *Political Anatomy of the Body. Medical Knowledge in Britain in the Twentieth Century* (Cambridge: Cambridge University Press, 1983); *idem, A New History of Identity: A Sociology of Medical Knowledge* (Basingstoke: Palgrave, 2002).

[23] G. Jones, *Social Hygiene in Twentieth Century Britain* (London: Croom Helm, 1986).

[24] J. Lewis, *The Politics of Motherhood. Child and Maternal Welfare in England, 1900–1939* (London: Croom Helm, 1980).

inner city slums, where unsanitary living conditions prevailed. Yet public health doctors and civil servants tended to see maternal and child health as a question of providing health visitors, personal services, and health education. Mothers were encouraged to breastfeed and to achieve higher standards of domestic hygiene. The possibility of rising living standards and real wages during the First World War may have had more impact on the infant mortality rate.[25] But public health came increasingly to mean the delivery of personal health services. The maternal arguments we will see resurfacing within public health and smoking in the 1970s.

This focus on the personal and the medical ownership of the area meant that what public health doctors did was less distinctive. How did public health doctors differ from general practitioners (GPs)? The local authority clinic, home of the MoH, seemed to many GPs to be offering only what they could also provide through their individual practices. At the same time, when local government took on the administration of Poor Law hospitals after 1929, many public health doctors found themselves running hospitals. The range of services under the public health umbrella in these interwar years was huge—especially in London, where the municipal hospital system was one of the most extensive in the world. It was argued at the time—and some historians have underlined this conclusion—that this administrative expansion was achieved only at the expense of the 'community watchdog' role of the MoH.[26] Recent research has shown the variability of what was achieved at the local level.[27]

Increasingly, the cutting intellectual edge of public health lay outside the discipline—in particular through the work of academics in social medicine, who remained distinct from public health practitioners. These were to be of crucial importance for the post-war history of public health ideology and for smoking. The goals of social medicine were developed through an international exchange of ideas and beliefs in the interwar years. Soviet social hygiene influenced intellectuals and public health leaders like Arthur Newsholme, the Chief Medical Officer (CMO) to

---

[25] D. Dwork, *War is Good for Babies and Other Young Children. A History of the Infant and Child Welfare Movement in England, 1898–1918* (London: Tavistock, 1987).

[26] C. Webster, 'Healthy or Hungry Thirties?', *History Workshop Journal*, 13 (1982) 110–29; Lewis, 'Origins and Development of Public Health in the U.K.'

[27] A. Levene, M. Powell, and J. Stewart, 'Patterns of Municipal Health Expenditure in Interwar England and Wales', *Bulletin of the History of Medicine*, 78(3) (2004), 635–69.

the Local Government Board, Henry Sigerist, later to be Director of the Johns Hopkins Institute for the History of Medicine, and René Sand, first professor of social medicine in Belgium. The International organizations like the Milbank and Rockefeller Foundations were important means for the transfer of ideas.[28] In Britain, the work of John Ryle at Oxford in the Institute of Social Medicine established during the war aimed to create a new type of medicine, while a committee of the Royal College of Physicians decided in 1942 that this would be the way forward for a new type of medical practice.[29] The aim was to be a holistic view of medicine: doctors were to be interested in the causes of ill health and their prevention as well as in the treatment of disease. Medicine was to be rehumanized in contrast to the technological determinism of specialist practice. This was a wide-ranging vision which attracted reformist doctors, those involved in the Socialist Medical Association and other reforming organizations pre-war.[30] It also attracted eugenists distancing themselves in the late 1930s from Nazi social policy. These were typified by Richard Titmuss, whose work with Jerry Morris during the war aimed to use statistical and other forms of social research to reshape health policy and medical practice.[31] Titmuss' work saw the use of the social survey as a means of collecting wider information about health which could be used in planning, another legacy which was to be developed post-war.

THE PRE-HISTORY OF SMOKING

Social medicine translated into a different style of public health: to understand this, first let us look at how smoking started to come

---

[28] D. Porter, *Health, Civilization and the State* (London: Routledge, 1999), 293; L. Murard, 'Atlantic Crossings in the Measurement of Health; from U.S. Appraisal Forms to the League of Nations' Health Indices', in V. Berridge and K. Loughlin (eds.), *Medicine, the Market and the Mass Media. Producing Health in the Twentieth Century* (Aldershot: Routledge, 2005), 19–54.

[29] D. Porter, 'Changing Disciplines: John Ryle and the Making of Social Medicine in Britain in the 1940s', *History of Science*, 30 (1992), 137–64; D. Reisman, *Richard Titmuss: Welfare and Society* (London: Heinemann, 1977); D. Porter (ed.), *Social Medicine and Medical Sociology in the Twentieth Century* (Amsterdam: Rodopi, 1997).

[30] J. Stewart, *'The Battle for Health': A Political History of the Socialist Medical Association, 1930–51* (Aldershot: Ashgate, 1999).

[31] A. Oakley, 'Making Medicine Social: The Case of the Dog with Two Bent Legs', in Porter (ed.), *Social Medicine and Medical Sociology*, 81–96.

into the picture. Here there is a body of work on the history of tobacco.[32] The post-war period, however, has been the province of policy science accounts or of journalist history.[33] The most sustained historical input in recent years has been the considerable amount of research on tobacco industry documents which has been published by 'activist' public health researchers: this has expanded our knowledge of the role of an increasingly globalized industry, in particular in the decades since the 1980s.[34] There are histories of US smoking policy but there the involvement of historians in writing tobacco history has been complicated by their involvement, on both sides of the fence, in the lawsuits by which US policy tends to proceed.[35] The high profile of the industry history and of those lawsuits has meant that the post-war history of smoking policy has itself become a globalized phenomenon. An international story which has been applied to all countries without much understanding of national differences has developed. The story has been American led; and the history of US developments in smoking policy has been seen as universal. The deficiencies of this type of analysis, and of the internationalized histories of public health will be discussed in the relevant sections of the book.

Smoking is now such a central part of modern public health discourse that it is surprising to realize how recently this issue has assumed centre stage. Edwin Chadwick was concerned with sanitation, not with smoking. At mid-nineteenth century, tobacco was consumed in pipes and cigars, not cigarettes; these came on the scene in the 1880s through technological innovation, the invention and use of the Bonsack machine.

[32] V. Berridge, 'Science and Policy: The Case of Post War British Smoking Policy', in S. Lock, L. Reynolds and E. M. Tansey (eds.), *Ashes to Ashes: The History of Smoking and Health* (Amsterdam: Rodopi, 1998), 143–63; R. B.Walker, 'Medical Aspects of Tobacco Smoking and the Anti-tobacco Movement in Britain in the Nineteenth Century', *Medical History*, 24 (1980), 391–402; J. Welshman, 'Images of Youth: The Problem of Juvenile Smoking', *Addiction,* 91(9) (1996), 1379–86 ; M. Hilton, *Smoking in Popular British Culture, 1800–2000* (Manchester: Manchester University Press, 2000); J. Goodman, *Tobacco in History. The Cultures of Dependence* (London: Routledge, 1993), among others.
[33] M. Read, 'The Politics of Tobacco', PhD thesis, University of Essex, 1989; M. Read, 'Policy Networks and Issue Networks. The Politics of Smoking', in D. Marsh and R. A. W. Rhodes (eds.), *Policy Networks in British Government* (Oxford: Oxford University Press, 1992); M. Read, *The Politics of Tobacco. Policy Networks and the Cigarette Industry* (Aldershot: Ashgate, 1996).
[34] See Glantz et al, *Cigarette Papers.*
[35] This has been an intensive controversy in the American historical profession. See D. J. Rothman, 'Serving Clio and Client: The Historian as Expert Witness', *Bulletin of the History of Medicine,* 77 (2003), 25–44.

Nineteenth-century public health paid little attention to smoking as a health hazard, and its health dangers were little discussed. Its health benefits were more central and were recognized to include alleviation of stress. Manufacturers submitted cigarettes to the *Lancet* for medical approval.[36]

The movements against smoking which did exist, the British Anti-Tobacco Society, the Anti-Tobacco Legion, and others, had more in common in terms of membership with the main temperance organizations. The pledge taken by some temperance supporters also included a commitment not to smoke. But the support for anti-tobacco organizations was limited; they were seen as 'faddist' and rather beyond the pale. Like opposition to drinking alcohol and taking drugs like opium, tobacco formed part of a distinct moral movement which stressed reformation of the individual rather than the environmental reform central to mainstream public health. These substances and their control were not part of contemporary public health movements and, indeed, have remained distinct until quite recently. It is one of the tasks of this book to analyse how and why they have moved closer to public health in recent years.[37]

Although tobacco was linked to alcohol in these organizations, it did not form part of the moves to develop disease theories, theories of inebriety, in the last quarter of the century. There was no discussion of treating or institutionalizing tobacco smokers in the way there was for non-criminal inebriates and drug takers. When the topic was occasionally brought up, it was laughed out of court; the smoker might be weak willed but he was not diseased.[38] This lack of a disease or addiction history was to have implications in the post-1945 years.[39]

The main period of concern came in the early 1900s when a number of anti-smoking organizations were founded to oppose smoking in children.[40] These included the British Lads Anti-Smoking Union, the

[36] R. Elliot, ' "Destructive but Sweet": Cigarette Smoking among Women, 1890–1990', PhD thesis, University of Glasgow, 2001.

[37] V. Heggie, 'Reimagining the Healthy Social Body; Medicine, Welfare and Health Reform in Manchester, 1880–1910', PhD thesis, University of Manchester, 2005; B. Harrison, *Drink and the Victorians. The Temperance Question in England, 1815–1872* (London: Faber and Faber, 1971).

[38] For example, N. Kerr, *Inebriety* (London: H. K. Lewis, 1888).

[39] Discussed below in chapter 9.

[40] Welshman, 'Images of Youth'; M. Hilton, ' "Tabs", "Fags", and the "Boy Labour Problem" in Late Victorian and Edwardian Britain', *Journal of Social History*, 28 (1995), 587–607.

International Anti-Cigarette League, and others. Through the youth issue, smoking was part of the debate about physical fitness and national deterioration which followed the revelations about working-class physique during the Boer War. Smoking by young boys was linked with fear of the residuum, of the out of control urban hooligan whose propensities for reproduction threatened to overwhelm civilized society.[41] This concern, like that about children in pubs, ultimately passed into law in the 1908 Children's Act, which prohibited the sale of tobacco to children and its sale in sweetshops. The image of smoking was largely male, although concern about the independence of the 'new woman' also focused on the issue of smoking and smoking in public.[42]

It was during the inter-war years that scientific evidence about the dangers of smoking began to become clearer. Statisticians like the American Raymond Pearl, working for the insurance industry, began to link smoking to reduced life expectancy and to cancer. Smoking was also the subject of scientific investigation in the 1930s in Nazi Germany, where concerns about racial hygiene and bodily purity led to scientific and policy interest in areas which came to be associated with public health and its redefinition post-1945 in other countries. There was an anti-smoking programme, with health education, bans on advertising, and restrictions on smoking in public places. German scientists were among the first to link smoking to lung cancer.[43]

In Britain in these interwar years, there was little connection between formal public health and opposition to smoking. Local MoHs were more concerned with running local hospitals and health services and it was widely assumed that any national health service would be based on local government, would be rate funded, and would be run by the MoH. MoHs worked to contain infectious disease, even if their efforts in that direction can be criticized, as in their slowness to adopt diphtheria immunization in the interwar period.[44] Changing individual habits like smoking were not part of this mindset at all.

[41] G. Pearson, *Hooligan. A History of Respectable Fears* (Basingstoke: Macmillan, 1983).
[42] R. Elliot, *Women and Smoking in Britain 1890–2000* (Abingdon: Routledge, forthcoming).
[43] R. Proctor, *The Nazi War on Cancer* (Princeton, NJ: Princeton University Press, 1999); G. Davey Smith, S. A. Strobele, and M. Eggar, 'Smoking and Health Promotion in Nazi Germany', *Journal of Epidemiology and Community Health*, 48 (1994), 220–3.
[44] Lewis, 'Origins and Development of Public Health in the U.K.'

THE HISTORY OF PUBLIC HEALTH IDEOLOGY, 1945–2000

Yet in the period after the war, public health underwent a fundamental reorientation so that the potential regulation of habits like smoking, eating, and drinking became central. Dorothy Porter has commented that social medicine ideas, privatized and repackaged, re-emerged in the 'healthy body' ideology of fashionable society in the 1980s and after.[45] This book subjects that new public health style to scrutiny. It was part of, but also strangely separate from, the professional and service-related activities which have dominated the historiography so far. Jane Lewis' work has shown how social medicine ideas remained academic and failed to penetrate the public health profession through the MoH. Public health, she argues, failed to develop a distinctive rationale and typically defined itself around whatever activities it undertook at the time.[46] The relocation of the MoH as the consultant community physician within the health service after the local government and health service reorganization of the early 1970s was part of the Titmuss/Morris vision. This also saw the emancipation of the social work profession from the MoH in local government. For public health, renamed as community medicine, the occupational relocation became a search for professional status within medicine, accompanied by the wrangling over the establishment of the Faculty of Community Medicine in the early 1970s.[47] Sociologists and other social scientists were excluded from the new Faculty and regrouped within the Society for Social Medicine, which developed an interest in research and ultimately a focus on the randomized controlled trial.[48] This is the occupational history of the change: but there was also a conceptual reorientation which is discussed in this volume.

Analysts of post-war public health like Walter Holland and Jane Lewis have identified twin polarities, technician manager and activist, in

[45] Porter, *Health, Civilization and the State*, 297–309.
[46] J. Lewis, *What Price Community Medicine?* (Brighton: Harvester, 1986).
[47] M. Warren, *The Genesis of the Faculty of Community Medicine* (Canterbury: Centre for Health Service Studies, University of Kent, 1997); V. Berridge and S. Taylor (eds.), *Epidemiology, Social Medicine and Public Health* (London: Centre for History in Public Health, 2005).
[48] M. Jefferys, 'Social Medicine and Medical Sociology, 1950–1970: The Testimony of a Partisan Participant', in Porter (ed.), *Social Medicine and Medical Sociology*, 120–36.

their professional role.[49] Such distinctions could also be applied to the ideology and role of public health post-1945. Social medicine bifurcated into two broad but overlapping strands: *evidence-based medicine* and *lifestyle public health*. These became clear by the 1970s, but the roots lay earlier as this book will indicate. The evidence-based strand saw the rise of the randomized controlled trial, associated in the 1930s with R. A. Fisher and agricultural research at Rothampstead and with the statistical work of Greenwood and Hill at LSHTM, and also with the MRC and its Therapeutic Trials committee. The post-war trial of streptomycin for TB is conventionally seen as the origin of the 'modern' trial. But the use of trials was also important in demands articulated by the social medicine supporter Archie Cochrane for more effective use of medical resources. His Rock Carling lecture, published as *Effectiveness and Efficiency* in 1971, was part of an international movement with particular input from Canada and the United States.[50] The lifestyle strand, on the other hand, was located in the post-war rise of chronic disease and the rise of risk factor epidemiology. The public health focus on these 'diseases of affluence' was what lay behind the reorientation of ideology which is the focus of this book. The 'delay' of central government in the 1950s which has been criticized by activist historians was in part located in an accommodation to this fundamental reorientation of public health and to the new role for government which it entailed. Governments had not been used to persuading their citizens to alter their personal habits and the electoral implications of that were worrying. It was not until the 1970s that cultural change was sufficiently advanced for governments to assume a more active role. Smoking and related lifestyle issues brought a new style of health activism into public health. Single-issue organizations developed science-based campaigns: the role of the mass media in public health initiatives became central, as a tool to be used, or as a mode to be attacked when used by others.[51] The 1962 report on smoking produced by the Royal College of Physicians was the harbinger of a

[49] Lewis, *Community Medicine*; W. W. Holland, 'A Dubious Future for Public Health?', *Journal of the Royal Society of Medicine*, 95 (2002), 182–8; W. W. Holland and S. Stewart, *Public Health, the Vision and the Challenge* (London: Nuffield Provincial Hospitals Trust, 1998).

[50] For the rise of the RCT, see Berridge, Christie, and Tansey (eds.), *Public Health in the 1980s and 1990s*; also J. Daly, *Evidence Based Medicine and the Search for a Science of Clinical Care* (Berkeley: University of California Press, 2005).

[51] V. Berridge and K. Loughlin, 'Smoking and the New Health Education in Britain, 1950s to 1970s', *American Journal of Public Health*, 95(6) (2005), 956–64.

new media-based role for medicine. Science, initially epidemiology, was central to the focus on lifestyle and risk. A population-level style of argument nevertheless placed its emphasis on modifying the behaviour of individuals. Health economics, psychology, and the social survey, outgrowths of social medicine, became the standard tools of this new public health. Discussions of evidence-based medicine often focus on the history of the randomized controlled trial, but the incorporation of the social sciences was also significant.

This new style of public health was developing while the MoHs became community physicians within the health service. But public health practice at the professional level seems strangely detached from the engines of public health in terms of ideology and activism. The changed outlook also paralleled and stimulated new relationships with government—networks or policy communities interlinked. Government gave financial support to activist groups which could then press it in turn to take more stringent action. Action on Smoking and Health (ASH) for smoking was one of the first of the new pressure groups. Mechanisms like the expert committee were reformed to bring science into closer relationship with policy making. At the policy level, this new style was represented in policy documents like *Prevention and Health, Everybody's Business* (1976), criticized at the time for adopting a 'victim blaming' approach.[52] The 1970s was a key decade: it saw a 'state-funded activism' develop, while both Conservative and Labour governments (through ministers such as Sir Keith Joseph and David Owen) developed technocratic models of science/policy exchange for public health and smoking, Joseph through his cross-government enquiry in the early 1970s and Owen through his attempt to bring tobacco and tobacco products under the aegis of medicines control. Such developments paralleled the rise of customer–contractor relationships between government departments and researchers more generally, and the initial rise of the 'evidence-based' model. [53]

By the 1970s activist public health had an agenda of abstention so far as smoking was concerned and a growing hostility to industry. But this was not the only public health agenda. There was still a strong strand of what would now be called harm reduction—risk reduction or 'safer smoking' in the terminology of the time, which had its public health

---

[52] *Prevention and Health, Everybody's Business: A Reassessment of Public and Personal Health* (London: HMSO, 1976).
[53] Berridge, *Making Health Policy*.

adherents. Moderation is a concept which has been much discussed in relation to alcohol and other substances. For smoking, its implications were to bring 'substance use' closer to public health from the 1990s and after.[54] Alcohol, illicit drugs, and tobacco moved closer together conceptually in a way which some scientists had tried to achieve in the 1970s.

From the 1970s came two further developments in public health: health promotion and the new public health, different but overlapping. Webster and French have related these developments to the influence of social medicine in the United States and at WHO and to radical critiques of medicine—Cochrane, but also Thomas McKeown, Ivan Illich and Thomas Szasz. The shortcomings of health services and hospital-based models were revealed, especially in developing countries. Health care costs were escalating, with a particular impact from the rise in oil prices by the OPEC states at the end of 1973.[55]

This was an international history of the rise of health promotion and of primary care, with its 'milestones' in the 1974 Lalonde Report on Canada, the 1978 Alma Ata Declaration, *Health for All* from the World Health Organization (WHO) in 1981, and its 38 targets for the European region in 1985. The Ottawa Charter for Health Promotion followed in 1986. The Healthy Cities project was launched in 1987.[56] The international health promotion movement also began to stress the environmental and structural determinants of health and the need for 'healthy public policy', rather than simply encouraging individual behaviour change. Britain in the 1980s saw a new version of public health. The sharpness of the political impact of the new Conservative government on some of the health politics of the late 1970s was mirrored in scientific change. A different scientific agenda emerged. The 'new environmentalism' based on the individual came into the

[54] For discussion of the crossover between the substances see V. Berridge and T. Hickman, 'History and the Future of Psychoactive Substances', position paper for the Foresight Brain Science, Addiction and Drugs Project: <http://www.foresight.gov.uk>.

[55] C. Webster, and J. French, 'The Cycle of Conflict: The History of Public Health and Health Promotion Movements', in L. Adams, M. Amos, and J. Munro (eds.), *Promoting Health. Politics and Practice* (London: Sage, 2002), 5–12.

[56] M. I. Roemer, 'Henry Ernest Sigerist: Internationalist of Social Medicine', *Journal of the History of Medicine and Allied Sciences*, 13 (1958), 229–43; E. Fee and E. T. Morman, 'Doing History, Making Revolution: The Aspirations of Henry E. Sigerist and George Rosen', in R. Porter and D. Porter (eds.), *Doctors, Politics and Society: Historical Essays* (Amsterdam: Clio Medica, 1993), 275–311; Berridge, 'Historical and Policy Approaches'.

smoking story through the rise of passive smoking. Passive smoking promoted what Peterson and Lupton have called the concept of the 'environmental citizen', the rational consumer protecting him- or herself from environmental risks.[57] This new environmentalism also carried with it a revival of the fear of infection which found its apogee in the impact of HIV/AIDS in the later 1980s.[58]

HIV/AIDS symbolized a revival of communicable disease in public health, later to be confirmed by BSE, SARS, and bird flu. But AIDS was also a lifestyle disease par excellence in its initial incarnation, and the response to it in the UK epitomized the key tenets of that style of public health, with the emphasis on behaviour modification and individual responsibility. In the 1990s came a further stage of public health termed 'pharmaceutical public health': this categorization draws on drug and vaccine responses to public health issues, on relationships with the pharmaceutical industry, and also on 'new' genetic insights into health.[59] The 'rise of addiction' for smoking symbolized these developments. Addiction and its adherents for smoking created new networks in public health but also drew on some of the developments of the 1970s. Epidemiology was coming under increasing criticism as an inadequate explanatory tool; the laboratory again entered the equation with biological markers being used as part of population-based studies. Dependence transmuted into addiction and psychopharmacology succeeded in gaining policy salience for a concept which psychiatry had earlier failed to establish.

In the early twenty-first century there were thus two distinct but also overlapping styles in public health: on the one hand the environmentalists, inheritors of the coercive tradition, who favoured the regulation of public space and criminal sanctions for individuals and companies: on the other, the harm reducers, inheritors of the systematic gradualism tradition, with a strong pharmaceutical input into treatment and prevention and industry connections. Public health had taken on drugs, alcohol, and smoking and had drawn closer to a regulatory and criminal justice agenda, but its 'backstage' was the medication of high-risk populations.

[57] Peterson and Lupton, *The New Public Health*.
[58] V. Berridge, *AIDS in the UK. The Making of Policy, 1981–1994* (Oxford: Oxford University Press, 1996).
[59] Berridge, 'Historical and Policy Approaches'.

WRITING THE CONTEMPORARY HISTORY
OF PUBLIC HEALTH

The book is a study in contemporary history, a subject about which I have written previously.[60] It is worth making some more comments on the topic to explain the methods and stance. Times have changed since I first wrote about contemporary history, and the areas analysed herein are 'hot topics', smoking in particular. Public health discussion of its own history has also been acrimonious, but has concentrated on the issue of professional ownership and the medical–non-medical divide, subjects I am not dealing with here.[61] Questions of methodology and historical positioning are, however, relevant to my approach in this book and also to the different styles adopted by other researchers in this area. I have used the standard historian's toolbox of archives, interviews, and published primary and secondary sources (with the overlap between the latter two which one finds in contemporary history—a secondary source can also be a primary one and vice versa). For HIV/AIDS, a previous area of research, interviews were important, and the interplay between oral history and archive was part of the methodology. The same has been true for this book, and my oral history interviews have been enriched by my 'living among the tribe', being an historian in a public health setting, with strong connections with the addiction field.[62] It is surprising how few contemporary historians in the health arena use interviews in this way. Historians of science have written about the use of interviews as a tool for the study of elites, but mostly oral history has not moved on from its 'life history' 'history from below' focus.[63] The dilemmas of the interview and 'getting beyond the official line' are important issues, and the rise of ethics has complicated the use of

[60] V. Berridge, 'Researching Contemporary History: AIDS', *History Workshop Journal*, 38 (1994), 227–34.

[61] Some of this is reflected in two witness seminar transcripts, V. Berridge and S. Taylor (eds.), *Epidemiology, Social Medicine and Public Health* (London: CHIPH, 2005) and Berridge, Christie, and Tansey (eds.), *Public Health in the 1980s and 1990s*.

[62] See V. Berridge 'History in Public Health: Who Needs It?' *Lancet*, 356 (2000), 1923–5.

[63] S. de Chadarevian, 'Using Interviews to Write the History of Science', in T. Soderquist (ed.), *The Historiography of Contemporary Science and Technology* (Amsterdam: Harwood Academic, 1997), 51–70.

interviews for contemporary historians.[64] Nevertheless interviews can still give a sense of the networks in the field, of the tensions and the scientific debates, which does not emerge from the official documents.

Archives are now a different matter. When I wrote about contemporary history a decade ago in relation to HIV/AIDS, I made much of the difficulties of access to archives and the need for what I called 'archives on the run', behind-the-scenes donations of material from key players. This access is still invaluable but, in the interim, more formal archives have become openly available. In Britain, the Open Government initiative of the 1990s allowed myself and colleagues to request material from the government from within the 'thirty-year rule' formal cut-off period. Some of that material, in particular from the Department of Health, has been used in this book. Freedom of Information came into operation just as the book was being written and the initial assessment is that it is formalizing procedures which we had used informally for quite a few years. But it is also throwing light on the poor archival practices of some government departments and this will have implications for the way in which history is written in the future.[65]

A key event in the interim, so far as tobacco is concerned, has been the opening up of industry archives and much work has stemmed from that access. However, their use presents methodological problems which have so far been little discussed. Easy availability online has led many users, often unaware even that there are other archives, to access only that source: a standard historical methodology would be to 'triangulate' and assess a number of sources against each other.[66] Thrilling titles like 'lifting the veil' and 'peering through the keyhole' encourage the view that here are secrets, although uncovering previously unknown material is what historians do with most archives. The provenance of the industry archival material—where it came from, its location within the parent

[64] V. Berridge, 'The Sources Bite Back: Oral History and the Study of Elites in Contemporary Health History', lecture given to Department of History, University of Auckland, 2005; K. Duke, 'Getting beyond the "Official Line": Reflections on Dilemmas of Access, Knowledge and Power in Researching Policy Networks', *Journal of Social Policy*, 31(1) (2002), 39–59.

[65] For another study, on drug user groups, we were given ready access to Department of Health material from the 1980s. However, the Home Office was unable to find the material we wanted, on its Voluntary Sector Unit, because the material had not been listed in a way which would have made it easily accessible in the time allowed for a search by the Act. Journalists appear to be having some success with the Act and this may be because they are more specific in their requests.

[66] Discussions with users of the archives have indicated that they are unaware of archives not online, or indeed that such possibilities and different styles of research exist.

organization, and thus its significance to the parent organization—is also rarely discussed, in part because the circumstances of deposit have not made standard archival practice possible. In this book, for example, I show, through my work on the Royal College of Physicians (RCP) archives, that the industry work on nicotine habituation was presented to the RCP committee, which discussed it with industry representatives in the 1960s. This is not the picture of 'hidden discovery' which emerges when industry archives alone are used.

While drafting this book, I carried out a test exercise: I tracked an organization I had already researched through other avenues in an online keyword search in industry archives. This revealed a document (a report from a US visitor to the UK), which was useful for my research. It underlined conclusions about the role of the British industry I had already drawn from other material, but gave greater detail and colour. In addition it provided me with material which was not unique and was available in other locations. The archives could be valuable for the post-war years (1950s to 1970s) when more of this material is made accessible. So far most research has been on documents relating to the period since the 1980s when industry–public health relationships had changed. There is gold in these archives, but studies will need to develop a more sophisticated assessment of the provenance of the material and of the cross-national differences in policy and government–public health–industry relationships and how these have changed over time.[67] They will also need to draw on a wider range of archival material. BAT, the main source of UK-based documents, mostly operated outside the UK. Imperial was the main UK company and its relationships with government and with the public health community were quite different from the US model—again until the late 1970s. A pilot study of the Wills tobacco archive, material deposited in a local record office, illustrated some of those corporate relationships, which are discussed in this book.[68] The enthusiasm for online industry archives is an interesting phenomenon. We are seeing a new type of family history, a Whig history revived and a rediscovery of 'the document' whose main role is to play to the policy objectives of the anti-tobacco field. The industry research

[67] A recent LSHTM student project using Guildford material has shown how differences about strategy operated between BAT and Phillip Morris in relation to the industry response to the draft 2001 EU Tobacco Directive. See S. Mandall, *Tobacco Industry Efforts to Influence the 2001 Tobacco Products Directive*, LSHTM MSc student project, 2006.
[68] This research was carried out by Dr Penny Starns.

is also raising technical and methodological issues of which the historical profession should be more aware as online archives expand as historical sources.[69] One problem with the tobacco archive history is the impetus for 'global history' (usually in the US mould), which takes little account of national differences. As a result, analyses of the documents have overlooked the significance of material in them which relates to the different nature of British policy making.[70] As an historian who has been characterized as a 'policy cool' I find a particular danger in the impetus to heroes and villains, unifactorial history.[71]

One of my historical characters agreed. In the ASH archive (not yet used by online researchers) a similar view is cogently expressed. In the 1970s William Norman, an American journalist, interviewed a number of 'key players' in the UK for a study of smoking policy. One of his interviews was with the politician Enoch Powell, who chided Norman over his partisanship about smoking. The two were discussing the differences between the regulation of tobacco and that of alcohol. Powell thought Norman's strong views blinded him.

You are saying 'should': you should sayd (error in transcript) 'there are arguments for penalising one which do not apply to the other' …
I would say that I think you will write a better book, and a more useful book, … if you can contrive to detach your own intention from it. I think at the moment you are liable to miss aspects of the subject because of the impatience of your own inclination one way or another. I think you would understand more and see more if you approached it at first rather more clinically.[72]

That is the intention in this book.

---

[69] The issue raised by research and its management by digitized and online documents is one such issue. At a more conceptual level are the opportunities for collective interpretation offered by the research methods used. Colleagues at LSHTM working on these documents will only publish document-based interpretation which all the team agree on: there is no competing historical interpretation because of legal requirements but also because of the collective process of the document research itself.

[70] In *The Cigarette Papers,* 272–3 for example, the authors note a visit in 1971 by Sir Derrick Dunlop, chair of the Medicines Committee, and Frank Fairweather: and there is also a reference to the Dawkins committee. These are significant people and organizations in the British context, and their roles relate to the different nature of British policy making, which is discussed in the current book. But to assess that significance would have needed much wider research outside the industry archives—and so the US text does not discuss these people and is not aware that they are historically significant.

[71] D. T. Courtwright, 'Drug Wars: Policy Hots and Historical Cools', *Bulletin of the History of Medicine,* 74 (2004), 440–50.

[72] Wellcome Library for the History and Understanding of Medicine, ASH archive SA/ASH R.27, Norman collection Box 79, Interview with Enoch Powell.

1

Public Health in the 1950s: The Watershed of Smoking and Lung Cancer

Richard Doll always maintained that discovering the link between smoking and lung cancer was a surprise:

we began our study without any expectation that tobacco was likely to be an important cause of the disease and we included questions about its use primarily because the consumption of tobacco and particularly the consumption of cigarettes had increased at a possibly appropriate interval before the increase in mortality began to be recorded. For my part, I suspected that if we could find a cause it was most likely to have something to do with motor cars and the tarring of the roads.[1]

Doll was questioned by the historian Roy Porter after he had made this statement. Porter asked how surprised he was by these findings: Doll said, 'Very'.[2] Such narratives of discovery are commonly observed in the history of science. Here was a new form of scientific discovery in the post-war period, a discovery of statistical correlation and its impact, rather than a microbe or bacteria causing disease and observed in the laboratory: but the language used to describe its unveiling was the same.

The early history of the smoking and lung cancer connection is well known and has been recounted in a number of different histories.[3] Concern was roused by the gradual increase in the incidence of cancer;

---

[1] Sir R. Doll, 'The First Reports on Smoking and Lung Cancer', in S. Lock, L. Reynolds, and E. M. Tansey (eds.), *Ashes to Ashes: The History of Smoking and Health* (Amsterdam: Rodopi, 1998), 130–40, 133. See also 'Conversation with Sir Richard Doll', *British Journal of Addiction*, 86 (4) (1991), 365–77.

[2] Doll 'First Reports on Smoking and Lung Cancer', 141.

[3] For example, J. Austoker, *A History of the Imperial Cancer Research Fund, 1902–1986* (Oxford: Oxford University Press, 1988), 186–99; C. Webster, 'Tobacco Smoking Addiction: A Challenge to the National Health Service', *British Journal of Addiction*, 79 (1984), 8–16.

a change in the balance of the sexes, towards men; and the increasingly important role of lung cancer. The greatest increase in lung cancer came in males over forty-five, where the incidence increased sixfold between 1930 and 1945. At first it was thought that these changes might be due to improved diagnosis and better recording and registration. Research had been carried out in the 1930s by Sir Ernest Kennaway, Professor of Experimental Pathology at the Chester Beatty Institute in London and famous for his late 1920s work on the carcinogenic potential of 3,4-benzpyrene. A detailed examination of post-mortem certificates had been published in 1947, and had helped to eliminate occupational and environmental factors. Kennaway pointed to a connection with cigarette smoking, but his work, based on statistical correlations, carried little weight in the context of the time, when such correlations were not seen as central to scientific proof. Laboratory studies also tended to support the connection. Research had also been undertaken before the War in Nazi Germany and by the American biometrician Raymond Pearl, for the insurance industry.[4] The issue became more urgent post-war and discussions between the Ministry of Health and the Medical Research Council (MRC) led to the council convening an informal conference on cancer of the lung in February 1947. The MRC agreed to initiate a large-scale statistical study of the past smoking habits of those with cancer of the lung and of two control groups. Who would take the work forward was a matter of discussion: both the Social Medicine Unit under Professor Jerry Morris and Patrick Lawther, who subsequently ran the Air Pollution Unit at St Bartholomew's Hospital, were under consideration.[5] This was the origin of the work carried out in the Statistical Research Unit at the London School of Hygiene and Tropical Medicine (LSHTM) by Professor Bradford Hill and Dr Richard Doll. The results, published in the *British Medical Journal* (*BMJ*) in 1950, concluded that there was a 'real association' between carcinoma of the lung and smoking and that smoking was a factor, and an important one, in the production of carcinoma of the lung. Work by Wynder and

---

[4] G. D. Smith, S. A. Strobele, and M. Egger, 'Smoking and Health Promotion in Nazi Germany', *Journal of Epidemiology and Community Health*, 48 (1994), 220–3; R. N. Proctor, *The Nazi War on Cancer* (Princeton: Princeton University Press, 1999), 173–247.

[5] L. Berlivet, '"Association or Causation?" The Debate on the Scientific Status of Risk Factor Epidemiology, 1947–c.1965', in V. Berridge (ed.), *Making Health Policy. Networks in Research and Policy after 1945* (Amsterdam: Rodopi, 2005), 39–74; interview with Pat Lawther by Virginia Berridge and Suzanne Taylor, February 2003.

Graham in the United States, published just before, had come to similar conclusions. Later prospective studies carried out by Doll and Bradford Hill and by Cuyler Hammond and Horn in the United States appeared to implicate cigarette smoking even further.

In the UK context, the work of Doll and Hill was the watershed. This was a case control study based on twenty London hospitals. With its talk of 'almoners' administering a 'set questionary' the text now has a period air. The conclusions were cautious. Then in 1956 came the results of a prospective study which Doll and Hill had started in 1951. The study related the deaths of doctors occurring since October 1951 to non-smoking, present smoking, and ex-smoking groups as constituted at that date. It concluded that the death rate for lung cancer increased as the amount smoked increased; and, conversely, that there was a progressive and significant reduction in mortality with the increase in the length of time over which smoking was given up. Further results from this British doctors study came at intervals over the next forty years. Results from the follow-up were published in 2004, just before Doll's death the following year.[6]

PUBLIC HEALTH IN FLUX IN THE 1950S

At this stage, the analysis of events could continue with the story of smoking and lung cancer and how the smoking issue fared over the next decade. This is a story which has been recounted within the different theoretical and ideological frameworks for the relationship between science and policy which were discussed in the Introduction: we will return to those and to the smoking story. But our main initial purpose is to set that story within its 1950s public health context. Smoking was the exemplar of what came to be the main style of post-war public health. Such a style emphasized the role of individual behaviour, legitimated through population-based epidemiology, as the dominant focus. It

---

[6] R. Doll and A. B. Hill, 'Smoking and Carcinoma of the Lung. Preliminary Report', *British Medical Journal*, 2 (1950), 739–48; *eidem*, 'The Mortality of Doctors in Relation to Their Smoking Habits. A Preliminary Report', *British Medical Journal*, 1 (1954), 1451–5; *eidem* 'Lung Cancer and Other Causes of Death in Relation to Smoking. A Second Report on the Mortality of British Doctors' *British Medical Journal*, 2 (1956), 1071–81; R. Doll, R. Peto, J. Boreham, I. Sutherland, 'Mortality in Relation to Smoking: 50 Years' Observation on Male British Doctors', *British Medical Journal*, 328 (2004), 1519–33.

stimulated new attitudes on the part of government in relating to the
public on matters of health and a heightened significance for research-
based surveillance. It was thus a key component of the establishment of
Beck's 'risk society', which was also a 'scientized society'. Public health
in that decade was in a state of flux—as an occupation, but also in terms
of its animating ideas and theories and modes of scientific explanation.
The response to smoking highlighted these tensions. The following
section will examine the state of play of public health as an occupation,
but also its disease focus, ideology, and the technical tools it came to
utilize.

It is not surprising that most historical attention has concentrated on
the occupational disarray of public health during these years. In many
respects, however, the occupation of public health post-war had little to
do with the rethinking of public health. As an occupation, it had failed
to capitalize on the coming of the National Health Service in 1948. The
Medical Officer of Health (MoH) could have been the unifying force
within local government in the tripartite structure of health services.
But the service was differently structured, through the nationalization
of the hospitals. It was funded through central government taxation
rather than local government rates, as had been expected. The pre-war
public health 'empire' in the local authorities had seen public health
doctors running hospitals and a wide range of services. But this empire
began to disintegrate post-war. Lewis has argued that MoHs bear some
responsibility for this outcome, having previously been happy to extend
their activities in whatever direction offered, without a distinct vision
of what 'public health' was all about.[7] Much clinic work began to pass
from local authorities into general practice, which was also redefining
its role in this period. In addition, the position of the MoH in the local
authority became increasingly uncertain as ancillary health occupations
defined their own professional competencies. Sanitary inspectors claimed
autonomy in the 1950s and were renamed public health inspectors in
1956.[8] The social work profession was also emergent as a separate
entity. Money spent on social welfare services in local government
grew considerably during this period.[9] This created further tensions as

    [7] J. Lewis, *What Price Community Medicine? The Philosophy, Practice and Politics of
Public Health since 1919* (Brighton: Wheatsheaf, 1986), 17–18.
    [8] V. Berridge, *Health and Society in Britain since 1939* (Cambridge: Cambridge
University Press, 1999), 44.
    [9] R. Baggott, *Public Health: Policy and Politics* (Basingstoke: Palgrave, 2000),
45–6.

increasingly social workers in local government saw medical control as inappropriate.

It would be a mistake to assume that there was no innovation or vitality in local public health practice. We know relatively little about the nature of public health work at this level. Recent research has revealed that the local dimensions of interwar public health practice were very variable, but there has so far been little in-depth research into the work of the MoH in the 1950s and 1960s.[10] Loughlin's work shows how some boroughs were appointing health education officers in the 1950s and that a distinctive localized style of group health education was emerging with professional concerns developing through an Institute of Health Education.[11] In Leicester, a reasonably progressive local authority, the role and work of the MoH in the 1950s was uncertain. Leicester appointed a health education officer to work within local government under the MoH. Work in community care for the elderly and the mentally ill expanded. However, the public health department remained remote from newer developments, such as the use of psychological techniques in the School Medical Service, and it was wedded to outdated concepts of 'the problem family' which had undertones of pre-war eugenics, rather than the newer case work approaches pioneered by the Family Service Units.[12] Individual MoHs moved towards new approaches. One trend, also underlined by the work of the health education officers, was towards the more effective use of communications strategies. The work of McQueen in Aberdeen before and during the 1964 Aberdeen typhoid outbreak illustrated the use of 'modern' technologies of mass communication within the context of the local remit of the MoH.[13] Here was one option for future public health directions. The work of another MoH pioneered a different approach—'evidence-based' health service research focused activity. The work of R. 'Paddy' Donaldson on Teesside in the 1960s developed research-based screening activities. But Donaldson handed

[10] A. Levene, M. Powell, and J. Stewart, 'Patterns of Municipal Health Expenditure in Interwar England and Wales', *Bulletin of the History of Medicine*, 78(3) (2004), 635–69.

[11] Kelly Loughlin's research on developments in health education in the 1950s is being drawn upon here.

[12] J. Welshman, *Municipal Medicine: Public Health in Twentieth Century Britain* (Oxford: Peter Lang, 2000).

[13] L. Diack and D. Smith, 'The Media and the Management of a Food Crisis. Aberdeen's Typhoid Outbreak in 1964', in V. Berridge and K. Loughlin (eds.), *Medicine, the Market and the Mass Media. Producing Health in the Twentieth Century* (Abingdon: Routledge, 2005), 79–94.

over such activities to the local general practitioners, a transfer which symbolized the continuing and growing overlap between the activities of the two professional groupings. Donaldson was the father of the current chief medical officer (CMO), Sir Liam Donaldson: his father's development of screening also symbolized public health's search for a technocratic role related to health services.[14]

The changed organization of health services under the NHS was in part responsible for this search for new roles. But so, too, was the changing pattern of disease. The traditional focus of public health had been the outbreak or the epidemic: public health practitioners looked back to the great days of environmentalism and the fight against cholera and typhoid in the mid-nineteenth century. But this pattern of disease and disease-related mortality began to change in the middle of the twentieth century. Between the 1840s and 1971, three-quarters of the improvement in death rates had been due to the decline in infectious disease, with non-infectious conditions accounting for the remaining quarter. But this pattern changed after the Second World War. The old 'public health' diseases like TB or diphtheria were in decline. For TB effective chemotherapy, and mass radiography, virtually eliminated the need for treatment by the mid-1950s. This accelerated a longer-term decline in TB rates which predated the advent of BCG vaccination introduced in the 1950s.[15] As the population lived longer, so non-infectious causes of death such as heart disease, strokes, and cancer grew in importance. The connection between smoking and lung cancer was one of the earliest instances of research-led discussion of the new patterns of disease. It also underlined a reorientation of chest medicine: after the 1950s this specialty no longer had TB as its major concern and sought a new role. Most of the increase in the 'chronic' diseases was relative, because of the decline of other causes and the survival of more people to ages at which those diseases occurred, but some also was thought to rise from an absolute increase in incidence.[16] These changes in the

[14] R. J. Donaldson, *Off the Cuff. Reminiscences of My Half Century Career in Public Health* (Richmond: Murray Print, 2000); S. McLaurin and D. F. Smith, 'Professional Strategies of Medical Officers of Health in the Post-war Period—2: "Progressive Realism": The Case of Dr R. J. Donaldson, MoH for Teesside, 1968–1974', *Journal of Public Health Medicine*, 24(2) (2002), 130–5.

[15] L. Bryder, *Below the Magic Mountain. A Social History of Tuberculosis in Twentieth Century Britain* (Oxford: Oxford University Press, 1988), 262.

[16] See A. Gray, 'The Decline of Infectious Diseases: The Case of England', in A. Gray (ed.), *World Health and Disease*, Health and Disease series, Book 3 (Milton Keynes: Open University Press, 1993), 75; K. McPherson and D. Coleman, 'Health', in A. H.

patterning of disease were important for the new role of public health, for they, along with the modes of explanation, prefigured the important changes in the nature and focus of public health activity in the next half-century. They ultimately brought with them a considerable focus on the role of the individual and what individuals could do to avoid the onset of 'self' as opposed to 'environmentally' induced disease.[17]

Social medicine had been the main ideology working for change in public health in the interwar and wartime years, becoming an international movement with an exchange of ideas and models, derived in part from Soviet social hygiene experiments after the Revolution.[18] Its influence extended to the United States, Latin America, and European countries like Belgium, where René Sand took the chair of social medicine in 1945, a post established with funding from the US Rockefeller Foundation. Rockefeller was also instrumental in the international promotion of social medicine in Latin America. In many countries the goals of social medicine were overtly linked to programmes of political reform.[19] In Britain, the ideas of social medicine were taken up by academics in medicine and the social sciences and the ideas developed as part of the more general discussion of health planning and reconstruction during the war. Jane Lewis notes that the term was not widely used in the UK until the early 1940s, and social medicine was sometimes confused with socialized medicine and the planning for integrated health services. After the establishment of the chair in social medicine at Oxford University in 1942, a chair taken by John Ryle, the development of the concept, so Lewis argues, was conditioned by its location within the universities and a search for academic credibility which led it further away from policy concerns.[20] The concept of

[17] M. Jackson, 'Cleansing the Air and Promoting Health. The Politics of Pollution in Post-war Britain', in Berridge and Loughlin (eds.), *Medicine, the Market and the Mass Media*, 221–43, sees the clean air activities of the 1950s as precursors of later environmentalism in relation to health. However, he recognizes that the environmental revival took place from the 1960s initially largely through single-issue pressure groups.

[18] For further discussion of pre-war social medicine and the post-war change, see D. Porter (ed.), *Social Medicine and Medical Sociology in the Twentieth Century* (Amsterdam: Rodopi, 1997) and her chapter 'The Decline of Social Medicine in the 1960s', 97–119.

[19] M. Cueto, *Missionaries of Science: The Rockefeller Foundation and Latin America* (Bloomington: Indiana University Press, 1994); D. Porter, *Health, Civilization and the State. A History of Public Health from Ancient to Modern Times* (London: Routledge, 1999), 293.

[20] Lewis, *What Price Community Medicine?*, 37.

social medicine remained vague. Although to Ryle it symbolized the combination of social conscience with clinical medicine, other leading proponents like Richard Titmuss and J. N. Morris attached importance to the involvement of social science, the use of epidemiology, and the study of health policy.[21] Its major practical impact during the 1940s was in the search for a new type of medical curriculum, but even there it failed to have the impact which it had hoped. Departments of social medicine were not generally established in the medical schools as two mid-1940s reports had proposed.[22] The new creed was also rejected at the level of practice, by the MoHs, who saw it as too clinical and too interested in social pathology rather than health. Thus began a division between theory and practice which continued to mark the public health field over the ensuing decades and which also underpins the developments analysed in this book.

Social medicine also intersected directly with the smoking and lung cancer story, for it was the social medicine networks which initially took the smoking issue forward. The tenets of social medicine in the 1940s were close to the interests of the Socialist Medical Association, of which Richard Doll was a prominent member.[23] The Medical Research Council set up a Social Medicine Unit under Jerry Morris at the Central Middlesex Hospital in 1948 and this hospital was where Doll also came to work on gastroenterology with Francis Avery Jones.[24] The Social Medicine Unit was one of those originally considered for the location of the smoking and lung cancer research. Dr Horace Joules, medical superintendent of the Hospital, was a member of the Socialist Medical Association; the hospital became a powerhouse of social medicine sentiment. Networks which would be of importance for post-war public health were beginning to form.

The key to the new post-war public health would be a revised epidemiology which dealt with chronic rather than infectious disease. This focus on epidemiology was part of the post-war transmutation of social medicine. In the mode of explaining social problems,

---

[21] Lewis, *What Price Community Medicine?*, 40.   [22] Ibid. 44.

[23] J. Stewart, *'The Battle for Health': A Political History of the Socialist Medical Association, 1930–51* (Aldershot: Ashgate, 1999), 39.

[24] S. Murphy, 'The Early Days of the MRC Social Medicine Research Unit', *Social History of Medicine*, 12(3) (1999), 389–406; C. C. Booth, 'Smoking and the Gold Headed Cane', in C. C. Booth (ed.), *Balancing Act: Essays to Honour Stephen Lock* (London: Keynes Press, 1991, 49–55.

tensions arose between the social scientific and the quantitative and also between an emphasis on class and occupation and that on individual behaviour as explanatory concepts. Social medicine in its Oxford variant and also in Birmingham under the leadership of Thomas McKeown increasingly came to mean medical statistics and here it intersected with the MoHs' traditional interest in local statistics and field studies. Murphy and Davey Smith's analysis of articles published between 1947 and 1951 in the *British Journal of Social Medicine* show that most dealt with the health of populations in traditional social medicine style, but that they did this through quantitative rather than qualitative methods. The majority of the papers were concerned with the biological causes of disease and what could be called clinical epidemiology.[25]

The work of Doll and Hill in the smoking and lung cancer studies took these epidemiological studies further. Their work established or refined new technical developments in epidemiology—large population-based surveys, case control and prospective studies. The concept of 'relative risk' was first introduced in the smoking and lung cancer work, replacing an earlier focus on the importance of childhood in adult disease by an emphasis on risk factors for specific diseases. Such approaches fitted with changes in patterns of disease but were by no means uncontroversial or uncritically accepted either by traditional laboratory scientists or by other branches of statistics, as we will see below. They also came at a time when the nature of the 'social' in social medicine investigations was changing.

Here was a major change away from explanation in terms of social structure, economic inequality, occupation, or environment. Smoking and lung cancer epitomized this pending change and helped to accelerate it. Earlier studies had emphasized the role of class and of occupation as for example in Morris and Titmuss' wartime study of rheumatic heart disease.[26] Those interested in diseases of the lung would have typically concentrated their investigation on the role of environment or of occupation. This emphasis continued in the 1950s: in 1954, as President of the Socialist Medical Association, Joules

[25] S. Murphy and G. Davey Smith, 'The British Journal of Social Medicine: What Was in a Name?', *Journal of Epidemiology and Community Health*, 51 (1997), 2–8.
[26] J. N. Morris and R. M. Titmuss, 'Epidemiology of Juvenile Rheumatism', *Lancet*, ii (1942), 59–63; V. Berridge, 'Jerry Morris', *International Journal of Epidemiology*, 30 (2001), 1141–5.

established a special committee on Clean Air and Diseases of the Lung which drew together medical experts on industrial diseases and representatives of the engineering, mining, and tobacco workers' unions.[27] But this focus on occupation and environment was also in flux. In 1950, Doll had demonstrated the relationship between infant mortality, tuberculosis, and poor housing conditions, calling on the government to build an extra 400,000 houses a year.[28] Such a focus was in contrast to the emphasis on individual responsibility which emerged from the smoking work. The rise of the local social survey—another aspect of statistical development in the 1950s—saw explanation in terms of social structural inequality replaced by an emphasis on social behaviour. Personality and mental health issues like neurosis also started to enter the framework. Porter's analysis of articles in the *British Journal of Social Medicine* shows that the psychosomatic nature of disease and the role of stress in the aetiology of the diseases of modern life came increasingly to preoccupy the journal by the middle of the 1950s.[29]

Developments in social medicine were an important context for the new epidemiology. The distinctively British statistical tradition was also a significant influence, more important in the late 1940s and 1950s than the US–UK epidemiological connections which developed later. The 'pre-history' of British statistics has been underplayed as a precursor of the developments in epidemiology after the War. Yet it was an important dimension. Places were beginning to give way to populations as the main focus. Edward Higgs points out that the work in the late nineteenth and early twentieth centuries of Francis Galton, Karl Pearson, George Udny Yule, R. A. Fisher, and their colleagues on correlation and regression analysis, goodness of fit, sampling, and statistical error had given science new techniques of measurement and also undermined its certainties.[30] Eileen Magnello traces a 'family tree' of statistical influence from Pearson through Greenwood and Percy

[27] P. Palladino, 'Discourses of Smoking, Health, and the Just Society: Yesterday, Today, and the Return of the Same?', *Social History of Medicine*, 14 (2001), 313–35.

[28] Stewart, '*The Battle for Health*', 202.

[29] D. Porter, 'From Social Structure to Social Behaviour in Britain after the Second World War', in V. Berridge and S. Blume (eds.), *Poor Health. Social Inequality before and after the Black Report* (London: Frank Cass, 2003), 58–80.

[30] E. Higgs, 'Medical Statistics, Patronage and the State: The Development of the MRC Statistical Unit, 1911–1948', *Medical History*, 44 (2000), 323–40.

Stocks, who were Pearson's students, to Bradford Hill.[31] In the interwar years, as Rosser Matthews has shown, Pearsonian statistics were little understood by medical practitioners of any persuasion and the mode of analysis had little legitimacy within medicine.[32] But the networks were developing. Higgs locates the institutional embedding of statistics in the personal networks formed in the interwar years between Major Greenwood, who developed close links with the MRC and the Ministry of Health (MH) as the London School of Hygiene and Tropical Medicine's (LSHTM) first professor of epidemiology and vital statistics, and Walter Morley Fletcher, secretary of the MRC. Greenwood's influence on a generation of British medical statisticians was profound; and post-war it was Charles Fletcher, Morley Fletcher's son, and Bradford Hill, statistician son of Leonard Hill, head of the MRC's interwar department of applied physiology, with whom Greenwood had worked, who took these developments further. But the transformation in epidemiology towards concepts of multiple causation and away from bacteriological models took place in the first quarter of the twentieth century, before the shift in patterns of disease. It was Greenwood, whose *Epidemics and Crowd Diseases* was published in 1935, who pioneered these developments and whose influence came to fruition in the post-war developments in public health.[33] The central powerhouse was the MRC Statistical Research Unit at LSHTM in the 1940s and 1950s. Its work had a profound impact on international medicine. The Unit conducted the first statistically rigorous clinical trial, that of the effects of streptomycin on tuberculosis, and was the location for the smoking and lung cancer studies. The role of the School as the institutional embedding of academic public health, and of personal networks and tactical alliances in the context of British statistics is an important part of the story.

So the research on smoking and lung cancer impacted on a period of change within public health and its way of analysing disease. Public health was 'on the cusp' between different ways of looking at health and illness in society. Legitimizing the smoking and lung cancer link was the

[31] E. Magnello and A. Hardy (eds.), *The Road to Medical Statistics* (Amsterdam: Rodopi, 2002), 95–123.

[32] J. Rosser Matthews, *Quantification and the Quest for Medical Certainty* (Princeton: Princeton University Press, 1995), 87–149.

[33] D. Roth, 'The Scientific Basis of Epidemiology; an Historical and Philosophical Enquiry', PhD thesis, University of California at Berkeley, 1976.

first stage in the establishment of society focused on individual health and obsessing over the concept of risk.

DENIAL AND DELAY? THE RESPONSE IN THE 1950S TO THE SMOKING–LUNG CANCER CONNECTION

Austin Bradford Hill came from the British statistical tradition outlined earlier, whereas Richard Doll's radicalism and move into statistics from medicine epitomized some of the interests of social medicine. Let us return now to the early 1950s and the publication of the Doll–Hill work to analyse its reception. The social medicine–public health context was important in that response: but so, too, was the view from government of what the implications of the research might be. Smoking and lung cancer impacted on public health in a state of flux, but it also highlighted a set of choices for a government just emerging from the wartime years. The policy response in the 1950s has often been categorized as one of 'denial and delay', of government failing to respond immediately because of the economic importance of tobacco duty and the political influence of the tobacco industry. Those issues were important: but there were also wider concerns about the proper role for government in advising its citizens about health risk. The government response was itself part of the gradual reorientation of society towards a focus on the idea of individualized health 'risk' and the marketing of such an ethos to the population.

Charles Webster has shown in detail how the particular issue of smoking and lung cancer fared over the seven years after the first results were published.[34] A written parliamentary answer from Ian Macleod as Minister of Health in the Conservative government in February 1954 accepted that there was a connection but that it was not a simple one.[35] When the MRC issued its own report on smoking and lung cancer in June 1957 the Ministry of Health adopted the argument more fully. The Parliamentary Secretary to the MH on 27 June 1957 expressed for the first time unambiguous support for the conclusions reached by Doll and Hill in 1950. Webster locates this sequence of events in the

[34] Webster, 'Tobacco Smoking Addiction'.
[35] Hansard. Parliamentary Debates. 12 Feb. 1954, 523, cols. 173–4. Written answer from Iain Macleod, Minister of Health.

machinations of the powerful and complex advisory machinery which stood between the MRC and the MH. The main advisory body was the Cancer and Radiotherapy Standing Advisory Committee, reporting to the Central Health Services Council, which in turn advised the MH. Horace Joules of the Central Middlesex Hospital, a member of both bodies, was the only person within the advisory committee machinery consistently to press the issue. Palladino has recently related his stance to a continuing Christian Socialist tradition.[36] The initial government response also in June 1957 was a MH circular encouraging local authorities to develop health education campaigns on smoking. The 1950s saw a fluid policy situation in which the government response was conditioned by a number of factors, not all of them directly smoking related. The economic and financial importance of smoking to the exchequer was important and the tobacco industry was a valued partner of government. But also in play were the contested nature of the evidence; changes in the nature and role of public health; the role of air pollution as a contentious political issue; the central government politics of health education; and the general culture of smoking with its electoral implications. Let us look at each of these issues.

The rise of a new style of epidemiology in the post-war years and the way in which social medicine was increasingly developing a statistical and epidemiological bent has already been discussed. But this had yet to establish legitimacy as an acceptable mode of scientific proof in wider public and political circles. The nature of the evidence which the epidemiological studies presented in the 1950s has been much discussed by American historians in recent years. Allan Brandt and John Burnham have seen the smoking–lung cancer 'discovery' and subsequent events as a major watershed in the acceptability of chronic disease epidemiology to provide legitimate forms of scientific explanation; this was a major paradigm shift towards epidemiology and statistical modes of explanation and causation at the expense of laboratory science.[37] Mark Parascandola has pointed out that the conflict was more within statistics, a controversy between biostatisticians and epidemiologists and has also related these discussions to the politics

[36] Palladino, 'Discourses of Smoking, Health, and the Just Society'.

[37] A. Brandt, 'The Cigarette, Risk and American Culture', *Daedalus*, 119 (1990), 155–76; J. Burnham, 'American Physicians and Tobacco Use: Two Surgeons General, 1929 and 1964', *Bulletin of the History of Medicine*, 63 (1989), 1–31.

of the National Institutes of Health (NIH) in the 1950s.[38] Talley et al. have argued that there was a legitimate scientific controversy over smoking and lung cancer in the 1950s and early 1960s which reached its denouement and codification in the Surgeon General's report of 1964.[39] However, these historical positions have been complicated by the involvement of historians in the litigation through which US smoking policy primarily proceeds.[40]

The British situation was not the same as that in the United States and there were distinct national differences in the process of scientific discovery. Social medicine and British medical statistics were of course lacking as a context in the United States. The research also filtered through different health systems and different governmental routes. In the UK politicians and bureaucrats in the central state were directly involved in pronouncing on science, and needed convincing: this was not the case in the United States. The links between researchers in the two countries also were slight at this stage. In the 1940s, Doll and Hill were not aware of the parallel research being carried out by Wynder and Graham, but in the 1950s contacts between British and American epidemiologists developed rapidly. It was significant that Hill gave the first presentation of his postulates, which gave the ground rules for establishing causation, at a lecture at Harvard in the 1950s. As in the United States, the conflict in Britain was within statistics, where a key opponent to the smoking and lung cancer hypothesis

[38] M. Parascandola, 'Cigarettes and the US Public Health Service in the 1950s', *American Journal of Public Health*, 91 (2001), 196–205, and *idem*, 'What Is an Epidemiologist? Biostatistics and Epidemiology at the National Cancer Institute', unpublished manuscript; *idem*, 'Skepticism, Statistical Methods and the Cigarette', *Perspectives in Medicine and Biology*, 47 (2004), 246–61.

[39] C. Talley, H. I. Kushner, and C. E. Sterk, 'Lung Cancer, Chronic Disease Epidemiology, and Medicine, 1948–1964', *Journal of the History of Medicine and Allied Sciences*, 59 (2004), 329–74.

[40] Brandt has recently changed his view in testimony given in a legal case in the United States against the Phillip Morris tobacco company. In this testimony, he argues that in the United States scientific consensus about the smoking and lung cancer relationship was reached without a doubt in the mid-1950s and that controversy was only kept alive by the tobacco companies through public relations activity. US District Court for the District of Columbia, United States of America versus Philip Morris USA Inc. United States written direct examination of Allan M. Brandt, PhD, <http://www.usdoj. gov/civil/cases/tobacco2/20040920%20Allan%20M%20Brandt%20Ph.D520Written %20Direct.pdf>, accessed 23 November 2004.

Talley and Kushner have worked for the tobacco industry defence law firms but have withdrawn their support for US industry legal positions and have declared that their article is not intended to provide any support for the industry's legal case.

was the statistician Ronald Fisher, who had played a central role in the development of the randomized controlled trial.[41] Ronald Fisher has been criticized because of his role as adviser to the Tobacco Manufacturers Standing Committee, set up in 1956 to assist research. More important was his eugenic worldview, which at the time that the Doll–Hill research was first published was still a dominant tendency within British statistical explanation, although subsequently it fell out of fashion. Recent evidence has thrown more light on the nature of this controversy. Fisher's opposition arose in part from statistical issues; correlation should not be taken as proof of causation. But it also emanated from his libertarian views, which meant that he was strongly against anti-smoking publicity. He thought people should be given the data and draw their own conclusions: he criticized Doll and Hill only after an article in the *BMJ* had stated that people should be discouraged from smoking. This view of what was termed 'propaganda' was common at the time and informed the early health education responses.[42]

The issue of inhalation also divided the researchers, since, paradoxically, fewer smokers who inhaled developed lung cancer.[43] There were threats of libel. Bradford Hill had offered data from the 1952 study he and Doll had carried out, not from the 1950 study. Fisher accused the researchers of suppressing evidence. His view was that he had requested these papers through the medium of Doll, but that Doll did not pass the request on to Bradford Hill and hence the dispute escalated. Doll's recollection was that he had not spoken to Fisher on the matter.[44] This controversy was played out in a number of publications and was also taken up by other authors. The closure in favour of the causal

[41] R. A. Fisher, 'Dangers of Cigarette Smoking', *British Medical Journal*, 2 (1957), 43 (in the same volume, see also 'Alleged Dangers of Cigarette Smoking', 297–8); *idem*, 'Lung Cancer and Cigarettes', *Nature*, 182 (1958), 108; *idem*, 'Cancer and Smoking', *Nature*, 182 (1958), 596; *idem*, *Smoking, the Cancer Controversy: Some Attempts to Assess the Evidence* (Edinburgh, 1959); J. B. Fisher, *R. A. Fisher: The Life of a Scientist* (New York, 1978).

[42] V. Berridge and K. Loughlin, 'Smoking and the New Health Education in Britain, 1950s to 1970s', *American Journal of Public Health*, 95(6), (2005), 956–64.

[43] This was the view at the time, although subsequently it was shown that all cigarette smokers inhaled, even if unconsciously. Thanks to Walter Holland for a comment on this point.

[44] This sequence of events is detailed in I. Chalmers, 'Fisher and Bradford Hill: Theory and Pragmatism?', *International Journal of Epidemiology*, 32 (2003), 922–48, the proceedings of a conference which included recollections from Walter Bodmer, Fisher's ex-student, and Sir Richard Doll. This evidence emerged in response to a question from the author of this paper and was subsequently elaborated by research in the Fisher papers carried out by Peter Armitage and Ian Chalmers.

hypothesis came through Bradford Hill's postulates, published in 1965 when Hill was President of the Section of Occupational Health of the Royal Society of Medicine. Hill had first begun to develop the criteria for cause and effect and association in the late 1930s and had expanded them in a lecture at Harvard in the 1950s. Their publication in the 1960s formalized guidelines for causal inference and marked the closure of the main period of controversy. In a recent paper, Luc Berlivet has taken the British story and looked at the controversy around smoking and lung cancer and its key role in the formation of the modern science of epidemiology. He argues that

there was more to criticism of supporters of the 'causal hypothesis' than just a reaction of rear guard scientists and vested interests plotting to undermine a promising, if young, scientific practice ... The controversy stirred up by the publications on the relationship between tobacco and lung cancer was eventually transformed into a highly positive retrospective story. This is a process which reminds us of other famous episodes of 'discovery' in the history of science.[45]

This was an important debate within statistics and epidemiology, but it was also a debate which civil servants and others had to deal with. This scientific debate impacted on the policy response of civil servants and others in government. After the publication of the second Doll and Hill report in December 1952, the Imperial Tobacco Company, the main British tobacco company, entered the fray and papers from both sides were circulated to the Standing Advisory Committee in February 1953. As a result, the conflicting evidence, from Doll and Hill and from Geoffrey Todd, assistant manager in the statistical department of the Imperial Tobacco Company, was submitted to a committee chaired by the Government Actuary, Sir George Maddox, later that year. The civil servants in the MH were uncertain. Sir John Charles, the CMO, told Percy Stocks, Chief Medical Statistician to the Registrar General's Office, 'As regards the evidence, I am in general agreement with what you say, but what I was looking for was evidence apart from the analogous or purely statistical. So far as I am aware, there is no *purely* pathological evidence of this long incubation period in lung cancer'.[46] Neville Goodman, a MH civil servant, cited in an internal minute the tobacco industry's opposing research report; the failure of attempts to show a carcinogen in tobacco; and other causes of the rise in lung cancer

---

[45] Berlivet, ' "Association or Causation?" ', 39–74.
[46] London, National Archives, Ministry of Health papers, MH55/1011. Sir John Charles to Percy Stocks, 18 February 1953.

such as smoke pollution.[47] Doubts about the scientific objectivity of Wynder, who visited the Ministry in 1953, also compounded the issue:

He is a young man 'far gone in enthusiasm' for the causal relationship between tobacco smoking and lung cancer. (I had been told when I was in New York this spring that he was the son of a revivalist preacher and had inherited his father's antipathy to tobacco and alcohol. The American Cancer Society was very suspicious of his early work for this reason.)[48]

The statistical panel reported in November 1953 that a 'real association' had been established, with a 'strong presumption' that the real association was causal. It might also be dependent on co-factors such as the urban–rural difference and occupational matters; the report therefore treated with great reserve the death rates which had been calculated by Doll and Hill through a section on estimated risks in the 1952 paper. The Cancer SAC accepted this conclusion, recommending that young people should be warned about the risks of smoking. The government assessment of the state of scientific opinion was beginning to become clearer; and it was this development in opinion which led to the first MH statement in the House of Commons in February 1954, followed by a press conference. Macleod as Minister of Health promised no further action; there was a need for further research.[49] The parliamentary discussions of the time show similar fluidity in the political appreciation of the health risk. In an adjournment debate held in March 1953, MPs from across the political spectrum expressed uncertainty or opposition. Harmar Nicholls, Conservative MP for Peterborough, expressed the then common view of the dangers of arousing 'cancer phobia', the fear of cancer could be worse than cancer itself; the report 'is more a report of statisticians than a medical report'. Bessy Braddock, Labour MP for Liverpool Exchange, favoured an environmental explanation, and therefore found the urban–rural divide a barrier to acceptance of the smoking–lung cancer connection. 'In view of the fact that cigarette and pipe smoking goes on all over the country, it is folly to say that it is the main cause of lung cancer.'[50]

[47] Ibid., Minute from Neville Goodman to Mr Gregson, 12 March 1953.
[48] Ibid., Note by Goodman to Gregson, 28 October 1953.
[49] Ibid., Smoking and Lung Cancer, Report of the statistical panel appointed by the Chief Medical Officer, Ministry of Health, 6 November 1953; Minutes of Standing Advisory Committee, 22 December 1953; Draft memorandum to Cabinet Home Affairs Committee, 26 January 1954.
[50] Hansard. Parliamentary Debates, 19 March 1953. Lung cancer (smoking) adjournment debate, cols. 333–50.

Expert opinion was also related to another issue: the role of the tobacco industry. Here there had been a long history of cooperation in Britain and a government–industry relationship different to that in the United States. Tobacco was a key import during the Second World War and its duty a major source of government revenue. During the War the industry had been under strict government control and the Board of Trade appointed Sir Alexander Maxwell, who before the War had been a leading leaf merchant, as Tobacco Controller. The industry, in its relationships with government, was different from the US tobacco industry, which had no such continuing corporate tradition.[51] Both Maxwell and Sir John Partridge of the Imperial Tobacco Company had close and continuing access to government. Imperial dominated the industry–government relationship in the UK until the late 1970s. The Imperial Board had been astonished by the Doll–Hill studies and saw its role as working with government, as it had done during the War, to produce a cleaner product. The US industry, by comparison, was distant from government, and concentrated from the start on public relations exercises to counteract the perceived dangers of smoking.[52] In the late 1970s, with changes in the ownership of the industry, Imperial's dominance faltered and the role of the US companies in the UK became more significant.[53] But in the 1950s the close relationship was marked by efforts to deal with the health issue.

The industry provided an alternative source of scientific expertise, in particular through its own statistician, Geoffrey Todd, whose report had been submitted to the Cancer SAC. The industry also planned to fund research, and had approached both the MRC and the MH in 1953. Sir Alexander Maxwell, chairman of the Tobacco Advisory Committee, in a secret memo to Harold Himsworth, Secretary of the MRC, stated his lack of belief in any true association between smoking and lung cancer. In order to investigate the true causes of lung cancer the committee wished to covenant £250,000 over a period of seven

[51] B. W. E. Alford, *W. D. and H. O. Wills and the Development of the U.K. Tobacco Industry 1786–1965* (London: Methuen 1973), 399–428.

[52] Brandt's legal testimony gives much detail on this public relations stance. USA vs Philip Morris USA Inc., United States written direct examination of Brandt.

[53] V. Berridge and P. Starns, 'The "Invisible Industrialist" and Public Health: The Rise and Fall of "Safer Smoking" in the 1970s', in Berridge and Loughlin (eds.), *Medicine, the Market and the Mass Media*, 172–91.

years. Discussions between the Treasury and the Ministry of Health resulted in a compromise whereby the tobacco company's gift was to the government, which would then allocate it to the MRC. This avoided charges of the impropriety of the Council accepting money from an interested body. The gift was for research into smoking and lung cancer, but also into the means of removing the harmful elements from the tobacco, when they were identified. This was the origin of a long programme of 'product modification' research which was of particular significance in the 1970s and also fuelled the work on nicotine carried out in the 1980s and 1990s. The gift was to be made, so John Boyd Carpenter at the Treasury wrote to the Lord President, the Marquess of Salisbury, for research into smoking and lung cancer, and 'presumably of the means of removing the elements in the tobacco which may have this effect'.[54]

A visit paid to Europe by Dr C. C. Little in 1956 to survey the state of play on tobacco research and funded by the Tobacco Industry Research Committee, an American industry organization, provided an outsider's view of the relationship between the British industry and government. Those connections were very different from those developed in the United States, where the industry took a public relations stance from the outset with a view to possible future legal action,[55] The British industry, he reported, had no knowledge at all of what had been funded through its MRC benefaction; industry was not seeking to influence the course of research. In the course of his visit, Dr Little moved easily between the scientific cancer research community, the Ministry of Health, where he met the CMO, Sir John Charles, and the Imperial Tobacco company offices and laboratories in Bristol. He advised the British industry that it should follow the US model and set up a coordinating committee to fund research. His idea was that it could be a MH advisory committee. In the event the manufacturers set up in 1956–7 the Tobacco Manufacturers Standing Committee, subsequently renamed the Tobacco Research Council, which opened its own laboratories in Harrogate in 1962 after the MRC benefaction had come to an end. None of these relationships were secret. The industry did not make a secret of its connections and referred to

[54] London, National Archives, Ministry of Health papers, MH55/1011, Letter from John Boyd Carpenter to Marquess of Salisbury, 8 February 1954.
[55] Little to Hartnett, 25 April 1956, Council for Tobacco Research Collection, <http://legacy.library.ucsf.edu/cgi/getdoc?tid=dqf1aa00&fmt=pdf&ref=results>.

the US industry research committee in its first published report.[56] However, there clearly also were differences in approach between the two industries, and there was criticism of the US industry from the British side which seemed uneasy with the American public relations approach.[57]

The role of the industry was also of concern at a broader level within government because of its revenue implications. In February 1954 Macleod as Minister of Health made a statement to the Commons which relayed the advice given by the Cancer SAC. This statement was made, as Herbert Brittain of the Treasury put it, 'in language which was in no way dangerous or embarrassing to us from the revenue point of view'. Macleod himself had commented with cheery cynicism in a letter to Boyd Carpenter at the Treasury in January 1954, 'we all know that the Welfare State and much else is based on tobacco smoking.'[58] Tobacco tax was an important part of government revenue (16% of central revenue in 1950) and signs of further movement on the causal hypothesis later in the 1950s evoked Treasury anxiety. A supplementary answer given by Robin Turton from the Ministry of Health on 5 March 1956, where he said there was a causal connection, brought forth enquiries from the Treasury; had there been more developments since 1954? Sir John Hawton, the MH Permanent Secretary, replied soothingly

needless to say, we are very conscious of the close Treasury interest in this subject and that is one of the things which governs the guarded sort of statements which we have so far made ... If there is any question of our being driven to say more than we already have on this subject, we shall of course only do it in consultation with you or your people ... I have a strong feeling that we are going to be put under more and more pressure to give more positive warnings to the public—and particularly from our own Central Health Services Council and its Medical Committee ... Until then I don't think there is anything we need do and I think that the best policy is to keep the subject as quiet as we are allowed to.[59]

[56] Tobacco Manufacturers Standing Committee, *First Annual Report for the Year Ended 31 May 1957*, refers to the close links with the US Tobacco Industry Research committee, 3–4.

[57] Duncan to Hartnett, 15 May 1956, Council for Tobacco Research Collection, <http://legacy.library.ucsf.edu/cgi/getdoc?tid=xpf1aa00&fmt=pdf&ref=results>.

[58] London, National Archives, Ministry of Health papers, MH55/1011, Letter from Ian Macleod to John Boyd Carpenter, 29 January 1954.

[59] London, National Archives, Ministry of Health papers, MH55/2232, Sir John Hawton to Hubert Brittain, Treasury, 15 March 1956.

But the matter was not allowed to remain quiet. Referred to the full Cabinet, it was decided that Turton should make a restrained statement in the Commons. Macmillan as Chancellor of the Exchequer wanted this held back until after the Budget. His diary entry for 19 April 1956 read, 'Cabinet 11.45, Singapore, British Guiana; medical views on the dangers of smoking. If we lose Singapore, it's a terrible blow to all our Far Eastern interests. If people really think they will get cancer of the lung from smoking it's the end of the Budget!'[60] Politicians at this period were generally cynical about the whole smoking issue, apart from its economic implications. Macleod told a House of Commons questioner who wanted an American report on smoking and lung cancer published as a White Paper that dozens of reports, all claiming to be authoritative, were being published. 'If my hon. Friend is a heavy smoker and is concerned about the connection between cancer of the lung and smoking, I would recommend him to give up reading.'[61] Macmillan commented about the statement to be made in 1956 by the minister of Health, 'Cabinet approved a statement to be made by the minister of Health about Tobacco and cancer of the lung. It was a much better draft than the original one. I only hope it won't stop people smoking!'[62]

Economic issues were not the only political consideration. Smoking was politically difficult for government, but so too was air pollution, with which the smoking–lung cancer issue intersected. This intersection came in two ways—through scientific uncertainty about the responsibility for the causation of lung cancer and through the political implications of air pollution. Scientific uncertainty was represented by Bessie Braddock's comment in the Commons debate. If lung cancer mortality was highest in urban areas how could smoking be the only factor implicated, when this did not have an urban–rural divide? The text of a TV broadcast on the subject in 1953 after publication of the Doll–Hill research on smoking and lung cancer in 1950 gives a sense of the focus on both individual and environment. Introduced by Charles Fletcher, later famous for his pioneering *Your Life in Their Hands,* the programme was

---

[60] H. Macmillan, *The Macmillan Diaries. The Cabinet Years, 1950–1957,* ed. P. Catterall (London: Macmillan, 2003), entry for 19 April, 1956, 551.

[61] Hansard. Parliamentary Debates 15 July 1954. Macleod himself gave up his sixty-a-day habit, not because of the scientific evidence, in which he firmly believed, but because he 'got bored with a messy habit'. He smoked three or four small cigars daily, in line with the health advice of the time, until his death. R. Shepherd, *Iain Macleod* (London: Hutchinson, 1994), 91–3.

[62] Macmillan, *Diaries,* entry for 23 May 1956, 556.

called *Matters of Medicine*. Dr Guy Scadding, taking part, expressed the views clearly:[63]

smoking cannot be called the cause of lung cancer, since non-smokers also get the disease, and moreover the increase in cigarette smoking is not likely to be the only cause of the increase in the lung cancer death rate. The effect of smoking cannot explain the difference in mortality between town and country dwellers. Perhaps the effect of air pollution is another factor. If the effects of smoking and general pollution of the air are ... if they reinforce each other, I think that most of the known facts about the incidence of lung cancer can be explained.[64]

This scientific uncertainty also caused difficulties at the political level, in the negotiations which took place in 1957 between the Cabinet committee on cancer of the lung, which was appointed in that year, and the Medical Research Council, which planned to issue a statement on the causes of lung cancer. This committee was operating just after the passage of the Clean Air Act in 1956, which had come about in part in response to the 'great smog' of 1952. The government's legislation had been delayed until after the general election of 1955 because of fears of how the public might react to restrictions on long-standing habits of open fire domestic heating; and the resultant legislation had also been criticized for dealing only with those habits and not with air pollution from industry.[65]

The MRC, so it was reported to the Cabinet committee, had for the first time come to the conclusion that the smoking of tobacco had a direct causal relationship to lung cancer and therefore there was no alternative but to publicize their conclusions. It was the proposed

[63] For the significance of this programme, see K. Loughlin, ' "Your Life in Their Hands": The Context of a Medical–Media Controversy', *Media History*, 6 (2000), 177–88.

[64] *Matters of Medicine*, 3, 12 January 1953. In an interview, Dr Scadding later recalled how Doll had put him up to make this broadcast because he did not want to do it. Scadding was the 'respectable front', a comment which indicates the status of issues round this scientific claim. Guy Scadding, interview with Sir Gordon Worstenholme, London, Royal College of Physicians, RCP/Oxford Brookes video interview collection.

[65] For the response at this stage, see Jackson, 'Cleansing the Air and Promoting Health', in Berridge and Loughlin (eds.), *Medicine, the Market and the Mass Media*; R. Parker, 'The Struggle for Clean Air', in P. Hall, H. Land, R. Parker, and A. Webb (eds.), *Change, Choice and Conflict in Social Policy* (London, 1975: repr. Aldershot: Gower, 1988), 371–409. See also Roy Parker's comment and oral history in the transcript of the witness seminar on the smog of 1952 in http://www.lshtm.ac.uk/history. V. Berridge and S. Taylor (eds.), *The Big Smoke: Fifty Years after the 1952 London Smog* (London: Centre for History in Public Health, 2005).

inclusion in the MRC statement that up to 30% of lung cancer might be caused by air pollution which caused the greatest political alarm. This would give air pollution, the minutes record, 'unwarranted prominence'. The committee thought that Professor Bradford Hill and Dr Doll had failed to show any substantial difference in risk among non-smokers in greater London and in rural areas. So the politicians asked the MRC to re-examine their statement. Both statements, so it was commented, had obvious political implications.[66] On 31 May 1957, Lord Home, the Lord President of the Council (responsible for the MRC), reported back on the changes made in the statement. The MRC had re-examined their draft and proposed to modify the references to atmospheric pollution which implied that it might be responsible for up to 30% of such deaths. The section would read instead, 'on balance it seems likely that atmospheric pollution plays some part in causing the disease, but a relatively minor one in comparison with cigarette smoking.' A further section was modified to read, 'A proportion of cases, the exact content of which cannot yet be defined, may be due to atmospheric pollution.'[67] The pollution issue was effectively headed off.[68] This episode showed that, although government was wary about the smoking and lung cancer case as a policy issue, it was infinitely preferable to air pollution. That was the issue which government did not want reopened.[69]

Also involved were the politics of health education. Health education had traditionally been conducted by the successor of the British Social Hygiene Council, renamed the Central Council for Health Education (CCHE) in 1927. During the War publicity had been a central responsibility of the Ministry of Information but after the War responsibility was again passed back to the local authorities who were to fund out of local rates the CCHE's work. Central government had no wish to resume funding of these activities as discussions of smoking publicity

---

[66] London, National Archives, Cabinet papers, CAB 130/127/GEN 588, Minutes of first meeting of the Cabinet Committee on cancer of the lung, 7 May 1957.

[67] Ibid., Memorandum by Secretary of State for Commonwealth Relations and Lord President of the Council, 31 May 1957.

[68] Parker, 'The Struggle for Clean Air', 371–409. See also Berridge and Taylor (eds.), *The Big Smoke*.

[69] In 2002, at a conference of European environmental epidemiologists held on the fiftieth anniversary of the 'great London smog' members of the audience informed the author that it was almost impossible to research air pollution and lung cancer because it would be seen as undermining the smoking and lung cancer case. This was not an issue of government funding, rather the 'climate of opinion' about research priorities which prevented such initiatives.

made clear.[70] But there were also other reasons why there was reticence about health education. An MH statement in May 1956 explained why central publicity would not be the right thing.

The considerations on publicity concerning smoking and lung cancer differ slightly from those on cancer publicity generally in that the special point—that people might give up smoking—is not a matter of reporting symptoms. It does however concern an individual decision which involves others to a very much smaller extent than the subjects of past central public health campaigns.[71]

Smoking, it argued, was not a 'disease' in the way cancer, or indeed infectious disease was. It might lead to disease, but not for many years. The notion of long-term 'risk', as we have seen, was not yet central to public health in the 1950s. Publicity would be asking people to curtail a habit which was at this stage deeply embedded in everyday culture. It might also raise public fear about cancer, which the Ministry had been concerned to damp down. Unfounded cancer phobia might generate a demand for services at a time when NHS costs were becoming a political issue.[72]

Conservative politicians were concerned about the implied role of the state. R. A. Butler, Lord Privy Seal, commented in May 1956, 'From the point of view of social hygiene, cancer of the lung is not a disease like tuberculosis; nor should the government assume too lightly the odium of advising the general public on their personal tastes and habits where the evidence of the harm which may result is not conclusive.'[73] This is a theme which emerged consistently throughout the political discussions. Politicians were worried about the implications of the 'nanny state'. As the minutes of the Cabinet committee on smoking record, 'The Government should not seek to intrude into the sphere of an individual's personal responsibility. It was, however, important to stress this element of personal choice since direct government action was excluded.'[74] The focus was also quite different from traditional public

[70] London, National Archives, Ministry of Health papers MH55/2203, Public health propaganda; smoking and lung cancer: publicity policy, 1957–60.
[71] London, National Archives. Ministry of Health papers MH55/2220, Tobacco smoking and cancer of the lung, Brief for adjournment debate, 1 March 1957.
[72] E. Toon, 'Cancer Education in the 1950s', paper given at the NIH conference on cancer, November 2004, forthcoming in the *Bulletin of the History of Medicine*.
[73] London, National Archives, Ministry of Health papers, MH 55/2232, Memorandum by Lord Privy Seal, 1 May 1956.
[74] London, National Archives, Cabinet papers, CAB 130/127/GEN 588, Minutes of second meeting of Cabinet committee on cancer of the lung, 3 June 1957.

health campaigns. One civil servant pointed out that any campaign would have to be directed to men (who were the majority of smokers) rather than women and children, who were the more usual objects of public health attention.[75] It was much easier on many political grounds to leave this to the local authorities.

Lying behind this discussion was the cultural normality of smoking and its embedment in a range of social customs and practices. This was far from the simple continuation of the liberal individualism of the gentlemanly culture of smoking which Hilton has ascribed to this period.[76] Tobacco tokens for old age pensioners were issued by government in the 1950s. The possibility of extra tobacco concessions for the disabled was discussed.[77] Smoking was also a cross-class activity with its own rituals embedded in social norms. The public health researcher Walter Holland in an interview recalled that for many years after the smoking–lung cancer research had been published, Bradford Hill would keep a box of cigarettes in his room at LSHTM. When Holland asked him why this was so, Hill was incredulous; it would be so impolite not to offer visitors a cigarette.[78] Norman Brook as Cabinet Secretary was equally amazed at a suggestion that government should be involved in trend setting. 'Does this mean that Prime Ministers should not smoke—or at least should not be seen smoking in public?', he wrote incredulously in 1962.[79] In the 1970s, when the researcher Nicholas Wald wished to trace the changes in tar levels in cigarettes since the 1940s, he was deluged with cigarette stubs and cigarette cases containing tobacco which grieving widows had kept as mementos of their dead husbands. 'His last cigarette' had a cultural significance which has become 'hidden from history' with the subsequent marginalization of smoking.[80] The cultural aspects of post-war smoking have been surprisingly little researched.[81] Anti-smoking attitudes did exist among

[75] London, National Archives, Ministry of Health papers, MH 55/2220, Minute to Mr Pater on new MRC statement, 1 April 1957.

[76] M. Hilton, *Smoking in British Popular Culture, 1800–2000* (Manchester: Manchester University Press, 2000), 234.

[77] London, National Archives, Ministry of Pensions and National Insurance papers, PIN 12/112, 1947, consultation with Treasury and other bodies about extension of token scheme to the totally disabled.

[78] Interview with Walter Holland by Virginia Berridge, 6 March 1997.

[79] London, National Archives, Cabinet papers, CAB 21/4878, Norman Brook to Prime Minister, 11 July 1962.

[80] Interview with Nicholas Wald by Virginia Berridge, 4 July 1996.

[81] Rosemary Eliot of the University of Glasgow has been carrying out oral history interviews with men and women smokers. Other evidence comes from research carried

the general population, but these, too, were not unproblematic in terms of the 'new epidemiology'. When Ann Cartwright and Fred Martin, along with other LSHTM researchers who had moved to Edinburgh with John Brotherston in the 1950s, carried out a survey of attitudes to smoking there after one of the first local authority-led publicity campaigns, their results were surprising. Even in the late 1950s they found no general acceptance of the connection between smoking and lung cancer. A substantial minority did believe smoking was personally harmful, however; but many thought that smoking would affect the health of other people. If they gave up smoking it was largely for financial rather than health reasons.[82] With the Labour governments of the 1960s the continuing normality of smoking had political implications which will be discussed below.

'Denial and delay' does not seem adequate as an explanation of the responses to smoking in the 1950s. Economic interests and the role of the industry were important; but the industry was an important post-war ally of government at this stage, no different from other such interests. There were other political considerations, like air pollution and health education's funding and role. The scientific evidence was indeterminate and cultural normality was centre stage: there was no interest group or 'policy community' round the issue. Apart from key individuals like Joules, no significant lobby was pushing the anti-smoking case, nor indeed was there any consistent policy position. Nor were the researchers themselves activists, another significant difference from later developments. Although Bradford Hill had worked within government during the War, he had advised Doll that it was best to steer clear of the political dimensions of the research. It was his view that a young researcher's career could be tainted by an apparent lack of scientific objectivity.[83] Hill was concerned that Doll's radical past might put him at a disadvantage at a time when political attitudes were

out by social scientists, for example the pioneering and controversial research by Hilary Graham on lone mothers smoking. H. Graham, 'Women's Smoking and Family Health', *Social Science and Medicine*, 25(1987), 47–56. There is also underused material in the Ministry of Health files on responses to the 1950s government campaign on smoking.

[82] A. Cartwright, F. M. Martin, and J. G. Thomson, 'Health Hazards of Cigarette Smoking. Current Popular Beliefs', *British Journal of Preventive and Social Medicine*, 14 (1960), 160–6; *eidem*, 'Distribution and Development of Smoking Habits', *Lancet*, 2 (1959), 725–7.

[83] 'Conversation with Sir Richard Doll', *British Journal of Addiction*, 86 (1991), 365–77; Interview with Sir Richard Doll by Max Blythe, December 1986, RCP/Oxford Polytechnic video archive.

hardening away from the left-wing stance of the wartime years. Hill remarked towards the end of his life that he had made Doll passionate about statistics as a replacement for left-wing politics.[84] Doll's socialist convictions were known and he remained a member of the Communist Party until 1957.[85] Morris at the Social Medicine Unit was affected by this change of view in the MRC.[86] Thus policy in the 1950s was being formed in a very different situation from that which operated later on. As Doll himself stated in evidence to the Commons Health Committee in 1999–2000,

In retrospect, it may be surprising that resistance to the idea that smoking caused so much disease was initially so strong. Three factors, at least, contributed to it. One was the ubiquity of the habit, which was as entrenched among male doctors and scientists as among other men and had dulled the sense that tobacco might be a major threat to health. Another was the novelty of the epidemiological techniques, which had not previously been applied to any important extent to the study of non-infectious disease. The findings were consequently undervalued as a source of scientific evidence. A third was the primacy given to Koch's postulates for determining causation. The evidence that lung cancer also occurred in non-smokers was consequently taken to show that smoking could not be the cause and the possibility that it might be a cause was inappropriately doubted. The manner in which lung cancer was linked to smoking was not, however, unique. All the other major diseases related to smoking were found to be so by epidemiological enquiry and laboratory evidence of physiological effects that provided plausible mechanisms by which smoking might cause them was obtained only later and, in some instances, is still awaited.[87]

The initial political assimilation of the new scientific fact was taking place at a time of change within health structures and modes of research, as we have discussed previously. Health trends showed the increased importance of chronic, rather than infectious or epidemic disease. The social medicine movement, which had been important both before

[84] Interview with Bradford Hill by Max Blythe, 1990, RCP/Oxford Polytechnic video archive.

[85] Letter from Chris Birch, the secretary of Doll's CP branch, *The Guardian*, 27 July 2005.

[86] See Murphy, 'Early Days of the MRC Social Medicine Unit'.

[87] Sir R. Doll, 'Tobacco: A Medical History', Appendix 1, Memorandum by Health Education Authority, Minutes of Evidence taken before the Health Committee, 18 November 1999, p. 26, House of Commons, session 1999–2000, Health Committee, *Second Report, The Tobacco Industry and the Health Risks of Smoking*, vol. ii, Minutes of Evidence and Appendices (London: HM Stationery Office, 2000), 27–II.

and during the War, as a possible 'new avenue' for medical practice, was changing its emphasis in the 1950s to a reliance on chronic disease epidemiology. This epidemiological technique was to become the foundation of a 'new public health' in the 1960s and 1970s when public health practitioners were relocated in health services and out of the local authorities where they had established their pre-war empires.[88] It marked the beginning too of a public health which would focus on single-issue campaigns and on issues of lifestyle rather than of occupation or class.

Smoking was the pioneer issue, but others followed. The connection between diet and heart disease began to be outlined in the 1950s.[89] Exercise and fitness also started to come on to the agenda. Jerry Morris' paper of 1953, which showed, through epidemiological methodology, the differential susceptibility to heart disease of sedentary bus drivers and active conductors, was symbolic of the old and of the new—an occupational study which showed the importance of lifestyle factors.[90] Morris' key text *Uses of Epidemiology*, published in 1957, set the tone for the emergence of the new scientific approach and the new role for public health: the text used smoking extensively as its exemplar.[91] Morris' Social Medicine Unit began to focus its studies on coronary heart disease and this became an international object of study—with the Framingham study in the United States.[92] Air pollution work also continued and a unit was funded at Barts out of the tobacco benefaction money given to the MRC and began its work in 1955. Its Director, Patrick Lawther, commented in an interview in 2003, 'Joan Faulkner (the MRC civil servant who became Doll's wife) told me that who took fags and who

[88] For discussion of these changes, see Lewis, *What Price Community Medicine?*; Porter (ed.), *Social Medicine and Medical Sociology in the Twentieth Century*; Berridge, 'Jerry Morris'.

[89] M. W. Bufton, 'British Expert Advice on Diet and Heart Disease *c*.1945–2000', in Berridge (ed.), *Making Health Policy*, 125–48. Horace Joules was one of the people who first alerted the British government to the fat and heart disease connection. See note 38 of Bufton.

[90] J. N. Morris, J. A Heady, P. A. B. Raffle, C. G. Roberts, and J. W. Parks, 'Coronary Heart Disease and Physical Activity of Work', *Lancet*, ii (1953), 1053–7 and 1111–20.

[91] J. Morris, *Uses of Epidemiology* (Edinburgh: Livingstone, 1957).

[92] For Framingham, see Berlivet ' "Association or Causation?" '; W. G. Rothstein, *Public Health and the Risk Factor: A History of an Uneven Medical Revolution* (Rochester: University of Rochester Press, 2003), 279–85; L. A. Reynolds and E. M. Tansey (eds.), *Cholesterol, Atherosclerosis and Coronary Disease in the UK, 1950–2000*, Wellcome Witnesses to Twentieth Century Medicine, vol. xxvii (London: Wellcome Trust Centre for the History of Medicine at UCL, 2006).

took air pollution was decided on the toss of a coin.'[93]Smoking and air pollution, bronchitis and lung cancer occupied a common conceptual space at this time. Charles Fletcher recalled in an interview how the MRC had set up a Bronchitis Research Committee after the 1952 great smog. His own research (with the occupational focus of the time—it was on post office workers) led him to the conclusion that both tobacco and smog caused the hyper-secretion of mucus that led to emphysema. He started to ask about smoking habits after the Doll–Hill work was published.[94] The fluidity of the smoking science was thus embedded in a more general period of reorientation both within public health and in the ideology and the technical tools of the field. Environmental concerns were changing to population ones and to the focus on risk. The scientific advocates were not anti-industry at this stage but would become so in the course of time. The culture of positive health was still to be established, as the cultural ramifications of smoking indicate. But the events of the 1950s nevertheless foretold a sea change in scientific and medical attitudes towards health and engagement with the public.

[93] Interview with Patrick Lawther by Virginia Berridge and Suzanne Taylor, February 2003.
[94] 'Conversation with Charles Fletcher', *British Journal of Addiction*, 87(4) (1992), 527–38.

2

Medicine and the Media: Marketing Public Health in the 1960s

In April 1963, one D. Kelly wrote to the Ministry of Health about an idea he had had in his head for quite a while about anti-smoking publicity. After discussion with a German doctor friend, he suggested

A rhyming poster might work ... 'THE MODERN BLOKE—DOESN'T SMOKE' ... The ladies are less of a problem—but a growing one. What about 'CONTEMPORARY HAGS ABHOR FAGS' with a similar illustration of modern witches refusing temptation.

K. Norman Reynolds had written in the previous month. He enclosed a poster he had originally designed for a competition, but was 'alas' 'too late in entering it'. 'The word "Cancer" is spelt in cork tipped cigarettes, which gets across a point as well as adding to the eye appeal. This unfortunately hasn't come out in this print.'[1] In the early 1960s, the Ministry was the recipient of 'puffing poems', drawings, the results of a National Society of Non-Smokers essay competition for children, as well as anti-smoking ideas that poured in from members of the public.

These suggestions, now yellowing in their folders in the National Archives, are testimony to the change which occurred in the 1960s and 1970s in public health, and, indeed, in the relationship between medicine and society more generally, for the talk of posters and home-made publicity efforts represented the last gasp of an older tradition of public education. A new era of mass media education and health consciousness was dawning. It repositioned itself in relation to government and to society and 'the public', marketing health. It is argued here that the report on smoking published by the Royal College of Physicians in 1962, *Smoking and Health,* was a key catalyst of the new modernized and mediatized medicine and public health.

---

[1] These suggestions are contained in National Archives, Ministry of Health files MH 151/23, Smoking and lung cancer: publicity suggestions.

The repositioning and its implications are central to two areas of historical debate—to reassessments of 'the permissive society' of the 1960s; and to the historiography of public health, which is the central focus of this book. For the former, commentators such as the health policy analyst Howard Glennerster have noted that a new social policy agenda was emergent in Britain in the 1960s and 1970s, which removed criminal sanctions round abortion and sexuality and was hostile to state intervention in such matters.[2] But others have noted that criminal forms of regulation were replaced by medical ones, and that 'permissiveness' in sexuality was dependent on new forms of medical surveillance.[3] The 'myth' of 1960s permissiveness has come under scrutiny in a wider range of more recent work.[4] That revision of view has not considered the changes in public health in that decade which this chapter argues were also central to the new permissiveness.

That historical debate needs to incorporate consideration of the 1962 Royal College Report and the rise of an ethos of public health not tied to health services, MoHs, or community physicians. The 1962 Report was highly significant for the history of smoking policy, but its significance was also a wider one. Firstly, it signified a new willingness on the part of medicine to speak to the public and to use the media to do so. The media became central to public health. Doctors reoriented their role so that they spoke to the public, not just to the rest of the profession. The role of the media also became central to debates within public health. On the one hand mass media campaigns were increasingly important as a strategy and began to focus on the role of individual risks to health, to urge the reformation of behaviour. On the other, control and even prohibition of advertising deemed detrimental to health was to become an important public health strategy. The wartime and immediate post-war emphasis on responsibility and citizenship gave way to an emphasis on propaganda and persuasion using consumerist techniques. Secondly it marked the emergence of a 'policy community' round public health linking civil servants within government with medical experts outside. This model of health policy making was, with variations, to dominate

[2] H. Glennerster, *British Social Policy since 1945* (Oxford: Blackwell, 1995), 96.

[3] J. Weeks, *Sex, Politics and Society. The Regulation of Sexuality since 1800* (London: Longman, 1981), 267–8.

[4] See, for example, the review by James Obelkevich of Arthur Marwick's *The Sixties: Cultural Revolution in Britain, France, Italy, and the United States, c.1958–c.1974* (Oxford: Oxford University Press, 1998) in *Twentieth Century British History*, 11 (2000), 333–6.

the process of British health policy formation into the twenty-first century. British government acted in a policy-balancing act in which the role of insider–outsider organizations and formal interconnections with scientific expertise were increasingly important. Thirdly, it emphasized at the public and policy levels the role of individual behaviour, legitimated through population-based epidemiology, as the dominant focus of public health endeavour in post-war Britain. The report gave public significance to the new type of public health and to different scientific ways of studying it. The new epidemiology of the 1950s and the new focus on the risk of chronic disease translated into a wider public and policy agenda. Fourthly, it stimulated new attitudes on the part of government in its role in relating to the public on matters of health and a heightened significance for research-based surveillance. Medicine and consumerism were allied through a focus on the role of the individual in society and through a new emphasis on individual persuasion. At the same time research and the social survey began to outline a new view of 'the public' and to establish a relationship between medicine and the social sciences, one which built on the alliances within social medicine but also turned them in a new consumerist direction.

The report therefore signified a new style and outlook for public health which was emergent at around the same time as the organizational and professional changes, but which was, in many respects, separate from them. The smoking activists were not MoHs or even the new community physicians: a new style and outlook for 'public health' was emergent distinct from the profession and its service role. This was research and 'evidence-based' using the social sciences as technical tools. Such developments also invite reflection about the nature of the permissiveness of the 1960s and the roots of the 'health tyranny' which journalists have criticized.[5] The health discussions of the 1960s were marked by contradictory tendencies, in one sense the very antithesis of permissiveness, in another by a new style of 'coercive permissiveness' in health.

The background to these developments was the rise of post-war consumer society and the removal of wartime restrictions on the economy and on consumption, together with the impact of these changes on the media and on advertising.[6] One such change which impacted directly on the tobacco industry was the 1956 Restrictive Trade Practices

---

[5] See discussion of this critique in the Introduction.

[6] J. Obelkevich, 'Consumption', in J. Obelkevich and P. Catterall (eds.), *Understanding Post War British Society* (London: Routledge and Kegan Paul, 1994), 141–54.

Act. This opened the industry up to the possibility of giving cigarette coupons again after the Martin Agreement of 1933 had outlawed coupon brands and maintained retail prices.[7] Newsprint restrictions were dropped and advertising began a rapid rise; advertising of cigarettes expanded. Television advertising became particularly important. In the 1950s the proportion of overall advertising expenditure which went to television shot up from 1% in 1955 to over 20% in 1959.[8] Increased competition for this essential source of revenue was accompanied by the development of market research, which encouraged a redirection in advertisers' money. The idea of what the public wanted became important and new commercial research techniques and surveys were used to find out. Vance Packard's seminal advertising text, *The Hidden Persuaders,* was first published in 1957 and appeared in a paperback version in 1960.[9] American advertising techniques began to filter into the British scene.

This was a time of radical change in the media and in what media sociologists have called the 'circuit of mass communication', the circuits which linked news gathering, news making, and provision. These were developing in the 1950s and 1960s and health was a particular example of these new approaches.[10] The traditional print media expanded, but it was television and the advent of commercial television which had particular influence. In 1946 the overtly propagandist Ministry of Information, which had controlled the flow of information during wartime, was replaced by a new Central Office of Information.[11] The creation and rapid expansion of information machinery at the heart of government drew fierce criticism from politicians and sections of

[7] B. W. E. Alford, *W. D. and H. O. Wills and the Development of the U.K. Tobacco Industry 1786–1965* (London: Methuen, 1973); see also National Archives, Cabinet papers CAB 130/185 GEN 763, minutes and papers of the Cabinet committee on smoking and health; meeting of 11 January 1963 where the Ministry of Health calls attention to the growth of coupon trading for cigarettes.

[8] J. Tunstall, *The Media in Britain* (London: Constable, 1983), 72–3.

[9] V. Packard, *The Hidden Persuaders* (London: Penguin, 1960). The book was reprinted six times between 1960 and 1967.

[10] The following section is based on the research of Kelly Loughlin. See K. Loughlin, 'Networks of Mass Communication: Reporting Science, Health and Medicine in the 1950s and 1960s', in V. Berridge (ed.), *Making Health Policy: Networks in Research and Policy after 1945* (Amsterdam: Rodopi, 2005), 295–322.

[11] J. Tulloch, 'Managing the Press in a Medium Sized European Power', in M. Bromley and H. Stephenson (eds.), *Sex, Lies and Democracy: The Press and the Public* (London: Longman, 1998), 63–83; Sir Fife Clark, *The Central Office of Information* (London: Allen and Unwin, 1970); M. Ogilvy-Webb, *The Government Explains: A Study of the Information Services* (London: Allen and Unwin, 1965).

the press, fearing it would constrain journalistic freedom.[12] The idea of 'propaganda' directed at the home audience during peacetime was seen by some as more akin to dictatorship than democracy. Relations between the media and democratic processes were also at the fore in Britain's first Royal Commission on the Press (1947–9), and the Beveridge inquiry (1949–51) into the future of the British Broadcasting Corporation (BBC). Beveridge recommended the 'democratisation of broadcasting' and the BBC's television monopoly ended in 1955 with the introduction of commercial television; the BBC acquired a second channel in 1963. In the ten years from 1950 to 1960 the percentage of the adult population owning a television set rose from four to eighty.

An expansion in government information services proved useful to the incoming post-war Labour government and the implementation of its social reforms. The government made extensive use of the media, especially broadcasting, in the publicity campaign to accompany the introduction of the National Health and National Insurance schemes (1948).[13] Some individual government departments had developed their own information services during the interwar years. These developments were sporadic. For example, on its inception in 1919 the Ministry of Health had instituted an information section, headed by a journalist, but after four years it closed due to financial retrenchment. Indeed the government had been involved in publicity campaigns before the war, such as the 'Use Your Health Services' campaign undertaken by the Ministries of Health and Education in 1937.[14] However, the publicity that launched the post-war National Health Service (NHS) re-drew accepted relations between the government and the media. Throughout the interwar period these relations had been restricted by ready accusations of publicity seeking or of using government position to promote party-political interests. The NHS was very much a party-political issue, and one that can be seen as distinct for the way it was effectively advertised and introduced through use of the Central Office of Information and the media.

[12] Tulloch 'Managing the Press', 69–72. See also T. Wildy, 'From the MoI to the CoI—Publicity and Propaganda in Britain, 1945–1951: The National Health and Insurance Campaigns', *Historical Journal of Film, Radio and Television*, 6 (1986), 3–16.

[13] Wildy, 'From the MoI to the CoI'; K. Loughlin, 'Spectacle and Secrecy: Press Coverage of Conjoined Twins in 1950s Britain', *Medical History*, 49 (2005), 197–212.

[14] M. Grant, *Propaganda and the Role of the State in Inter-War Britain* (Oxford: Oxford University Press, 1995).

The expansion and more extensive use of government information resources heralded a change in the culture of political communication. Television broadcasting also began its first incursions into 'domestic news', at the time the traditional territory of the press and to a lesser extent radio. Party-political broadcasts also emerged in the early 1950s, and Independent Television News first covered a local by-election in 1958.[15] Ultimately this led to an expansion of outlets for domestic news and the development of new formats like the political interview and current affairs programmes.[16] Politicians themselves who had been reluctant to be 'on the air' and who had tightly controlled political discussion began instead actively to seek out publicity. This change became particularly marked with the Conservative government under Macmillan in the late 1950s.[17] Programmes like *Panorama* began actively to make news and the dropping of the Fourteen-Day rule, whereby the media could not cover anything coming before Parliament within the next fortnight, made coverage easier. The media itself was becoming part of the message.

Health and medicine were caught up in these new developments. At the end of the war, the British Medical Association (BMA) appointed a press officer and renamed its Propaganda Committee the Public Relations Committee. One outcome of the BMA's battle over the NHS was the creation of its highly organized press and information service. Established in 1947 as the information section of the PR Department, by 1950 it was receiving around one hundred telephone calls a week, plus correspondence and personal enquiries, mainly from the press. None of the Royal Colleges, the Medical Research Council, or Royal Society of Medicine had press offices at this time. Although press and PR work at the BMA separated in the 1960s and thereafter, the role of the press department remained of key importance.[18] The specialism

---

15 M. D. Kandiah, 'Television Enters British Politics: The Conservative Party's Central Office and Political Broadcasting, 1945–55', *Historical Journal of Film, Television and Radio*, 15 (1995), 265–84. On Independent Television News, see G. Cox, *Pioneering Television News* (London: John Libbey, 1995).

16 B. Winston, 'The CBS Evening News, 7 April 1949: Creating an Ineffable Television Form', in J. Eldridge (ed.), *Getting the Message: News, Truth and Power* (London: Routledge, 1993), 181–208.

17 J. Betteridge, 'Post War Broadcasting and Changes in Political Public Life', seminar paper given at the media history seminar, Institute of Historical Research, 10 October 1995, notes that it was ITN which stimulated a fresh approach on the part of politicians.

18 K. Loughlin, 'Publicity as Policy: The Changing Role of Press and Public Relations at the BMA, 1940s–1980s', in Berridge (ed.), *Making Health Policy*, 275–94.

of health journalism also developed in these years. Some national newspapers like *The Times* and *Daily Express* had existing arrangements with practising scientists or doctors who supplied reports from 'our science correspondent' or 'our medical correspondent'. However, the specialists that came to prominence after the war were outsiders, in that they were full-time journalists, and many had no formal training in these fields. The *Manchester Guardian* appears to have taken an early lead with J. G. Crowther, who served as science correspondent from 1929 to the early 1950s. Ronnie Bedford, who began covering science and medicine at the *Daily Mirror* in 1950, was a self-made specialist, with a humble entry into journalism, sweeping floors and running errands at the *Wakefield Express*. A new kind of specialist joined their ranks in the 1950s. This was the health services correspondent. Medico-politics and the NHS was an area pioneered by John Prince, a former lobby correspondent at *The Times* who moved to take up the position of health services correspondent at the *Daily Telegraph* in 1957.[19]

THE FIRST REPORT OF THE ROYAL COLLEGE OF PHYSICIANS, 1962

Such was the commercial and health infrastructure emergent at the time of the developments around smoking. At the end of the previous chapter we left the story in 1957 at the time of the MRC's statement accepting the causal hypothesis and the instigation of a health education campaign at the local level. The next five years were to see considerable change. The Royal College of Physicians (RCP) was not the most obvious body to produce a report on the link between smoking and lung cancer and in fact it had already turned down the opportunity once.[20] In November 1956, Francis Avery Jones, the gastroenterologist from the Central Middlesex, with whom Doll had originally worked, wrote to

---

[19] Loughlin, 'Networks of Mass Communication'.
[20] The point about the RCP and the role of the media is also discussed in V. Berridge, 'Science and Policy, the Case of Post War Smoking Policy', in S. Lock, L. Reynolds, and E. M. Tansey (eds.), *Ashes to Ashes: The History of Smoking and Health* (Amsterdam: Rodopi, 1998), 143–63, and in *eadem*, 'Smoking and Public Health', in G. Davenport, I. McDonald, and C. Moss-Gibbons (eds.), *The Royal College of Physicians and its Collections. An Illustrated History* (London: Royal College of Physicians, 2001), 57–9. This point has been taken up by A. Briggs, *A History of the Royal College of Physicians, vol. iv* (Oxford: Oxford University Press, for the Royal College of Physicians, 2005), 1370–99.

the president of the College, Lord Brain, urging that the College put out a statement on the effect of smoking on health 'with particular reference to the rising generation'. Brain, a shy reserved man, took a month to reply, only to turn the proposal down. The reasons for his refusal were typical of the time in their dislike of giving advice:

The work of Richard Doll and Bradford Hill has received very wide publicity and must be known, I should imagine, to every doctor in the country, so it is difficult to see that the College could add anything to the knowledge of the existing facts.

If we go beyond facts, to the question of the giving of advice to the public as to what action they should take in the light of the facts, I doubt very much whether that should be a function of the College.[21]

Subsequently the College's attitude changed. In 1957 Robert Platt was elected president as successor to Brain. Platt had a modernizing agenda for the profession which smoking fitted admirably. Platt was first approached on the subject of smoking by Charles Fletcher, first director of the Medical Research Council's (MRC) pneumoconiosis research unit in Cardiff and who was then working as a respiratory physician in the Department of Medicine at Hammersmith Hospital. Invited to lunch by the deputy chief medical officer, George Godber, who was frustrated by the lack of activity within his Ministry, the two agreed to sound out Platt about taking on the smoking issue.[22] Godber was a member of the RCP's council and a close friend of Platt. Avery Jones also heard what was afoot and wrote again in January 1959 to urge the Royal College to action. The first informal meeting was held on 16 February 1959 and in April the comitia of the College agreed that a committee should be formed 'to report on smoking and atmospheric pollution in relation to carcinoma of the lung and other illnesses'. The first formal meeting was held at the College on 15 July 1959 at 5 p.m.[23]

This sequence of events was illustrative of wider changes in post-war medicine. Smoking was a chance for the Royal College to position

[21] Brain's response is quoted in C. C. Booth, 'Smoking and the Gold Headed Cane', in C. C. Booth (ed.), *Balancing Act: Essays to Honour Stephen Lock* (London: Keynes Press, 1991), 49–55.

[22] Fletcher continued this 'pressure from without' during the course of the committee. See his correspondence with Godber on what the Ministry was doing on lung cancer and on health education. In National Archives, Ministry of Health papers, MH 55/2226, 18 January 1960, Letter from Fletcher to Godber.

[23] Royal College of Physicians archive, Committee to report on smoking and atmospheric pollution, minutes volume one, 1959–63.

itself in relation to new agendas emergent in health. The earlier medical interests—symbolized by Fletcher's occupational work on miners' lung disease and his interest in air pollution and chest disease—were giving place to the new focus on chronic diseases of the individual brought on by habits like smoking. The networks which operated in this instance—Godber in the Ministry of Health working in relation to medical and health interests outside—were illustrative of the emergence of the 'policy community', the term used by political scientists to analyse how policy-making interests work, with interests within government forming alliances with those outside. These were to become important in the making of post-war health policy in particular in relation to the medical profession.[24] The role of the chief medical officer was important in relation to this 'politics of expertise'.[25] Platt's interests in medical modernization extended more widely—he was a leading figure behind the subsequent Todd committee on medical education in 1968 and was also important in new moves round genetic disease in Manchester.[26]

The membership of the RCP committee was also symbolic. Platt was in the Chair, but Fletcher as its secretary was the moving spirit of the committee's work. Fletcher was the son of Walter Morley Fletcher, former secretary of the MRC. He had 'all the confidence of the Old Etonian' and impeccable connections in medical circles, but also a social conscience and a commitment to communicating with the public through the media.[27] In 1958 his series *Your Life in Their Hands*, showing surgical procedures on television, had caused huge controversy. The series had been part of wider developments in medical broadcasting. The 1958 series had originated in an earlier set of programmes called 'Thursday Clinic' transmitted in 1954 and 1956, consisting of outside broadcasts from St Mary's hospital in Paddington. The work of NHS hospitals had been seen in earlier programmes such as *Matters of Life and Death* (1951) and *Matters of Medicine* (1952) and medical procedures were also shown in *The Hurt Mind* (1957), which dealt with new

[24] The extensive literature on policy networks is summarized in V. Berridge, 'Making Health Policy: Networks in Research and Policy after 1945', in Berridge (ed.), *Making Health Policy*, 5–36.

[25] S. Sheard and Sir L. Donaldson, *The Nation's Doctor. The Role of the Chief Medical Officer, 1855–1998* (Oxford: Radcliffe Publishing, 2005).

[26] P. A. Coventry and J. V. Pickstone, 'From What and Why Did Genetics Emerge as a Medical Specialism in the 1970s in the UK? A Case History of Research, Policy and Services in the Manchester Region of the NHS', *Social Science and Medicine*, 49(9) (1999), 1227–38.

[27] Comment made in interview with Roger Braban by Virginia Berridge, June 1996.

developments in the treatment of mental illness and in which Fletcher was also involved.[28] Such programmes, and the media controversy over cases on conjoined twins in the 1950s, had begun the reordering of relationships round medical confidentiality which had up until then been a constraining issue for public depictions of medicine.[29] Fletcher was a leading light in such developments. But other members of the committee were also closely involved in the new relationships between medicine and the media. Dr Guy Scadding, a member of the committee, had, as we saw in the previous chapter, appeared early on in *Matters of Medicine,* explaining the complexities of the interactions between lung cancer, smoking, and air pollution. Dr J. N. (Jerry) Morris, of the Social Medicine Unit, was also a member of the committee, and had given radio talks, including one in 1955 whose content was prescient of the new developments in public health which the RCP committee came to symbolize:

We are dealing with a different social situation. The nineteenth century epidemics, bred in poverty and malnutrition, arose from the failures of the social system ... But coronary thrombosis ... with its origins apparently in high living standards ... seems to be arising from what we regard as successes of the social system ... It is becoming clear that in the modification of personal behaviour, of diet, smoking, physical exercise and the rest, which look like providing at any rate part of the answer, the responsibility of the individual for his own health will be far greater than formerly. It will not be possible to impose from without (as drains were built) the new norms of behaviour better serving the needs of middle and old age. They will only come about in a new kind of partnership between community and individual.[30]

Morris' advocacy of media and advertising initiatives on the committee was strong and a continuing strand in his long career. In 2000 at his ninetieth birthday conference at London School of Hygiene and Tropical Medicine (LSHTM), leading epidemiologist Michael Marmot remarked that 'Jerry has always told me that I should watch more

---

[28] Fletcher's media work is discussed in K. Loughlin, ' "Your Life in Their Hands" : The Context of a Medical–Media Controversy', *Media History,* 6(2) (2000), 177–88.

[29] Loughlin, 'Spectacle and Secrecy', 197–212.

[30] BBC written archives, Caversham Reading, J. Morris, 'Twentieth Century Epidemic: Coronary Thrombosis', Transcript of BBC third programme talk, 1 December 1955. Printed version 'Coronary Thrombosis: A Modern Epidemic', *The Listener,* 8 December 1955, 995–6.

television rather than less.'[31] Others on the committee like Avery Jones, the gastroenterologist who had originally suggested action to the RCP, symbolized the new medical interest in smoking and chronic disease, while the presence of Sir Aubrey Lewis of the Institute of Psychiatry indicated the role which psychological insights were to play in the new developments in public health. The committee subsequently added Dr N. C. Oswald to its number. He was a smoker and all the rest of the committee were by then non-smokers. The committee also consulted experts including Doll and A. Haddow of the Chester Beatty, while Godber was also available, although not a member of the committee. Morris remembered that they tried also to involve an MoH with an interest in smoking but could not find one.[32] That comment was indicative of the gulf between academic and practice-based public health. The committee's membership underlined the networks forming round the new risk-based public health, and symbolized an alliance between Fletcher's prestigious medical connections and the clinicians and social medicine/epidemiologists who had lower status within the profession, not least through their original location at the Central Middlesex, a former LCC hospital and consequently of lower status compared to the prestigious teaching hospitals.[33]

The work of the committee proceeded through nine meetings between 1959 and 1961, often with long gaps between them. Much was done outside the committee with members preparing papers and gathering evidence. Early on it made two key decisions. The minutes of the fourth meeting on 17 March 1960 record that a discussion was opened by the president on how the Report should be presented. 'The usual College report had limited circulation among the medical profession.' The other point was its purpose and how it was to be achieved.

It was agreed that the Committee's report should have more publicity and a wider circulation than the usual College reports. It could not advise government on any course of action, but it could suggest lines of action.[34]

[31] V. Berridge and S. Taylor (eds.), *Epidemiology, Social Medicine and Public Health*, transcript of the witness seminar held on 21 July 2000 on the ninetieth birthday of Professor Jerry Morris (London: Centre for History in Public Health, 2005).

[32] Interview with Jerry Morris by Virginia Berridge, June 1995.

[33] Older colleagues at LSHTM remember how it was customary for the epidemiologists to wear white coats to show that they were real doctors, although they did not see patients. A photograph of Morris from 1978 shows him with a white coat. LSHTM archive, photographic collection. See Illustration 3.

[34] RCP archive, Committee to report on smoking and atmospheric pollution, minutes, 17 March 1960.

It also disposed of the air pollution connection. Although the comitia of the Royal College had wanted a report which combined discussion of both issues, the committee decided not to produce this:

It was agreed that the evidence would be of an entirely different quality and nature. It was pointed out that individuals could avoid the dangers of smoking but not those of pollution. It was also thought that a section on atmospheric pollution within the main report might detract from the main arguments on smoking and lung cancer.[35]

The committee did eventually produce a separate report on air pollution but this was not published until the early 1970s and without much sense of urgency. The committee recognized that the smoking and lung cancer issue was a much more clear-cut case where individual action could be stressed. It was thus moving towards a concept of health which focused more clearly on individual responsibility and which could be expressed by appealing to the public rather than the profession.

The areas of the committee's work were divided between members according to their own interests, so memos appeared through the meetings on diseases of the lung, on the chemistry and pharmacology of smoking, on smoking and the gastrointestinal tract. Its interest in consumer issues, on advertising and the media, and also on what the public thought and how it could be influenced was a significant thread of discussion. Early on Aubrey Lewis produced a paper on the psychological aspects which pointed out that there was no evidence that health education could discourage inveterate smokers. School-based prevention might be more effective but there was little information on projects undertaken.

Lack of information on these newer aspects of health interest was a theme throughout. Economic issues and consideration of the role of the media were to be of growing importance within the new ideology of public health. But in the late 1950s and early 1960s, the profession of health economics was still in the future and it was the social medicine interests which took up the economic and media issues. It was the social medicine pioneer Jerry Morris who was active throughout the life of the committee in investigating consumer expenditure and the role of tobacco advertising. His work showed the expanding importance of television advertising in the situation. The committee pressed for an official survey of smoking habits in

---

[35] Ibid.

children and enquired into advertising controls on television.[36] Morris also brought the issue of coronary heart disease into the committee's discussions, influenced by the early publications of the Framingham study which had investigated this in the US situation.[37] Fletcher drew together the final report, making it accessible to the lay public, but clearly other members of the committee played an important role: Morris' work was particularly important for the public, media, and consumerist emphasis. It was agreed that the report should include a section on the use of advertising against smoking: 'modern methods should be employed to combat modern methods'.[38] Public health at this stage had close relationships with the tobacco industry.[39] Building on those relationships, Geoffrey Todd, the Imperial Company lead statistician, and others from the Tobacco Manufacturers Standing committee provided information and statistics for the final report. The report was also shown informally to the Tobacco Manufacturers Standing Committee before publication.[40]

The report was finally published in March 1962. Surveying the history of smoking, the chemistry and pharmacology of tobacco smoke, and the latest scientific evidence about the relationship with cancer, gastrointestinal diseases, lung disease, and coronary heart disease, as well as the psychology of smoking, its form and nature and its presentation were significant. It laid out a possible seven-point agenda for action for government. Five of the seven were consumerist and media oriented: public education, restrictions on sale to children, restriction of tobacco advertising, tax increases, and perhaps differential taxation for less harmful pipes and cigars, information on the tar and nicotine content of cigarettes. Only two came from different traditions: the environmentalism of restrictions on smoking in public places, and the

[36] RCP archive, Committee to report on smoking and atmospheric pollution, minutes, 18 February 1960.
[37] Ibid., minutes, 17 March 1960. See also L. A. Reynolds and E. M. Tansey (eds.), *Cholesterol, Atherosclerosis and Coronary Disease in the UK, 1950–2000*, Wellcome Witnesses to Twentieth Century Medicine, vol. xxvii (London: Wellcome Trust Centre for the History of Medicine at UCL, 2006).
[38] Ibid., minutes, 4 January 1961.
[39] For the history of this relationship see V. Berridge and P. Starns, 'The "Invisible Industrialist" and Public Health: The Rise and Fall of "Safer Smoking" in the 1970s', in V. Berridge and K. Loughlin (eds.), *Medicine, the Market and the Mass Media: Producing Health in the Twentieth Century* (Abingdon: Routledge, 2005), 172–91.
[40] RCP archive, Committee to report on smoking and atmospheric pollution, minutes, 23 February 1961.

'medical model' of anti-smoking clinics.[41] The agenda for government thus largely dropped action on the environment (air pollution) and gave full rein to the new appeal to the public, to economic and consumerist trends.

The manner of the report's presentation and publication symbolized this. The College hired a PR consultant, Roger Braban, to manage the launch of the report and held its first press conference. Braban recalled,

I came in as PR consultant to the RCP a few months before the smoking report—they had never used a professional launch ... then they got a taste for it and used it for every report ... I spent a lot of time in finding the right team ... the President and Charles Fletcher, he was a popular figure with the media ... I timed it so that Ministers had the report before it was published—they feel they're party to something.[42]

Charles Fletcher later gave a flavour of that first press conference.

On the day before publication a press conference was held at the College and it was crowded. Many questions were asked. When one reporter quoted that the annual risk of lung cancer in heavy smokers aged 55 was only one in 23 the president asked him if he would fly with an airline only one in 23 of whose planes crashed he agreed he would not. Next day there was fortunately no big news and the report got major headlines, Robert Platt on the BBC and I was interviewed on ITV.[43]

The report was also marked by a *Panorama* programme, the flagship TV vehicle for current affairs, which was broadcast on 12 March just after the publication of the report. Fronted by the commentator Richard Dimbleby, the programme interviewed scientists (mostly laboratory based) and members of the public about their response and about giving up smoking. The centrepiece of the programme was an interview by the presenter Robert Kee with John Partridge, the Chairman of the Tobacco Manufacturers Standing Committee, and Sir Robert Platt. The stand-off between the two, with Platt robustly interrupting Partridge's defence of the industry, made good television.

KEE: Mr Partridge, would you agree that we must stop young people smoking?
PARTRIDGE: No I would not, and let me, just while I can, take up one point that Sir Robert made just now. The *Observer* had no right to make that

---

[41] Royal College of Physicians, *Smoking and Health* (London: Pitman, 1962).
[42] Interview with Roger Braban by Virginia Berridge, June 1996.
[43] C. Fletcher, 'The Story of the Reports on Smoking and Health of the Royal College of Physicians', in Lock, Reynolds, and Tansey (eds.), *Ashes to Ashes*, 203.

remark in its editorial yesterday, Sir Robert, and nor, with respect, have you
(INTERRUPTION) … about only a tobacco manufacturer could deny this.
KEE: Well that is the position we have here now isn't it?
PARTRIDGE: It is so, but the implication is some dishonest approach to this
problem, and that is not well founded (INTERRUPTION) … May I just
finish here?[44]

This was unusual television for the time: but it was a portent of the
future mediatization of health issues and the premium it put on conflict
and opposition.

The report was popular with the public. Originally the College had
only wanted 5000 copies printed and when Fletcher insisted on double
that number, it had required the committee pay for any unsold copies.
But the report sold out within a few days and a second printing was
needed. The report sold over 33,000 copies in the UK by the autumn
of 1963 and over 50,000 in the United States.[45] The following year
saw the publication of Fletcher's Penguin special *Common Sense about
Smoking*, which symbolically linked the medical evidence with a chapter
on economic effects and others on social implications and how to stop.
Here was a further attempt to appeal to the public, which brought
together what was to become a common combination in public health:
a review of the science coupled with a self-help guide to individual
reformation.[46]

THE GOVERNMENT RESPONSE; A NEW ROLE
FOR HEALTH EDUCATION

Governments of the period have often been criticized for inadequate
responses, reliant on health education rather than more stringent measures of control. The choice of health education as the main response
and change in the nature of that education was significant. Just as
medicine was also reorienting towards a public advice role, so we can
see in this period governments of both political persuasions, Labour
and Conservative, moving towards a new view of their role in relation

[44] There is a transcript of the programme in the Ministry of Health papers. See
National Archives, Ministry of Health papers, MH55/2204, Public health propaganda,
Cancer smoking and lung cancer, Publicity policy, 1961– .
[45] Fletcher's contribution in *Ashes to Ashes*, and RCP archive, Committee to report
on smoking and atmospheric pollution, minutes, 6 December 1961.
[46] C. Fletcher, *Common Sense about Smoking* (London: Penguin Books, 1963).

to the population and health matters, in line with the changed profile of disease. Governments assumed a new duty to advise and warn about health risk, to persuade their citizens rather than to assume that a sense of public duty inherent in the population would lead them to make up their own minds. They also began to assess the health of normal populations through surveys, a development which paralleled the increased emphasis on population-based epidemiology. This was an important change which again built on the wartime social surveys and gave a new role to research and also to quantitative social science.[47] The social science disciplines assumed heightened technocratic significance in relation to these developments: they were taking place at a time when medical sociology and psychology were also beginning to penetrate public health education.[48] The 1962 report was an important catalyst for the 'evidence-based' tendency within public health.

Let us look at how these responses developed in the 1960s. The main vehicle for the government response to the report was the Cabinet committee on smoking. Cabinet committees had been briefly formed in the 1950s at the time of the various parliamentary statements and had been chaired by the Home Secretary of the day. R. A. Butler as Home Secretary chaired the first meeting of the latest committee. But Harold Macmillan, the prime minister, did not want Butler in this role and Lord Hailsham, Lord President of the Council, took over. The ministerial committee was paralleled by one of officials which did the detailed work.[49] The officials moved swiftly. The first meeting of their committee was on 23 March, two further meetings followed, and a draft report was ready to go to the Lord President by the middle of April.[50] The report, preceded by a flurry of activity in the relevant departments, was relatively anodyne, placing its reliance on health education and on voluntary agreements for advertising. The officials came down against differential taxation (taxation graded according to the harm occasioned

[47] For the earlier history of surveys see M. Bulmer, K. Bales, and K. K. Sklar (eds.), *The Social Survey in Historical Perspective, 1880–1940* (Cambridge: Cambridge University Press, 1991).

[48] M. Jefferys, 'Social Medicine and Medical Sociology 1950–1970: The Testimony of a Partisan Participant', in D. Porter (ed.), *Social Medicine and Medical Sociology in the Twentieth Century* (Amsterdam: Rodopi, 1997), 120–36.

[49] Cary, the civil servant who chaired this committee, was reluctant to reveal its existence. See the note from him to the other officials on the committee, 27 April 1962, London, National Archives, Cabinet papers, CAB 21/4648.

[50] London, National Archives, Cabinet papers, CAB 130/185/GEN 763, minutes of third meeting, 13 April 1962.

by the product—so pipes and cigars, thought to be less harmful, would attract lower tax rates than those for cigarettes) and the taxation option in general. Taxation, it was argued, would penalize the poor, raise the cost of living, and have a serious effect on producer economies in the Empire such as Rhodesia. This view reflected the belief that more restrictive action could not be sustained without major change in public attitudes to smoking. Research in Edinburgh and the government's own pilot survey of public attitudes to smoking through the Central Office of Information (CoI) had confirmed that most people knew about the smoking and lung cancer link, but their views on why smoking was harmful to health were different from those of the scientists. The public view of smoking stressed the environmental nuisance aspects rather than the risk-based epidemiology.[51]

The politicians did not agree on the sales to children issue and also on differential taxation. The Treasury fought strongly against the latter and ultimately the committee could not agree. In the event education and voluntarism were the keynotes of the response and the committee decided not to make a statement. As Hailsham told Macmillan, a small publicity campaign would not be welcomed and interest anyway had abated for the present. He proposed to set up the machinery and start the campaign, perhaps issuing a statement later on. A meeting with the manufacturers might also result in an agreement to apply the TV restrictions voluntarily to other advertising so the government could then claim credit for that also.[52] At a subsequent meeting in the House of Lords with representatives of the Tobacco Advisory Committee (TAC), the main industry representative organization, the Lord President said the government accepted the scientific case as in the RCP report but was against compulsion and action which would lead to pressure for similar measures in respect of alcohol and even foods like chocolate. It was 'not the government's purpose to induce any catastrophic change in smoking habits'. The meeting resulted in a move towards overall agreement on advertising restrictions based on the code applicable to television. On 14 November, Hailsham wrote to Maxwell, Chairman of the TAC and previously wartime Tobacco Controller. He felt the informal way this matter had been dealt with was suited to other issues as they arose. But

    [51] For discussion of this point see National Archives, Ministry of Health papers, MH55/2203, Public health propaganda, Smoking and lung cancer: publicity policy, 1957–60.
    [52] London, National Archives, Cabinet papers, CAB 21/4878, Lord President to Prime Minister, 25 July 1962.

he was clear that he was no stooge for industry interests. Someone at Carreras had sent him a box of filter-tipped Piccadilly cigarettes. 'This was indeed bearding the lion in his den, but it was as ineffectual as the devil's attempt on St. Anthony.'[53]

The government response was thus muted and focused on the strategy of health education. The multiplicity of interests in government was a key factor. The Treasury view ultimately prevailed over the taxation issue but not before the implications had been fully aired at the political level. The role of the industry was important, although its representatives were called in after the political decisions had been taken. Also behind these decisions was a desire to achieve a balance in policy and the realization that, without a huge change in the social positioning of smoking, there was little point in initiating a major programme of activity. Discussion of health education strategies and organization was not the only way in which government considered the implications of the RCP report. The debates about differential taxation and other strategies also led to important developments both in smoking policy and in public health.[54] But health education was the main response.

THE CONTROL OF ADVERTISING

Advertising for health was part of the emergent media and consumerist focus of public health. But advertising was also an activity to be opposed where it was promoting harmful products. The same combination of economics and statistical evidence began to mark government activity against tobacco advertising. Control of advertising was the other key plank of the government response to the report, achieved in relation to public health interests and the industry. This new consumerist strand in policy was symbolized by another report which arrived in the Ministry of Health just after the publication of the RCP one. It was from the Advertising Inquiry Council, a body formed in March 1959 in order to

[53] Ibid., Hailsham to Sir Alexander Maxwell of the Tobacco Advisory Committee, 14 November 1962.
[54] For discussion of how the differential taxation question evolved see V. Berridge and P. Starns, 'The "Invisible Industrialist" and Public Health: The Rise and Fall of "Safer Smoking" in the 1970s', in Berridge and Loughlin (eds.), *Medicine, the Market and the Mass Media*, 172–91.

represent the interests of the consumer in advertising.[55] It was a study of expenditure and trends in sales advertising on tobacco, researched and written by an economist and a doctor, a significant combination for the future of public health. It looked at the rise in expenditure on tobacco advertising in the early 1960s: figures had risen by 50% in one year, 1960, and the public's expenditure on tobacco was also rising. Women's smoking was on the increase and the teenage market was growing. Filter cigarettes had taken off in popularity in the mid-1950s after their introduction in the late 1940s to save leaf and save smokers' money after increases in tobacco duty. The report noted that their sales now accounted for 20% of the cigarette market. The whole nature of tobacco and cigarette promotion had changed in recent years. The Council's report, which was mentioned in Parliament, added to fears already raised about trends within the tobacco industry: a Monopolies Commission report had drawn attention to its high degree of business concentration. Two firms, Imperial and Gallaher, accounted for over 90% of the market. Philip Noel Baker MP, Chairman of the Advertising Inquiry Council, was pressing Macmillan for an advertising ban.[56] Fletcher and Morris were also involved.[57] Advertising was an important component of the response to the 1962 report; the tobacco companies voluntarily offered the removal of all advertising on television before 9 p.m. But concerns later arose on their part about this voluntary concession. Partridge of Imperial told a Board of Trade official in June 1962 that Imperial and Gallahers had seen advantages in the concession. They had envisaged being able to reduce advertising expenditure by 50% because of the television restriction. But Rothman Carreras had increased their advertising and so the manufacturers were beginning to break ranks.[58]

[55] The report was widely circulated within government. See National Archives, Cabinet papers, CAB 124/1672, Tobacco smoking and health, Restrictions on advertising, 1962–5. For the Council see also M. Hilton, *Consumerism in Twentieth Century Britain. The Search for a Historical Movement* (Cambridge: Cambridge University Press, 2003), 200.

[56] National Archives. Cabinet papers, CAB 21/4878, 1962–3, 29 May 1962, Philip Noel Baker, MP to Harold Macmillan.

[57] Ibid., CAB21/5083, 1963–4, Smoking and health 16/2/3 part 4, 24 July 1963, Ministry of Health. Note of a meeting with the Advertising Inquiry Council to discuss cigarette advertising. Fletcher and Morris were present at the meeting along with Noel Baker, and representatives from the Baptist Union, the Methodists, and others. The Advertising Inquiry Council also met with the TAC and agreed to differ about advertising control, 13 May 1963.

[58] National Archives, Cabinet Office papers CAB21/4878, 1962–3, 15 June 1962, G. J. MacMahon of the Board of Trade to Fife Clark of the CoI.

Negotiations about further restrictions dragged on into the changeover to a Labour government in 1964—which took a stronger line.

HEALTH EDUCATION BEGINS TO CHANGE

Health education began to change in the 1960s. The 1962 report was a catalyst, together with the 1964 Cohen report on Health Education and the setting up of the Health Education Council in 1968. Both the nature of health education, its content and message, and the organization behind it were in flux. The older local 'information-giving' model was being superseded by persuasive messages produced by a centralized technocratic agency. In the late 1950s at the time of the MRC's statement on smoking and lung cancer, the response had been at the local level through the MoH. There was no lack of interest. After a Ministry of Health circular went out to the 129 English local authorities in 1958, of the 127 who replied, 118 accepted the need for local action and only 9 did not.[59] However, with the exception of Edinburgh, only modest campaigns of action were initiated. The attitude and personality of the local Medical Officer of Health (MoH) appeared to have influenced local action as much as anything else. Detailed reports on the local response showed variety, ranging from a prompt response to those where the relevant committee discussed anti-smoking publicity in a cloud of cigarette smoke, or where the Director of Education was a heavy smoker and it was recorded that there would be no health education in schools.[60]

The nature of health education was also significantly different from its later version. The message which came across in public education in the 1950s was equivocal. A 1957 pamphlet issued by the Central Council dealt with the adventures of the fictional Wisdom family under the title 'What—no smoking?' In this comic strip, a boy and his mother drew the attention of the smoking father to the risks he was running. Worried, he goes to see his general practitioner, Dr Brain, who presents the facts. One in every three hundred smokers gets lung cancer. If he gives up, he is three times as likely to get it; if he continues, he is seven times as likely. Dr Brain's advice is measured and calm. 'It still does not

---

[59] National Archives, Ministry of Health papers, MH 55/2225, Summary of local health authority replies to circular 17/58.

[60] Ibid., MH 55/2228 Publicity—action taken by local authorities 1957–8.

sound as if the risk is very great, so there's no need to get in a panic, whatever you decide to do.'[61] The idea of outlining specific courses of action to take was anathema to a society which associated 'propaganda' with wartime central direction and with earlier Nazi propaganda. Health education at this time placed its faith in the citizenship of its recipients.

So the report led initially to only small signs of change. An Advisory Group on Publicity was set up in the MH and a circular was issued to local authorities offering free publicity. Posters showing coffins and graphs of rising deaths were prominent; but there were also posters showing a teenage boy and girl hesitating before they started smoking. The economic dimension of smoking also came increasingly to the fore. Seventy pounds a year spent on smoking could have bought an annual holiday on the Continent, declared one 1963 leaflet.[62] A range of material was produced by other organizations, including the British Temperance Society. A record, 'No Smoking', was produced by Transatlantic Records of Edgware. 'A Scottish psychologist outlines colloquially and effectively the dangers of smoking.'[63]

The Central Council (CCHE) ran a van campaign in 1962–3 which disseminated anti-smoking propaganda throughout the country.[64] Four non-smoking male graduates were recruited to disseminate the message, finding a readier acceptance in schools than in youth clubs or factories. 'The girls enjoyed it, they were such charming young men!', wrote the head of one school in 1963. There were reports of a lecture to three thousand schoolchildren in September 1962 at the new Gallery Evangelical Centre in London's Regent Street. But the focus was still on the local authorities, where some MoHs took up the cause enthusiastically. Education on smoking among school children was also emphasized after the 1962 report. However, Devon education committee refused to allow leaflets supported by the pop stars Cliff Richard and Frankie Vaughan to be distributed in schools. They were in

[61] Health Education Authority leaflet archive (later Health Development Authority and currently part of NICE), *The Adventures of the Wisdom Family: No. 2, 'What—no smoking?'*, Central Council of Health Education leaflet, 1957. Illustrations.
[62] Wellcome Library for the History and Understanding of Medicine, Iconographic Collection, a young woman smoking, with silver coins representing the expense of buying cigarettes. Colour lithograph after Reginald Mount (London: Central Office of Information, n.d.). One of a pair with a similar poster of a man. Photo no. L24904. Illustrations 7 and 8.
[63] National Archives, Ministry of Health papers, MH 82/205, Correspondence re proposal for two mobile units.
[64] Ibid., MH 82/205, 206, 207, 208, 209. Files on the mobile unit campaign.

'beatnik language' objected a teachers' representative, and quite contrary to what was being taught.[65] There were also problems with the Joint Censorship committee of the Poster Advertising industry, which refused in 1963 to approve the display of posters with the words 'cigarettes cause lung cancer'. 'Cigarettes are a cause of lung cancer' was acceptable.[66]

Health education was in an interim phase. The posters prepared by Reginald Mount for the CoI and the van campaign focused on 'youth' and on persuasion, and used economic arguments. But techniques often still smacked of the temperance lecture. In the Ministry there was a emergent realization of a need for change. A memo from March 1960 had commented:

> It now seems apparent that local health authorities are not likely to be the most effective major agencies for conveying to the adult population information on smoking and lung cancer. Newspapers, magazines, radio and television are the main instruments for informing the public and these naturally look for their sources of news on this subject either to Government announcements or to scientific papers written by researchers in the field.[67]

This was the way of the future but in the mid-1960s, campaigns were organized primarily at the local level with some central input. The 1964 Cohen committee took the new tendencies further.[68] Its origin lay in lobbying from health educators who sought greater national organization and coordination; they formed an Institute of Health Education in 1962 which presented evidence to the committee.[69] The committee itself had a strong media membership. Its deputy chair came from the Consumers Association and from a BBC background, while there was also an advertising agency representative and the health editor

---

[65] Ibid., MH 151/18, Smoking and health campaign policy, *Daily Mail* report, 22 February 1963. Here is some of the language reported

> Always puffin' a fag—squares,
> Never snuffin' the habit—squares,
> Drop it, doll, be smart, be sharp!
> Cool cats wise,
> And cats remain,
> Non-smokers, doll, in this campaign

[66] Ibid., MH 151/14, Smoking and health poster policy.
[67] Ibid., MH55/2226, Paper to Mr Galbraith on smoking and lung cancer, 15 March 1960.
[68] Ministry of Health, The Central Health Services Council, The Scottish Health Services Council, *Health Education. Report of a Joint Committee of the Central and Scottish Health Services Councils* (London: HMSO, 1964).
[69] G. M. Blythe, 'A History of the Central Council for Health Education, 1927–1968', MLitt thesis, Oxford University, 1987.

of *Woman* magazine. The report wanted to drop the traditional health education focus, which had been on individual advice to mothers, on specific action like vaccination and immunization. It considered that more was needed on human relationships—sex education, mental health, the risks of smoking and being overweight, the need for physical exercise. These were difficult areas, where 'self-discipline' was required.

Moral and medical imperatives intermingled. Diseases such as chronic bronchitis could be prevented if individuals would modify habits such as smoking and if the government would accelerate its health promoting campaigns. What was needed was a greater degree of central publicity, using habit changing campaigns and social surveys, as well as strengthening the new profession of health educators. The models came from American social psychology. The new breed were to be trained in journalism, publicity, the behavioural sciences, and teaching methods. Training people would involve both imparting knowledge and inculcating self-discipline, a telling phrase. The new health educator was to be part salesman, persuading people to take appropriate action. Just knowing about the risks of cigarette smoking was not enough: Cohen called tobacco advertising 'propaganda' and it had to be countered in the same way. This was a major change from the even-handed response of health education in the 1950s. Persuasion was now the key.

The Cohen report emphasized the role of the mass media in health education—one TV programme could reach five million people, whereas it would take 250,000 group discussions of twenty people each to do the same. The report led to the establishment of the central government-funded Health Education Council in 1968, reconstituted in the early 1970s.[70] The change in approach was initially evident outside the health field as such. A nationwide campaign for the Ministry of Transport over the Christmas period in 1964, mounted by the government's CoI, sought to change public attitudes to drinking and driving, informing people of the dangers and penalties. This short-lived (six weeks) media blitz used press, television, and poster advertising, and was supported by research into public attitudes and responses before, during, and after the campaign.[71] Drink driving was in some sense a model for

[70] The Second World War and post-war history of health education up to the 1980s is surveyed in R. Smith, *Working Paper no. 66, The National Politics of Alcohol Education: A Review* (Bristol: School of Advanced Urban Studies, 1987), 1–21. Also Blythe, 'History of the Central Council'.

[71] The research was carried out by the Road Research Laboratory and the campaign organized by the Advertising Division of the CoI, which drew on the services of commercial advertising companies. See Clark, *The Central Office of Information*.

the later smoking and public health media model and one can trace a process of 'policy seepage' as well as one of 'policy transfer' from the United States. Here, an initiative developed in one government department, transport, influenced the model subsequently developed in another, health.

By the late 1960s, under the impact of these changes, the approach in smoking health education was very different. In October 1969, a major anti-smoking poster campaign was launched. There was research input, pre-testing, and market evaluation. The campaign was pre-tested on a statistically selected group of subjects and based on Ministry of Health research published in 1967. An advertising agency was used and the 'look' of the advertisements was quite different. We will see in Chapter 7 how these developments were taken further in the 1970s.

THE SOCIAL SURVEY, SOCIAL RESEARCH, AND THE NEW ROLE OF THE PUBLIC

What was also beginning to change in the mid-1960s was the view of 'the public' held by politicians and by officials: this was to be a crucial component of public health initiatives in future. The commercial techniques of market research expanded in the post-war years and government also began to assess the nature of public opinion and attitudes through the social survey. This surveillance of the population was part of a more general expansion of research and evaluation epitomized by the smoking issue. In 1962, a report from a public relations (PR) firm, Armstrong Warden, presented to the Ministry of Health's advisory group on publicity, had pointed out the long-term nature of trying to change public attitudes to smoking. The first job was to convince people that smoking did constitute a danger, and the effects of that should be measured by public opinion research.[72] As with the change of attitude towards the content of public education, government was edging towards this form of surveillance. A pilot social survey had been carried out in 1960 for the Home Affairs committee by the Social Survey division of the CoI. This had confirmed the impression given by earlier surveys carried out in Edinburgh to evaluate

---

[72] National Archives, Ministry of Health papers, MH 55/2237, April 1962, The Role of Publicity in the Smoking and Health campaign, Report for the CoI by Armstrong Warden Ltd.

a campaign led by the MoH there in the 1950s. Most of the population was aware of the association between smoking and lung cancer; only one person in the 1960 survey was not, an old lady of 87, who was a non-smoker. But both the Edinburgh and the pilot surveys showed that a smaller proportion of the survey population accepted that the association was proved and a negligible number had given up smoking because of it.

In the mid-1960s the surveillance of public attitudes went further. For the first time survey research and evaluation accompanied a campaign almost from the start and research into young people's attitudes to smoking was carried out. There was also research into medical students' attitudes to smoking. The research was carried out by Drs McKennell and Thomas of the Social Survey division and by the social psychologist John Bynner. Bynner's work on adolescent smoking was based on the smoking questions in a wartime survey by the CCHE of adolescent sexual behaviour. The wartime surveys of VD prefigured the peacetime developments.[73] The results of the McKennell survey, started in 1963 and first reported to the officials committee in 1964 when the American Surgeon General's Report was under consideration, emphasized the potential new role for government health education. 'The ethics or appropriateness of using such an approach in Government publicity needs to be faced. The use of somewhat devious, emotional rather than straightforward means of persuasion is of course, for better or worse, a characteristic of much successful commercial advertising.'[74]

Other survey research, carried out by social scientists and epidemiologists, increasingly focused on the young. During the 1950s and early 1960s the sociologist Margot Jefferys was involved in a study of Harlow New Town with other researchers from the London School of Hygiene. Her study of the impact of health education on children's attitudes towards smoking was one of the first academic publications in the field.[75] The choice of smoking and of children also indicated the reorientation of this type of 'community study' which had until then concentrated on the environment rather than individual issues. Jefferys as a key figure in the Society for Social Medicine in this period was

[73] L. Moss, *The Government Social Survey. A History* (London: HMSO, 1991).

[74] National Archives, Cabinet Office papers, CAB 130/185 GEN 763, February 1964, study by the Social Survey report to Cabinet committee on smoking.

[75] M. Jefferys and W. R. Westaway, ' "Catch Them Before They Start!" A Report on an Attempt to Influence Children's Smoking Habits', *Health Education Journal*, 19 (1961), 3–17.

also part of that transformation of social medicine into a new form of public health which the smoking work symbolized.[76] In the discussions of the ongoing research in the CoI and the Ministry of Health can be seen in embryo the emergent evaluative paradigm of 'relevant research', a precursor of later evidence-based tendencies in health research.[77]

THE ELECTORAL ARGUMENT DIMINISHES

The publication of the American Surgeon General's report in 1964 led to a further officials' report and to political interest. The American report extended associations between smoking and health risk to diseases other than lung cancer, but British officials did not feel this warranted further action. On 30 June 1964 the Cabinet committee approved the officials' suggestion of a modest extension of the government health education campaign. There was no support for a ban on TV advertising or on smoking in cinemas. Least opposition was attracted by packet warnings. Lord Hailsham wanted more action. On 6 April 1964, Hailsham wrote in response to his officials' lack of enthusiasm, 'I consider that the American Report, the American action and the Social Survey *have* strengthened the case for action, and that it is *not* too early to say that our limited campaign is failing and that unless we can bare our teeth nothing that we do *will* be taken seriously.' He also inserted a significant change in the inequality argument deployed by officials. Now the words 'it would bear more hardly on the poor than on the rich' were replaced by 'it could be harder for a poor man than for a rich man to continue his existing level of smoking and while this element of discrimination might be said to be more to the poor man's benefit, it would be unlikely to go uncriticised.'[78]

[76] Jefferys, 'Social Medicine and Medical Sociology', 120–36. Smoking among school children was also one of the early pieces of research carried out at St Thomas' where one of the first health services research units was set up by Walter Holland, a pioneer of such research in the UK. Interview with Walter Holland by Virginia Berridge, March 1997.

[77] The connection with smoking and research is not noted in J. Daly, *Evidence Based Medicine and the Search for a Science of Clinical Care* (Berkeley: University of California Press, 2005), 128–53, in her discussion of the lineages of evidence-based medicine, although she does make the connection between social medicine and the rise of health services research in Britain.

[78] London, National Archives, Cabinet papers, CAB 21/5083, Note from Hailsham, 6 April 1964.

But Hailsham's response in 1964 was unusual for the time. As he pointed out in the Commons adjournment debate on the Surgeon General's report, he was a non-smoker in a parliament of smokers, a Cabinet of smokers, and an electorate of smokers. His views did not at that stage represent either the cultural or the political norm.[79] Enoch Powell, the Conservative Minister of Health when the RCP report was published, had expressed his opposition to media strategies.[80] He wrote with characteristic vigour to denigrate the approach in November 1961:

The Government has it in its power, without prohibition or interference directly with anyone's freedom of choice, to cut cigarette smoking whenever and to whatever extent it pleases. Indeed, given the probable flatness of the demand curve, they could combine a big cut in consumption with no reduction, and possibly an increase in revenue. If duty were increased for explicitly public health reasons, the opprobrium would be much less than with ordinary increases of taxation, and it would be possible to use a cost of living index which excluded tobacco (or cigarettes). In my opinion if the Government is unwilling to use this power ... then health education and all the rest is merely humbug and will be felt and seen to be such. In any case, 'health education' has already gone a long way ... without producing the slightest effect, and I don't believe advertising makes any difference one way or the other.

The publication of the Report will excite temporary interest and for weeks afterwards we shall have to answer a shower of tiresome Questions about what the Government is not doing; but unless my colleague is prepared to use the fiscal weapon, I personally propose to indulge in as little humbug as I can get away with.[81]

Powell was subsequently criticized by Godber for his refusal to ban tobacco advertising while he was Minister of Health: this minute makes clear his rationale for his dislike of the advertising strategy. In an interview conducted in 1975, Powell was more forthcoming about the roots of his opposition. Governments did not like to reorganize taxation, and then there was the question of harm, which, in the case of smoking, was fluid and vague. Legislating against a widespread and common form of behaviour was very different from legislating against an uncommon and marginal form. Governments would be very foolish to act without overwhelming evidence and here the 1962 report, in

    [79] Hansard. Parliamentary Debates, 630, col. 522, 12 February 1964, Adjournment debate speech by Lord Hailsham.
    [80] London, National Archives, Ministry of Health papers, MH55/2227, Minute from Enoch Powell, 11 November, 1961.
    [81] Ibid.

his view, did make a difference to the clarity of the issue.[82] Kenneth Robinson as Labour Minister of Health in the mid- to late 1960s was more active against smoking, but his view of policy was also that it was constrained by public opinion, not by financial considerations. He also stressed that the main constraint on government had been that there was no public support for action against smoking. The answer, as he saw it, was to change the climate of opinion through health education, in particular with themes like smell and attractiveness which appealed to young people.[83] The Labour politician Richard Crossman's opposition to Robinson's proposed changes in smoking policy in the later 1960s was also prompted by electoral considerations.[84] But this argument began to change in the 1970s when politicians like the Conservative Keith Joseph and Labour David Owen and Denis Healey as Chancellor of the Exchequer saw dawning electoral advantage in anti-smoking measures.

The RCP report of 1962 was the forerunner of later College reports on smoking and a host of other health-related subjects, all of which were aimed at both government and public. The 'medical voice' developed important relationships with both government and the public in areas which would not previously have been considered the province of either. In the 1970s this insider–outsider relationship for medicine developed further into a host of expert committees with close relationships within government. The RCP report in 1962 was the catalyst for a new era in which the presentation of science to the public through the media with the authority of scientists and the medical profession became central. As consumerist trends in society consolidated, and medicine and public health both sought 'modernization', the old tradition of 'giving the facts' to citizens was transformed into warnings about health risk. The nature of public opinion and 'the public' was exposed to research-based surveillance. The techniques of social as well as medical science were brought into play. The roots of such changes were recognizably in some of the post-war transformations of social medicine, but they also incorporated new commercial techniques of persuasion and commercial ideas about research. The permissive society analysts have argued for

---

[82] Wellcome Library for the History and Understanding of Medicine, ASH (Action on Smoking and Health) archive, SA/ASH R.27 Box 79, William Norman papers, Interview with Enoch Powell.

[83] Ibid., Interview with Kenneth Robinson.

[84] R. Crossman, *The Diaries of a Cabinet Minister, vol. iii, Secretary of State for Social Services, 1968–1970* (London: Hamish Hamilton and Jonathan Cape, 1977), entry for 19 July 1968, 147.

a diminished state role for some health-related issues. But the case of smoking, and the new ideas within public health, show the influence of the state increasing, not diminishing. Such influence was exerted through new relationships with the medical profession and with research and through new agencies. The case of smoking and the RCP report shows how such ideas and interests were beginning to shape a distinctive post-war British public health ideology separate from the organizational base of the profession in health services and community medicine which has attracted most commentary. The report mediated between social medicine in flux and the new evidence-based medicine and public health.

3

Systematic Gradualism: Harm Reduction, Public Health, and the Industry, 1950s–1971

This chapter will trace the history of what Sir Peter Froggatt, Chair of the Independent Scientific Committee on Smoking and Health, writing in the 1980s, called the strategy of 'systematic gradualism' as a major public health and industry area of interest from the 1950s through to the 1970s.[1] By this term Sir Peter meant scientifically informed strategies to reduce risk and harm which also drew on relationships with industry. The history of this approach tells us about the nature of public health and the tensions between different strategic approaches to health risk in the post-war years. Techniques of persuasion exemplified in health education and the mass media were to be a central dimension of the 'new public health'. Another key component of that new public health which emerged during the 1960s and 1970s was to be hostility to industrial interests. In 2003, the ASH (Action on Smoking and Health) website commented:

Tobacco is unique: the only product that kills when used normally—120,000 deaths per year in the UK. ASH is leading the fight to control the tobacco epidemic and to confront the lies and dirty tricks of the tobacco industry.[2]

TV documentaries such as the *Tobacco Wars* or *The Secrets of Big Tobacco* told of the forty-year struggle to hold US tobacco companies to account for the damage caused by cigarettes. Journalist histories, such as *The Smoke Ring* or *Dirty Business: Big Tobacco at the Bar of Justice*, recounted a thrilling story of corporate greed and duplicity,

---

[1] P. Froggatt, 'Determinants of Policy on Smoking and Health', *International Journal of Epidemiology*, 18(1) (1989), 1–9.
[2] Text on ASH website, <http://www.ash.org.uk>, accessed January 2003.

of big business which cared little for the health of its customers.[3] Hostility to industrial interests now pervades the public health field: campaigners on obesity attack the food industry, and the drinks industry and its influence within government is reviled by some sections of the alcohol research community.[4] The malign and duplicitous role of industry is part of the 'denial and delay' argument which is discussed in Chapter 1.

This chapter shows how such attitudes are time specific and how different relationships prevailed earlier on. At the time these relationships were related to the perceived legitimacy of industry interests and to an agenda, shared by industry and by public health interests, of removing the harmful components from tobacco, of reducing harm from smoking rather than eliminating the habit. In the 1950s and 60s (and afterwards) some public health interests did work with 'the manufacturers', the term then used rather than the perhaps more pejorative 'industry'. We have already discussed how tobacco industry interests had an historically lengthy relationship with government: this developed into the strategy of voluntary agreements in the 1970s. But it is less well known that working with industry was also a strategy for some, although not all, public health interests. From the time of the manufacturers' benefaction to the Medical Research Council (MRC) to the middle of the 1970s—through the publication of the first two Royal College of Physicians (RCP) reports—industry, government, and public health interests operated in a policy-balancing act aiming to reduce harm from smoking. However, the events of the second half of the 1970s and the rise of a new militant public health effectively curtailed it as a major strategy for mainstream public health interests. The change in strategy also owed something to changes of ownership and influence within the tobacco industry in the late 1970s and the rise in influence of the US industry, alongside diversification on the part of Imperial.[5] This chapter traces the operation of this balancing act from the end of the MRC tobacco benefaction through the research in the industry's joint laboratories in Harrogate and the development of the 'safer cigarette'

---

[3] P. Taylor, *The Smoke Ring: Tobacco, Money and Multinational Politics* (London: Sphere Books, 1985); P. Pringle, *Dirty Business: Big Tobacco at the Bar of Justice* (London: Aurum Press, 1998).

[4] G. Edwards, P. Anderson, T. F. Babor, et al., *Alcohol Policy and the Public Good* (Oxford: Oxford University Press, 1994).

[5] Anon., *The Imperial Story, 1901–2001* (Bristol: Imperial Group plc, n.d. ?2001), details the problems encountered in particular during the 1970s.

by Imperial and other companies. Relationships between the industry and the Royal College of Physicians committee continued and focused on the role of nicotine, while the nicotine harm reduction research was openly published in major journals. The industry work on nicotine and habituation was known to the public health scientists. The 1950s and 1960s, when much of this activity was taking place, was a precursor to the reordering of relationships between scientists, industry, and the state which took place in the 1970s. Later on, as we will see in chapter 9, different industry–state relationships emerged in the 1990s, when the focus of attention shifted to the pharmaceutical industry, which inherited the tobacco substitute mantle through the development of nicotine replacement therapy.

THE MRC RESEARCH FUNDING

The Medical Research Council's tobacco benefaction-funded research programme was the responsibility of its committee on the etiology of lung cancer, which was set up in 1960. The industry benefaction funded lung cancer studies in the Carcinogenic Substances Research Unit at the Exeter, the Statistical Research Unit at the London School of Hygiene and Tropical Medicine (LSHTM), the Institute of Cancer Research, and the Cancer Research department of Glasgow Hospital. There were various other studies, including those on the chemical composition of tobacco smoke, and additional research by other organizations—the British Empire Cancer Campaign, the Imperial Cancer Research Fund, and the General Practitioner Field Research Unit, which was carrying out clinical trials of an anti-smoking preparation of lobeline.[6] Research was also occurring in the laboratories of the industry, especially those of the Imperial Tobacco Company Ltd. One scientist who was involved in tobacco-funded research at this time remembered,

The tobacco industry reaction to Doll and Hill was to provide half a million pounds to the MRC to solve the problem—they thought it could—just modify the smoke a bit. There were very few known carcinogens ... there was no concept of thousands of carcinogens waiting to be discovered and therefore many rather than one irritant ... The MRC didn't know what to do with it.

---

[6] London, National Archives, Cabinet papers, CAB21/4648, Medical Research Council brief for Lord President.

Professor James Cook was set up in a lab in Exeter and wasted a lot of it … the industry money was wasted.[7]

THE TOBACCO MANUFACTURERS STANDING COMMITTEE AND RESEARCH

After the initial contacts with the US tobacco industry in 1956 and Dr C. C. Little's visit, the UK manufacturers followed the advice to set up their own cross-industry research funding organization with a 'public education' component. In June 1956, the Tobacco Manufacturers Standing Committee (TMSC) was set up 'to assist research into smoking and health questions, to keep in touch with scientists and others working on this subject in the UK and abroad, and to make information available to scientific workers and the public'[8]. The Committee consisted of nine representatives of the home and export tobacco manufacturers; two representatives came from British American Tobacco and two from the Imperial Tobacco Company. At its first meeting Sir Alexander Maxwell was invited to become the chair. A technical committee consisting of the principal scientists in the constituent companies was also set up. The committee had two external scientific consultants, Sir Alfred Egerton, Emeritus Professor of Chemical Technology in the University of London, and the statistician Sir Ronald Fisher, who had continued his assessment of the relationship between statistical association and causation in terms of smoking and lung cancer. The research carried on in the participating companies, however, had been mainly technical and physiological in nature. Some considerable time was spent in developing a smoking machine which could reproduce the features of human cigarette smoking. The machine developed could smoke six cigarettes at a time and was adopted both by the industry and by others researching in this area. The machine, once developed, was used to investigate reports of the presence in cigarette smoke of 3:4-benzpyrene, 1:2:5:6-dibenzanthracene, and arsenious oxide. Research was carried forward into the mode of origin of benzpyrene and 'other substances in tobacco smoke are being separated.'

---

[7] Interview with industry scientist 1 by Virginia Berridge, 23 February 1998.
[8] Tobacco Manufacturers Standing Committee, (TMSC) *First Annual Report for the Year Ended 31 May 1957.*

This type of industry-sponsored research funding organization was a common model at that time. The Asbestosis Research Council was also founded in 1957 and funded a research programme mainly based at the Institute of Occupational Medicine at Edinburgh University.[9] During its first two or three years of existence the tobacco committee followed a similar path in funding external research. It decided on the focus of its research interests and began to fund research as well as to report on what the companies were doing. It kept in touch with the American Tobacco Industry Research Committee and made no secret of those links in its annual reports: its first reports mentioned the close links between the two. It had a potentially broad research agenda, it reported in 1959: factors affecting smoking habits; the chemical and physical properties of tobacco and tobacco smoke; principles of the smouldering process applicable to tobacco; the biological activity of tobacco smoke; factors affecting the increase of lung cancer and other diseases; and the physiological and psychological effects of smoking.[10] By then, it had published two reports, one on the statistics of smoking and the second on the reliability of statements about smoking habits. In both of these the statistician Geoffrey Todd of Imperial, who had taken over as secretary of the committee, was instrumental.[11] The committee also published an edited bibliography of the constituents of tobacco smoke.[12] Early psychological research was industry funded. After the chief medical officer's (CMO) report noted that emotional disturbances played a part in the development of cancer, the manufacturers' committee established a research post in psychosomatic medicine awarded to Dr D. M. Kissen, research associate in psychosomatic medicine at the University of Glasgow, while Mass Observation and Professor Eysenck of the Institute of Psychiatry carried out an enquiry designed to shed light on the personality of smokers.[13] A fourth research paper, *Cigarette*

---

[9] G. Tweedale, *Magic Mineral to Killer Dust. Turner and Newall and the Asbestos Hazard* (Oxford: Oxford University Press, 2000), 174.

[10] TMSC, *Report for the Year Ended 31 May 1959.*

[11] G. F. Todd, *Statistics of Smoking in the United Kingdom*, TMSC research paper no. 1 (London: TMSC, 1957); G. F. Todd and J. T. Laws, *The Reliability of Statements about Smoking Habits*, TMSC research paper no. 2 (London: TMSC, 1958). A supplementary report on the latter by Todd was published by the Tobacco Research Council, the successor to the TMSC, in 1966.

[12] H. R. Bentley and E. G. N. Berry, *The Constituents of Tobacco Smoke; an Annotated Bibliography*, TMSC research paper no. 3 (London: TMSC, 1959).

[13] The report is cited in the TMSC, *Report for the Year Ended 31 May 1960*, as published in the *British Medical Journal*, 1 (1960), 1456–60.

Smoke Condensate: Preparation and Routine Laboratory Estimation, was produced. This paper described the work undertaken to determine the conditions under which automatic smoking machines could be operated in preparing cigarette smoke condensate and to devise a reliable method for estimating the smoke condensate yield of cigarettes.[14]

By 1960, the committee was experiencing problems with its research policy and future directions. Egerton died, Fisher was abroad, and the MRC benefaction was entering its seventh and last year. Todd began to cast around for how to proceed. A note of a meeting with Sir Alexander Todd FRS at Cambridge in February 1960 shows a discussion of what the Committee should do next. Should it get into the biochemical field and if so, what fundamental research should it support? Sir Alexander Todd himself was not willing to be the consultant to the committee but suggested several other biochemists who might. Geoffrey Todd's note of the meeting indicates the twin objectives which animated the enquiry.

He (Alexander Todd) showed himself alive to the public relations implications of our research activity. We had to be honest, but we had to appear to be honest as well. In this connection, while all the research we were devoting to the cigarette itself was right and proper and was unlikely to be adequately pursued unless we did so, it still remained true that these items in our effort would not be getting us any nearer to the discovery of the central facts about cancer causation—what was happening to the cell and how it was happening. Indeed, if our labours were confined simply to the cigarette we might not be doing any more than showing if the cigarette was not guilty it ought to be! ... T.M.S.C., therefore, would be wise to get behind some chosen piece of fundamental research and in helping humanity it would be helping itself at the same time, for it could gain inside knowledge of the factors involved not only in causing but in preventing or curing cancer.[15]

The committee, after these feelers, decided to take a new direction. In November 1960, Sir Alexander Maxwell came to see the Secretary of the MRC and proposed the establishment of a biological research unit. This was to be located in York and to cost half a million pounds. It would mean that the manufacturers' contribution to MRC-sponsored research would come to an end. The broad objectives of the TMSC Research Unit were outlined in an attached paper. They were to see whether it were possible to put the measurements of biological activity in animals

---

[14] TMSC, *Report for the year Ended 31 May 1960*, 4.
[15] Legacy Tobacco documents library, Note on meeting with Sir Alexander Todd FRS at Cambridge, 1 February 1960, 19600204.

of cigarette smoke and of known carcinogens onto a sound quantitative basis, and to exploit experimental methods to discover which substances in cigarette smoke were important for lung cancer and whether rational means for improving cigarettes could be devised. Biological tests more reliable than skin painting were to be sought; and the committee aimed to study the general physical and pharmacological effects, especially in terms of the beneficial effects which smoking was believed to have. This research had not been attractive to academic departments, the paper noted.[16] In 1961, Dr Herbert Bentley, from the research department at Imperial, noted where research had got to. The real problem was that it was not possible to say what compounds in tobacco smoke were quantitatively significant for the causation of human disease. Requests had been received from outside investigators for supplies of standard smoke preparations for experiments and they had been able to lay down a standard procedure for sampling and testing cigarettes for tar yield which would allow realistic comparisons to be made. Three major collaborators had been Professor Blacklock at Bath, Dr T. D. Day at Leeds, and Dr F. J. C. Roe at the London Hospital Medical College. Now it was proposed to carry forward the chemical and bioassay work at laboratories in Harrogate, and it was also proposed to do work on the beneficial effects of smoking.[17]

THE WORK OF THE HARROGATE LABORATORIES

The Laboratories, which seemed to have been the initiative of Bentley ('he said we must do it ourselves', said one of the researchers involved), opened in September 1962 under the leadership of Dr Tom Day, Reader in Pharmacology at Leeds who had carried out earlier work for the TMSC. The industry had not conducted biological research before.

Scientists in industry were all concerned with quality control, there were no biological or pathological or medical people involved. The labs were built at

---

[16] National Archives, Ministry of Health papers, MH 55/2223, 3 November 1960, Note to Mr Emery from P. Hooper with attached paper from TMSC on TMSC Research Unit.

[17] Ibid., Research on smoking and lung cancer by the Tobacco Manufacturers Standing Committee. Paper by Dr H. R. Bentley, Research department, Imperial Tobacco Ltd., March 1961.

88   *Systematic Gradualism*

huge cost—Tom Day was … quite a character—he'd done biological work but it wasn't very good.[18]

The committee did not abandon its external funding, although the MRC benefaction came to an end. In 1963 it announced that it had agreed to give up to £500,000 over the next ten years to LSHTM for the establishment of a research programme on cardiovascular disease. The Department of Epidemiology under Dr Donald Reid was to be expanded to accommodate the study, whose Deputy Director would be Dr Peter Armitage, and the funding would allow for a permanent endowment for the development of epidemiological studies at the School. This funding supported the early work on the Whitehall study of British civil servants, whose long-running investigations and epidemiological data continue to inform policy. Other research was also funded in a variety of university departments.[19]

At Harrogate, the work fell into two main areas—studies on experimental animals to see whether changes in the constituents of cigarette smoke were desirable and possible; and research on the pharmacological effects of smoking, arising from the desire to discover the positive effects of smoking. Day led the laboratories overall, while the pharmacological research at Harrogate was under the direction of Dr Alan Armitage, a pharmacologist who had worked for the pharmaceutical company May and Baker and also at Kings College in London. The heyday of the laboratories was in the 1960s and early 1970s. One early researcher recalled, 'There was a relaxed atmosphere—one didn't feel one was working in a commercial environment.' In his view Harrogate, in those days, was a 'quasi university outfit'.[20] The main aim was to work towards the modification of tobacco so that harmful ingredients could be left out. There were inhalation studies and also skin painting work to try to induce tumours and study them. One scientist recalled that the laboratory animals were a problem due in part to some being of poor quality. An added problem was that the laboratories were funded on a consensus basis by the members of the committee in proportion to the companies' market share. The research used only experimental cigarettes which were produced on this proportionate basis. 'The companies kept

[18] Interview with industry scientist 1 by Virginia Berridge, 23 February 1998.
[19] Tobacco Research Council, *Tobacco Research Council, Review of Past and Current Activities* (London: Tobacco Research Council, 1963); Tobacco Research Council, *Tobacco Research Council. Review of Activities, 1963–66* (London: Tobacco Research Council, 1967), 17–27, review of the LSHTM research funding and other activities.
[20] Interview with industry scientist 2 by Virginia Berridge, 27 January 1998.

themselves to themselves and didn't want us working on their cigarettes. Science varied by commercial aspects was questionable because of this funny mix.'[21]

There were further problems. Some of the researchers had little research experience and conducted experiments with small numbers of mice which proved little. A statistician who joined the laboratories in 1966 recalled the tobacco smoke condensate painting on mouse backs. In the United States Wynder had demonstrated that this could produce tumours but the Harrogate research aimed to find out whether different types of tobacco would produce a different response. The aim was to find out through chemical fractionation what the carcinogenic bits were and to remove them. 'Each test took one and a half years to do—it was split in various ways but it was still a horribly complicated chemical mixture and no one knows to this day.'[22] The smoke inhalation studies on rats found it difficult to induce tumours. The problem was that it was difficult to get the rats to smoke enough, as they had learned how to hold their breath during the inhalation experiments. A scientist who arrived at the labs on an inspection visit in the early 1970s remembered,

The day I went they had their first papilloma produced by any tobacco product ... Day said we'll have cider and cakes—fortunately it was early closing day. The idea that the man in charge should be celebrating because we produced a tumour![23]

It was clear both to scientists working there and to visitors that the skin-painting people were 'on a limited leash—businessmen controlled it and really didn't want to know any bad news'.[24] The problems over publication were not entirely from the companies' point of view. One researcher produced little and had to be replaced after a visit from the committee's head office in London; the London office was asking for publication but little appeared for some years. [25] There was also a sense that the animal studies side of things was running out of ideas by the early 1970s and so there was a swing towards epidemiology.[26]

One area of research not constrained in the same way was that on nicotine, which arose from the aim of investigating the positive effects of tobacco. Here the Harrogate work about nicotine and its

[21] Ibid.
[22] Interview with industry statistician by Virginia Berridge, 12 March 1996.
[23] Interview with industry scientist 1 by Virginia Berridge, 23 February 1998.
[24] Ibid.   [25] Ibid.
[26] Interview with industry statistician by Virginia Berridge, 12 March 1996.

effects and the subsequent contacts with the RCP committee and public health researchers (discussed in this chapter and Chapter 9) show that the secrecy with which US tobacco activists have charged the US tobacco industry on this issue was not the case in the British context at this time. Glantz et al. have highlighted a 1962 conference in Southampton at which Sir Charles Ellis, of British American Tobacco (BAT), characterized nicotine as addictive; and various BAT-funded projects were underway with the Batelle Laboratories in Switzerland to develop nicotine delivery systems to avoid the toxicity of cigarettes.[27] This account emphasizes the secrecy of the research. At Harrogate, however, the nicotine research was the 'acceptable face' of the research activities. 'We were allowed to publish whatever we wrote up. That wasn't the case for the respiratory and skin painting work ... I was the good guy, studying the effect of nicotine on the brain, I was doing beneficial work but others didn't have the same freedom'.[28] The work used cats and the scientists involved were critical of the earlier, BAT-funded work that had been carried out in the Batelle Laboratories in Geneva. 'They didn't demonstrate at Batelle that nicotine was addictive ... it was poor work and incomplete. The contract labs are testers—they don't do creative work. They did a few tests and made up a story—they wanted more BAT money!'[29] Work emanating from the Harrogate research on nicotine was published in *Nature* in 1968 and was widely cited in the emergent scientific field of pharmacology.[30] The research showed the nature of the nicotine habit, that different people smoked for different reasons, and that the dose of nicotine could vary enormously. The research team at Harrogate was recognized as the cutting edge of research. 'By the 1970s we were invited to every key symposium and we were the leading researchers in the field.'[31]

But this preeminence did not last and the laboratories also were in a more difficult position by the end of the 1960s. Contract research laboratories like Huntingdon and Batelle started to do more research

[27] S. A. Glantz, J. Slade, L. A. Bero, P. Hanauer, and D. E. Barnes, *The Cigarette Papers* (Berkeley: University of California Press,1996), 60–70.

[28] Interview with industry scientist 2 by Virginia Berridge, 27 January 1998.

[29] Ibid.

[30] A. K. Armitage and G. H. Hall, 'Further Evidence Relating to the Mode of Action of Nicotine in the Central Nervous System', *Nature,* 214 (1967), 977; A. K. Armitage, G. H. Hall, and C. F. Morrison, 'Pharmacological Basis for the Tobacco Smoking Habit', *Nature,* 217 (1968), 331; and further references to this work in *Tobacco Research Council, Review of Activities, 1967–69* (London: Tobacco Research Council, 1970), 59.

[31] Interview with industry scientist 2 by Virginia Berridge, 27 January 1998.

and the companies started to look for more commercially applicable data. Harrogate then had to compete for funds with these other laboratories and became less useful to the companies. The laboratories were sold to a commercial operator, Hazelden, in 1973. The nicotine line of work there came to an end, although it continued elsewhere (as we will see in Chapter 9). The sense of disappointment was palpable. 'I ceased to be a scientist and became a businessmen—selling testing services to the pharmaceutical industry and the dentist industry, it was safety evaluation.'[32] The Tobacco Research Council was disbanded and became part of the Tobacco Advisory Committee in 1978.[33]

INDUSTRY AND PUBLIC HEALTH RESEARCHERS

Working with the industry was an important strategy for some key figures in the public alliance of the 1960s. Some, like Platt, and Godber, were always strongly opposed to the industry. In a letter to Keith Ball in 1968, Platt expressed a desire to expose the cigarette manufacturers. 'I think if the public realized that the cigarette manufacturers were evil they might be put off smoking—wonder if I'm right.'[34] Godber, too, made no secret of his dislike of the industry.[35] But Fletcher and others had good contacts; a key figure was Geoffrey Todd, the Imperial statistician who became director of the Tobacco Research Council and who was also trusted by the business side of the industry. Todd provided statistics and assessment of both the 1962 and 1971 RCP Reports and was seen by Fletcher as a 'valuable critic'. His colleagues within the Tobacco Research Council (TRC) did not always see him in the same way. One recalled, 'I didn't really like him— ... he produced draft after draft of papers and never divulged [*sic*] any power. But he was trusted by the business side of industry.'[36]

---

[32] Ibid.

[33] Tobacco Advisory Council, *Tobacco Advisory Council. Fifth Review of Research Activities, 1974–1984* (London: Tobacco Advisory Council, 1984).

[34] Wellcome Library for the History and Understanding of Medicine, ASH archive Box 19 (old system), Letter from 'Robert' [Platt] to Keith Ball, 31 January 1968. Platt suggested getting together a group at the House of Lords to discuss this, or else a group to discuss on TV.

[35] Wellcome Library for the History and Understanding of Medicine, ASH archive SA/ASH R.18, William Norman collection, Box 77, Interview with Godber, 8 February 1976.

[36] Interview with industry scientist 1 by Virginia Berridge, 23 February 1998.

Two specific areas demonstrated the interactive nature of the relationships between public health and industry at this stage: tar and nicotine and the labelling of tobacco products. The latter also showed tensions in the industry relationship with government and the need for scientific adjudication of 'risk'. The need for scientific adjudication also arose through debates on another policy issue: that of differential taxation. Meanwhile, both industry and public health scientists believed that harm and risk could be reduced: this was a mainstream strategy which informed industry moves to produce the 'safer cigarette'. The following sections of the chapter will deal with these initiatives.

Todd's main written and published commentary was on the statistics of tobacco smoking. But he was also the conduit for discussion of the implications of the tar and nicotine work. This interaction shows clearly the nature of the collaborative relationships with public health at this stage. In March 1967 Max Rosenheim, president of the RCP and chair of the ongoing committee on smoking and air pollution, and Fletcher were approached by members of the Tobacco Research Council for advice. Recent research conducted by the TRC at Harrogate had confirmed the carcinogenic nature of cigarette smoke and so they suggested that labelling of cigarette products with figures showing the tar and nicotine content of smoke might be started. This was something which Bentley, as part of the assessment of the 1962 RCP report, had originally opposed.[37] The TRC wanted advice on what guidance the public should receive on this and who should give it. Fletcher reported that the cigarette manufacturers were marketing cigarettes with a lower tar content by using more effective filters. This also reduced the nicotine content and the manufacturers did not want to market cigarettes which would not sell. They had contemplated increasing the nicotine content of cigarettes. The members of the committee agreed to meet the TRC 'and offer what help they could'.[38] A brief provided by the TRC for the meeting outlined their problems and a meeting of the committee with the TRC took place on 17 April 1967 at which Doll, Aubrey Lewis, and Platt were also present. The TRC aide-memoire for the meeting focused on issues round tar, nicotine, and volatile irritants. It included the questions 'Does

---

[37] H. R. Bentley, Note on the Recommendations for Labelling Cigarette Packets Legacy documents, American Tobacco collection, 1962, <http://legacy.library.ucsf.edu/tid/ujd01a00>.

[38] Royal College of Physicians archive, minutes of air pollution committee, 13 March 1967.

the Committee consider that nicotine, in the quantities absorbed by smokers, can have some helpful psychopharmacological effects? … How would the Committee view lower tar cigarettes in which nicotine was *not* reduced below a level that was satisfying to smokers when compared with existing cigarettes?'[39] At the meeting Todd circulated a paper showing the tar and nicotine content of the main brands. There was discussion about how much tar could be reduced without reducing the nicotine. Dr Oswald, a member of the RCP committee, asked whether extra nicotine could be added to a cigarette with a low tar content and Dr Bentley said this was a possibility they had in mind. The RCP committee at its following meeting on 2 May took the TRC memorandum and gave detailed responses. It confirmed the conclusion of the 1962 report that full protection could only come through abstention and was circumspect in its responses on nicotine and the potential hazards of low tar, low nicotine cigarettes. But it was clear from its response on nicotine that it was well aware of the issue of habituation.

The Committee was provided by the Tobacco Research Council with evidence confirming the implication in this question that habituation to smoking is probably attributable to nicotine absorption in that smokers claim less 'satisfaction' from cigarettes with lower than from cigarettes with higher nicotine content. If lowering nicotine content were to increase the number of lower tar cigarettes that were smoked the risk might be increased … Since, however nicotine itself cannot be absolved from blame, especially in relation to cardiovascular disease, a reduction of both nicotine and tar might be desirable if some other means (such as an appropriate increase in price) were adopted to discourage increased consumption of the modified cigarette.[40]

It gave support for the publication of information on these issues.

It seems that by 1967–8, the research emanating from Harrogate, despite its deficiencies, was beginning to produce a reassessment of industry strategies. The earlier optimism about removal of whatever was harmful was tempered by a growing realization of how difficult this was going to be. The TRC, representing the industry as a whole, wanted guidance and advice from the medical experts on the RCP committee. They also sought active government involvement in the strategy of labelling cigarettes with their contents. The policy-balancing

[39] Ibid., Tobacco Research Council aide-memoire, considered at meeting 2 May 1967.
[40] Ibid., Meeting 2 May 1967 response to TRC.

act continued into the late 1960s. But the issue of lists of tar and nicotine did not make progress within government. The reason why this was so tells us about the emergent tensions within public health between risk–harm reduction and a more absolutist strategy and also about tensions within the tobacco industry. It was the tobacco companies who pushed initially for labelling. Imperial Tobacco was pressing for tables in 1967 but no further action was taken then because of opposition from Gallahers and Carreras, the other main UK tobacco companies. At a meeting held in February 1968 chaired by Sir Arnold France, Permanent Secretary of the Ministry of Health (MH), it was agreed that the scientific evidence was still inconclusive and so such tables should be available to research workers rather than to the public. Imperial had asked the government to institute a new procedure—testing cigarettes for their tar and nicotine yield and publishing the results. Bentley stated in the *Financial Times* at the time that the Ministry had rejected the request. Later, in 1975, the chairman of Imperial, R. A. Garrett, told the journalist William Norman that 'tar has been progressively reduced by the industry, with the active discouragement of a previous Government'.[41] But there was more to this refusal on the part of government. W. G. Hammerton, a Department of Health and Social Security (DHSS) civil servant, explained to Norman in 1976 why the department had taken this decision. The Ministry did not know whether the cigarettes would be safe; it could lead to compensatory smoking, and they wanted to recommend people to stop. The industry strategy was not a Ministry one. Hammerton would not comment on whether Robinson had been involved, as Minister, in this decision.[42] Godber later checked the minutes of this meeting for Norman, at which he was not in the chair. The industry representatives had claimed that it was Godber who had stopped the publication of the tar tables, which he denied. At the meeting, so the note confirmed, it had been said from the Ministry of Health that in view of the evidence the Minister could not be recommended to say that a reduction in tar and nicotine would be beneficial. The position therefore was not that the Minister had refused to publish, but that he had refused to publish figures with the implications of claims for greater safety which might be made by

---

[41] Wellcome Library for the History and Understanding of Medicine, ASH archive SA/ASH Box 77, William Norman papers, Letter from Norman to Hammerton, 7 April 1976.

[42] Ibid., Hammerton to Norman, 4 June 1976.

the manufacturers.[43] As Godber commented to Norman, the problem was whether one could do more for people by emphasizing the less dangerous cigarette or whether one should spend money discouraging people from starting: in his view the correct strategy to follow was the latter. [44] Godber was a major representative and advocate of the new style of public health.

The low tar issue and its relationship to nicotine in cigarettes was an issue which was discussed with government in other ways. The relationship with Customs of one company, Gallahers, illustrated the ways in which thinking about risk reduction was developing. In 1967, Dr Tugan, scientific advisor to Gallahers, discussed problems with civil servants in Customs and Excise. His company was considering how to approach the problem of dealing with the noxious substances in cigarettes, but the problem was that reducing tar also reduced taste and flavour, as reducing tar contents also affected the nicotine content. Gallahers had conducted laboratory experiments and had found that it was practical to add nicotine to tobacco in such proportions as to maintain the normal nicotine content of smoke after filtration. They might, he reported, wish to commence experimental manufacture later in the year. But the civil servants pointed out that the addition of nicotine would be prohibited under the present law and in any case the results of the TRC research would be needed before any change could be contemplated.[45] When the report on nicotine was published later that year, the civil servants commented that 'it seems that the TRC are leaving the MH to decide what action if any should be taken in the light of their report. In the circumstances Gallaher are unlikely to want to jump in too quickly with firm proposals for the addition of nicotine to filter tipped cigarettes and I think we might leave ... in abeyance until they reopen the matter.'[46]

In general, however, the government had distanced itself more from the industry during this period. The easier relationships of the late 1950s, when the TMSC had consulted with the government about when to publish its first report in relation to the MRC statement of 1957, were over. The acceptance of money from the manufacturers

[43] Ibid., Godber to Norman, 14 February 1976.
[44] Ibid., Interview with Godber by Norman, 8 February 1976.
[45] National Archives, Customs and Excise papers, CUST 49/5632, Proposal to use nicotine in the manufacture of tobacco, Meeting held with Gallaher Ltd., 9 January 1967.
[46] Ibid., Hold to Christopherson, 25 May 1967.

for research was no longer a straightforward matter. When the issue of resumed industry funding was reopened in the mid-1960s, various possibilities came under consideration, including an MRC takeover of the Harrogate laboratories, but nothing came of the contacts. There were objections to asking the manufacturers for money since this would call into question the impartiality of the MRC's scientific judgement. It was suggested that money could be given and channelled through the MH as before, but nothing came of this.[47] Such requests were seen as calling into question government policy, including the banning of TV advertising of cigarettes.

The Royal College report had raised the question of whether government fiscal policy could be used to encourage safe smoking. This was a crucial question which was to bring the scientific analysis of tobacco centrally on to the policy agenda. The issue of differential taxation opened up another avenue for relationships between government, industry, and public health interests which ultimately led to the focus on safer smoking of the 1970s. The question of differential taxation was taken up within government. A committee of civil servants reporting to the Cabinet Ministerial committee on smoking and health on 15 May 1962 concluded that differential taxation would not be effective. The government ministers could not agree. Despite pressure on the Cabinet from the Lord President, Lord Hailsham, no action was taken. But the publication of the US Surgeon General's report on smoking in July 1964 revived interest. However, proposals from Members of Parliament for differential taxation were rejected by the Chancellor of the Exchequer in the Budget. The matter was discussed within the Treasury and a note prepared for the Economic Secretary in June 1964 pointed out that the introduction of differential rates would need a clear distinction between what was and was not harmful. Her Majesty's Customs was particularly opposed. It commented,

While the Royal College of Physicians and the US Surgeon General have condemned conventional cigarettes but have given cigar and pipe tobaccos a cleaner if not entirely clean bill of health, they have at no time indicated what it is about cigarettes (such as the paper wrapper, the nature of the tobacco used therein, the method of manufacture, or the method of packing) which makes them more dangerous than the other categories. In the absence of knowledge concerning the factors which create greater risks to health, the distinctions

---

[47] London, National Archives, Cabinet Office papers, CAB124/1686, letter from Herbert Bowden to Norman Buchan MP, 26 August 1965.

which would have to be drawn in deciding whether a particular product was, say, a cigar or a cigarette could make it appear that the Government had reached conclusions about the causes of the danger to health whereas on the basis of present statistical and medical evidence the distinctions would in fact be arbitrary, misleading and wide open to criticism as being unfair between one smoker and another and between one section of the trade and another.[48]

There was clearly a need to define what was harmful. The differential taxation discussions opened up the issue of how a change in taxation policy could be justified scientifically. In effect, it brought together health, scientific, and economic evidence at this stage in a way which anticipated the later alliances to be forged within the 'new public health' of the 1970s. Public health came to rely heavily on the discipline of health economics. A twin-track strategy developed within the overall emphasis on risk reduction, one which was supported at this stage by government, industry, and some public health interests. This aimed to modify cigarettes in ways which removed the harmful cancer-causing components; or to replace them entirely by some new smoking product which would be risk free.

HARM REDUCTION IN THE INDUSTRY: THE SAFER CIGARETTE

The Harrogate laboratories had contributed to the general expansion of knowledge about the properties of tobacco and what might be harmful or capable of removal. But it was thanks to the industry and a range of non-cigarette industrial partners that research on possible new products was developed in the 1960s and afterwards. This research and development was done at the company level: this part of the chapter will concentrate on the research carried forwards within the Imperial Group.[49] When the 1962 RCP report reaffirmed the links

---

[48] National Archives, Treasury papers, T 320/371, Customs and Excise brief, 26 June 1964.

[49] This section of the chapter is based on research carried out by Dr Penny Starns in the Wills archive in Bristol Record Office, funded by a pilot grant from the Wellcome Trust for which Virginia Berridge was Principal Investigator. The Wills archive is further analysed in V. Berridge and P. Starns, 'The "Invisible Industrialist" and Public Health: The Rise and Fall of "Safer Smoking" in the 1970s', in V. Berridge and K. Loughlin (eds.), *Medicine, the Market and the Mass Media: Producing Health in the Twentieth Century* (London: Routledge, 2005), 172–91.

between smoking and lung cancer it was the directors at Wills, the largest company within Imperial, who took the lead in formulating that group's reaction. They decided to adopt what they believed to be a responsible attitude towards the problem, and embarked on a policy of cooperation with the government. The RCP findings stressed the health risks associated with cigarette smoking rather than pipe tobacco and cigars. Subsequently the company stepped up its production of the latter products and the cigar trade boomed. The smoking public had also responded to the report by purchasing filter cigarettes in preference to ordinary cigarettes. To some extent Wills had predicted this trend, and by 1965 the company was the largest producer of tipped cigarettes in the country. Thus it was well placed to take advantage of the 'swing' in public preference.

Wills began to experiment with different types of cigarette filters in an attempt to make cigarettes 'safer'. In addition, large sums of money were invested in new machinery and research in order to produce a filter cigar. Code-named 'Pongo', the filter cigar was supposed to appeal to members of the public who were concerned about the health and smoking issue by offering a dual safeguard. In the event, despite the considerable investment 'Pongo' did not really get past the drawing board. As an experimental product 'Pongo' was probably the most expensive, but by no means the only failure.[50]

However, further research which concentrated on the development of a low tar and low nicotine cigarette blend was more successful. The research began almost as soon as the RCP report was published, though it was considered to be a long-term project. Code-named 'Wallflower' the research was shrouded in secrecy and information with regard to developments was only available on a 'need to know' basis. The product was considered to be a pre-emptive measure against further adverse publicity with regard to smoking and health. As the marketing minutes explained on 10 January 1966,

The project is under development to provide for the possibility that further smoking and health publicity may awaken consumer interest in cigarettes with low tar characteristics.[51]

---

[50] Bristol Record Office, Wills Archive, 38169, M/11/C, Marketing minutes, 13 February 1967, minute 3316; 15 May 1967, minute 3378; and 18 July 1967, minute 3402.
[51] Ibid., 10 January 1966, minute 3081.

Thus Wallflower as the name suggested was lying in wait for the right 'health climate' in order to be launched. Even five years after the publication of the 1962 report the company believed that 'smokers were not predisposed to seek out low tar and low nicotine cigarettes.'

A relatively long time span elapsed before Wallflower reached the market, during which time Wills conducted 'acceptability' experiments with the help of its workforce. By January 1966 internal tests were completed and a public relations firm, William Schlackman Ltd, was commissioned to carry out further consumer research. The fee for the research was estimated to be between £7000 and £8000 and the cost of the samples £6600. A proportion of smokers was selected to smoke the experimental Wallflower blend for a period of four weeks while a 'control' group smoked another brand, Embassy, for the same period.[52] In the meantime Wills employees were set another 'assessment' task. The company wanted help in carrying out tests on experimental dual-filter versions of Woodbine Filter and Escort. These experimental cigarettes also provided lower tar and slightly lower nicotine in-smoke yields than the existing mono-filter versions of the same brand. For the Escort brand employees were asked to assess the following three types of cigarettes:

A/Existing Escort which has a 24% retention mono-acetate plug and which yields 13 mgm. tar and 1.68 mgm. nicotine per cigarette. (control cigarette).

B/The existing Escort blend fitted with a 32% retention dual plug which is expected to reduce yields to 11.7 mgm. tar and 1.5 mgm. nicotine per cigarette.

C/An experimental blend with a 48% retention dual plug. This cigarette is expected to yield 10 mgm. tar and 1.5 mgm. nicotine per cigarette.[53]

Employee assessment of cigarettes was considered to be 'phase one' in any test of new tobacco, cigar, or cigarette blend. As usual the external tests were only carried out once these internal tests were completed. On the basis of the results of phase one William Schlackman Ltd carried out phase two, an external test on about two hundred smokers.[54] Thus employees provided Wills with essential information in terms of consumer research on a regular basis, and were more than willing to do so.

While the smoking and health issue flared up from time to time, Wills had not, at this stage, suffered any great economic loss as a

---

[52] Ibid., 3 January 1966, minute 3070.   [53] Ibid., 23 May 1967, minute 3379.
[54] Ibid.

result. Moreover the cigar trade was still booming in the late 1960s, and there was a quiet confidence amongst management personnel that new smoking materials would be found that would gain public approval. There were indications, too, that savings could be made as a result of health-prompted research. The production of low tar–nicotine cigarettes saved the company money because the rag length of the cigarette was shorter than that which was used in normal cigarettes. There were problems with consumer research, however, and consequently with the overall development of the Wallflower blend. Both in phase one and phase two of the Wallflower tests, consumers had expressed dissatisfaction with the draw resistance of the cigarette and the level of tar–nicotine. Eventually five different levels of tar and nicotine were tested, ranging from the Embassy cigarette, which was already on the market, down to the lowest Wallflower blend. Some of this research ran parallel to a programme initiated in 1967 by the Tobacco Intelligence Department (TID). The object of the TID research was to compile a short list of acceptable levels of nicotine and tar in cigarettes and measure as far as possible nicotine withdrawal tolerance by trying out 27 permutations of tar, nicotine, sugar, and draw resistance levels.[55]

The results of consumer tests were not conclusive across the country, and even in areas where they were, the results still posed a technical problem. In terms of the political climate which surrounded smoking and health, Wallflower was ready to come off the shelf, since the government had announced its intention to publish tar and nicotine figures in the near future. Wills intended to use the Wallflower blend to convert Embassy, its largest selling cigarette, into a very low tar–nicotine brand. But by this stage the sales of Embassy were already under threat from a proposed ban in coupon trading. Members of the Wills marketing committee feared that changes in the blend would have disastrous effects on sales when combined with a coupon ban:

Concerning tar/nicotine yields, there is evidence from the recent 'Wallflower' tests that yields of 1.2 mg and 9.5 mg. would probably be acceptable to Embassy smokers. We cannot, however, achieve these yields even with a 16 mm. plug without increasing the draw resistance of the cigarette above its present level. We do not know to what extent, if any, draw resistance could be increased without giving rise to adverse comment. It seems clear however, that within the

[55] Bristol Record Office, Wills Archive, 38169, M/11/C, Marketing minutes, 18 July 1967, minute 3403.

limitations imposed by 15 mm and 16 mm. plugs the critical factor in terms of consumer acceptance will be draw resistance rather than absolute tar/nicotine levels.

We therefore have to decide on the basis of judgment alone which will pose a greater risk to Embassy sales—a change in dimensions or tar and nicotine publicity. … Our experience in the past has indicated that a change in the product is more likely to have an adverse affect on sales than smoking and health publicity.[56]

The Wills company was proceeding with product development round the safer smoking option, with both consumer preference and health risk on the agenda. The idea of a replacement substance for tobacco also took hold and companies from within the chemical industry began to show an interest. These developments will be surveyed in the following chapter; they prefigured the involvement of a different sector of industry, the pharmaceuticals, in tobacco harm reduction in the 1990s and early twenty-first century (see Chapter 9).

This was a joint objective between industry–government and public health. The second Royal College report, *Smoking and Health Now*, published in 1971, in its section on 'less dangerous forms of smoking' included a reference to changing to pipes and cigars, but also addressed cigarettes with reduced nicotine and tar content in more detail. It wanted information on the packet and an authoritative medical statement on the significance of this analysis in relation to health risk. There should be a statutory upper limit for tar and nicotine. The production of 'less harmful' cigarettes was a more complex matter than at first envisaged, and so the MRC should sponsor some research.[57]

By the end of the 1960s the tobacco industry had invested considerable sums of money in research. Sir Peter Froggatt, commenting from the perspective of the late 1980s, thought that it had no desire to sell a harmful product and had invested heavily in R & D into tobacco toxicity as well as product acceptability. Along with the contribution of a quarter of a million pounds to the MRC and the employment of 250 staff at the research labs at Harrogate in their heyday, by 1969 the industry had spent six million pounds on extramural research above its in-house work. The industry was, he commented, in chorus with government, the smoking public, and the medical profession. All wanted safer smoking but for different reasons. But these interests were

[56] Ibid., 17 October 1967, minute 3426.
[57] Royal College of Physicians, *Smoking and Health Now* (London: Pitman, 1971).

in discord over anti-smoking objectives. The policy of harm reduction had worked in the 1950s and 1960s. There was the move towards filter cigarettes which brought a decline in the amount of tobacco actually smoked, and also the policy of developing alternative products through the rise of cigars and cigarillos.[58]

Politically, the climate was beginning to change by the late 1960s. Kenneth Robinson as Labour minister of Health and also a general practitioner by background was able to be more active against smoking, but his view of policy was also that it was constrained by public opinion, not by financial considerations. In the mid-1970s, in an interview, he stressed again and again that the main constraint on government had been that there was no public support for action against smoking. The answer, as he saw it, was to change the climate of opinion through health education, in particular with themes like smell and attractiveness which appealed to young people.[59] Robinson had Labour backbenchers like Laurie Pavitt, the MP who chaired the Labour Party health committee from 1964, pressing him for action. Pavitt brought in a bill on cigarette labelling in 1964.

Robinson's meetings of individual ministers on the smoking issue had caused alarm on the part of Burke Trend, the Cabinet Secretary, who diverted these through the Home Affairs committee in order to stop the proliferation of ad hoc ministerial committees on the boundaries of home and economic affairs. Trend also promoted the 'anti-nanny state' argument which had carried weight with Conservative politicians. All governments, he commented, had areas of behaviour in which they were entitled to intervene (if not bound to)—social diseases which were highly infectious (TB, VD, polio); industrial diseases contracted because of work; addictions—drink and drugs, by which a man lost his freedom of choice and became a social burden, at worst a menace to others. But, he went on,

on what grounds are the Government justified in intervening in those cases where a man's personal habits may damage only himself? And, if we accept that the Government are entitled to intervene in such cases, does this argument apply only to a man's physical habits, or does it extend also to his mental

---

[58] Froggatt, 'Determinants of Policy on Smoking and Health'.
[59] Wellcome Library for the History and Understanding of Medicine, ASH archive, SA/ASH Box 79 R.31, William Norman collection, Interview with Kenneth Robinson, 18 January 1976.

habits—i.e. to what he reads or watches on television? In short, where does the argument, if logically pursued, stop?[60]

But the nature of policy was changing. Robinson banned cigarette advertising from TV and promoted voluntary agreements on cigarette promotion.

But in the late 1960s, when Robinson brought forward to Cabinet a draft bill to outlaw cigarette coupons Richard Crossman's opposition, as overall Secretary of State, was based on electoral arguments. Crossman recorded that he

simply blurted out that this was another of those Bills which we simply couldn't afford to pass when we were running up to an election because bans of this sort made us intensely unpopular, particularly with children and families. If you're going to deal with the cigarette smoking problem, you should not try this kind of frivolous but intensely unpopular method. There was a tremendously violent reaction with everyone saying that here we must stand on moral principle. I heard it from Eirene White, Dick Taverne, and Edmund Dell, representing the Board of Trade which has switched its junior Ministers around, and, indeed, I only had two or three people on my side. However, I'm still just powerful enough to hold the thing up and finally I suggested that instead of forbidding coupons we should ration the amount of money to be spent on advertising and leave it to the cigarette manufacturers to decide how they should spend their money. I found this infinitely preferable. Harmony achieved.[61]

It was significant that Dell, as minister for the department with close links to the tobacco industry, supported restriction, not a 'pro industry' approach. Smoking's significance in terms of electoral implications was changing, although this was still a strong disincentive to action as this incident indicates.

Times were beginning to change also in terms of the policy-balancing act between government public health and industry. Sir Alexander Maxwell, long the link with government, retired in 1968 and Geoffrey Todd also left the TRC in the early 1970s. In a sense the late 1960s and 1970–1 period marked a turning point for the industry, for public health, and for government. The old corporate post-war relationships were beginning to break down and new structures to be put in their place. The 1950s and 1960s had shown a degree of collaboration

---

[60] London, National Archives, Cabinet papers, CAB 124/1686, Note from Trend to prime minister, 27 January 1965.

[61] R. Crossman, *The Diaries of a Cabinet Minister, vol. iii, Secretary of State for Social Services 1968–1970* (London, 1977), entry for 19 July 1968, 147.

between public health interests and the industry while both sought means to eliminate risk and harm from smoking. Labelling of tobacco products and the role of nicotine were two key areas of exchange of information and potential collaboration. This characterized the post-war public health outlook which still emphasized information rather than persuasion with the recognition that risk could be reduced rather than eliminated. That collaboration continued in the 1970s although increasingly under strain and already in the early 1970s, there were signs of a new and dominant public health agenda.

4

Technical Public Health: The 1971 Cross-Government Enquiry and the Rise of Economics

Change was in the air in other ways in the late 1960s and early 1970s. It was a period of transformation in medicine and public health but also within government. The way in which researchers related to government and the mechanisms which brought the two together became more formal and framed by government interests. The idea of rationality, that there could be a rational relationship between research and policy, was high on the agenda. This was a technocratic message. The 1970s was to be a distinctively modernizing period in the ideology of health, not least in the scientific disciplines considered appropriate and in the mechanisms for bringing research into a relationship with policy. The rise of the expert committee was a feature of this period. Also characteristic of this emphasis on the bringing of expertise into policy making were the moves to develop 'rational' policies on a cross-departmental basis, which are seen as characteristic of the late 1970s. The 'think tank' report on alcohol policy, produced in 1979 but only published some years later, was one such move. Public health partook of this rational technocratic impetus. This chapter, and the following one on the work of the Independent Scientific Committee on Smoking and Health, will show how this emphasis on science and policy making operated at the central government level. Smoking, through the four 'expert committees' which the chapters consider, was again emblematic of changes in the ideology of public health and the relationships between science and policy. The changes which took place in these years in public health as an occupation also threw up technocratic issues. Commentators such as Walter Holland have characterized public health at this time of change as divided between the roles of technician manager in health services and that of community activist.[1] In the Introduction, I discussed how social medicine bifurcated into evidence-based medicine and lifestyle public health. Let us first look at how this dichotomy played out within formal public health and in the rise of health services research and then return to the elaboration of mechanisms within central government which affected smoking.

The National Health Service went through a protracted reorganization which fundamentally affected the role of public health, which was also caught up in changes in local government. The Seebohm Committee of 1968 recommended the removal of social workers from local authority public health to separate social work departments. Both Seebohm and the Todd Commission on Medical Education in 1968 promoted a 'new vision' of public health as 'community medicine'. Richard Titmuss at the London School of Economics and J. N. Morris at the London School of Hygiene and Tropical Medicine (LSHTM) envisaged a new role for public health practice which capitalized on the Medical Officer of Health's (MoH) expertise in epidemiology, transforming him into a specialist whose knowledge and techniques would be available to colleagues in all branches of medicine. The Todd report called community medicine the speciality practised by epidemiologists and administrators of medical services. Morris described the community physician as responsible for community diagnosis, the analysis of the health problems of the population, and therefore providing the intelligence necessary for the efficient and effective administration of health services. Public health doctors found the idea of specialist status attractive and the Faculty of Community Medicine was established in 1972. Principles of non-medical eligibility were lost and the occupation of public health remained in the 1970s uncertain about whether its focus was the analysis of health problems or the administration of health services.[2] The changes presaged a technocratic era both in medicine and in government. The public health doctor was

[1] W. W. Holland, 'A Dubious Future for Public Health?', *Journal of the Royal Society of Medicine*, 95 (2002), 182–8. See also W. W. Holland and S. Stewart, *Public Health, the Vision and the Challenge* (London: Nuffield Provincial Hospitals Trust, 1998).

[2] These changes have been widely discussed, not least in J. Lewis, *What Price Community Medicine? The Philosophy, Practice and Politics of Public Health since 1919* (Brighton: Harvester/Wheatsheaf, 1986); D. Porter, 'The Decline of Social Medicine in Britain in the 1960s', in D. Porter (ed.), *Social Medicine and Medical Sociology in the Twentieth Century* (Amsterdam: Rodopi, 1997), 97–119; V. Berridge, D. A. Christie, and E. M. Tansey (eds.), *Public Health in the 1980s and 1990s: Decline and Rise?* (London: Wellcome Trust, 2006).

to become technician manager in this revised version of the social medicine vision.

Social medicine had a complex legacy. Its supporters were also active in the emergent critique of medicine in the 1960s and 1970s: but one result was greater emphasis on techniques such as the randomized controlled trial and on screening within health care, which also emphasized technology. Health services research (HSR) with its focus on the randomized controlled trial was also a legacy of social medicine in those new configurations.[3] The work of both Thomas McKeown and Archie Cochrane typified the 'technocratic turn' in social medicine. McKeown's critique of the part played by clinical medicine in the decline of mortality was presented to the public in his Rock Carling lectures, published in 1976, but had been known for some while previously.[4] Archie Cochrane's Rock Carling was published as *Effectiveness and Efficiency* in 1972. Cochrane had been taught statistics by Hill at LSHTM and drew on the same social medicine legacy as Morris and Doll; he was the first president of the Faculty of Community Medicine. His original view of the randomized controlled trial (RCT), formed during his work in the Medical Research Council's (MRC) Pneumoconiosis Research Unit in Cardiff, was as a means of analysing medical care in the community.[5] The movement spread internationally, building also on Canadian clinical epidemiology, and in the late 1970s and early 1980s became institutionalized in Oxford through studies of perinatal epidemiology.[6]

[3] J. Daly, *Evidence Based Medicine and the Search for a Science of Clinical Care* (Berkeley: University of California Press, 2005).

[4] T. McKeown, *The Role of Medicine: Dream, Mirage or Nemesis?* (London: Nuffield Provincial Hospitals Trust, 1976).

[5] A. Cochrane, *Effectiveness and Efficiency: Random Reflections on Health Services* (London: RSM Press, 1991) reprint of 1972 publication. See also A. R. Ness, L. A. Reynolds, and E. M. Tansey (eds.), *Population-Based Research in South Wales: The MRC Pneumoconiosis Research Unit and the MRC Epidemiology Unit*, Wellcome Witnesses to Twentieth Century Medicine, vol. xiii (London: Wellcome Trust Centre for the History of Medicine at UCL, 2002).

[6] H. M. Marks, *The Progress of Experiment. Science and Therapeutic Reform in the United States, 1900–1990* (Cambridge: Cambridge University Press, 1997); A. Yoshioka, 'Use of Randomization in the Medical Research Council's Clinical Trial of Streptomycin in Pulmonary Tuberculosis in the 1940s', *British Medical Journal*, 317 (1998), 1220–3; Ness et al. (eds.), *Population-Based Research in South Wales*; '50 Years of Clinical Trials, Past, Present and Future', *British Medical Journal* conference 29, 30 October, London, 1998; 'Beating Biases in Therapeutic Research: Historical Perspectives', conference at Osler-McGovern Centre, Green College, Oxford, 5–6 September 2002. Some papers and an edited transcript of the discussion at this meeting have been published in *International Journal of Epidemiology*, 32(6) (2003), 922–48.

Screening as a public health technology was another example of the technocratic impetus as public health practice. McKeown and Cochrane were involved in the Nuffield Provincial Hospital Trust's committee in the late 1960s on screening in medical care, which produced a report in 1968 sympathetic to the need for trials.[7] Public health screening for TB, established within the MoH empire in local government, became cervical screening in general practice in the late 1960s.[8] Some MoHs had actively assisted in these developments, in the transfer of responsibilities from public health into general practice. The work of Dr Paddy Donaldson (father of the current chief medical officer (CMO) at the time of writing) on Teesside was a particular example. Donaldson established his own health services research unit within the public health department before its demise, but also actively promoted the transfer of responsibility for screening to the general practitioner. [9] There was also pressure for a national breast cancer screening programme in the 1970s, although this did not come about until the 1980s.[10]

Government also went through a phase of technocracy and modernization. The connections with social scientists in particular began to be more formally drawn. Smith has characterized a period until the late 1960s in which social scientists were few in number, with an ad hoc influence on government.[11] The intellectual consensus which they represented largely corresponded to the political consensus, in particular over the management of the economy and the need for a welfare state. Research funding for the social sciences was minute in the early 1960s and the 'pool' of research and of researchers was small and close-knit, although the same was not true for mainstream science. The work of the Government Statistical Service, growing rapidly in the 1960s, represented a significant extension of activity in the field of social intelligence, while university teachers of social administration and

[7] Daly, *Evidence Based Medicine.*

[8] R. Baggott, *Public Health: Policy and Politics* (Basingstoke: Palgrave, 2000), 114.

[9] See R. J. Donaldson, *Off the Cuff: Reminiscences of My Half Century Career in Public Health* (Richmond: Murray Print, 2000); S. McLaurin and D. F. Smith, 'Professional Strategies of Medical Officers of Health in the Post-war Period—2: "progressive realism": the Case of Dr R. J. Donaldson, MoH for Teesside, 1968–1974', *Journal of Public Health Medicine*, 24(2) (2002), 130–5.

[10] Baggott, *Public Health,* 120.

[11] C. Smith, 'Networks of Influence: The Social Sciences in the UK since the War', in P. Wagner, C. Weiss, B. Wittrock, and H. Wollman (eds), *Social Sciences and Modern States. National Experiences and Theoretical Cross Roads* (Cambridge: Cambridge University Press, 1991), 131–47.

sociology, were translated into government advisors.[12] Research funding began to be channelled into social science research through the newly established Social Science Research Council (SSRC, established in 1965).[13] Research-linked government programmes of social intervention in education and community development embodied a commitment to evaluate social action, a tendency which was also increasingly marked in donor programmes in Third World countries.[14]

In the 1970s these developments took more government-oriented directions. In 1972, a report in the UK produced by Lord Rothschild on central government research and development clarified lines of accountability in Whitehall. The much publicized 'customer contractor' principle specified a more utilitarian view of research funding. 'The customer says what he wants; the contractor does it (if he can); and the customer pays.'[15] The implementation of this principle brought consequences for the science research councils as some of their funds were transferred to the relevant ministries; it led to more formalized research funding machinery within departments and across government, with the establishment of Cabinet machinery for the coordination of advice on the research and development activities of government, a process which was studied at the time.[16] A rational model of research and practice began to emerge in which quantitative models of research became the norm. Issues of costs in services, health in particular, became more important than ever after the oil crisis of 1973 and disciplines like health economics rose in significance. The numbers of health economists working in health services grew rapidly in this period.[17] Psychology and

[12] M. Bulmer, 'Social Science Research and Policy-Making in Britain,' in M. Bulmer (ed.), *Social Policy Research* (Basingstoke: Macmillan,1978); *idem*, 'The Policy Process and the Place in It of Social Research', in Bulmer (ed.), *Social Policy Research*, 3–30; *idem*, 'Social Science Expertise and Executive-Bureaucratic Politics in Britain', *Governance,* 1 (1988), 26–49; L. J. Sharpe, 'Government as Clients for Social Science Research', in Bulmer (ed.), *Social Policy Research.*

[13] A. Nicol, *The Social Sciences Arrive* (London: ESRC, 2001); ESRC, *SSRC/ESRC— The First Forty Years* (London: ESRC, 2005).

[14] For example the DHSS/SSRC programme on Transmitted Deprivation in the early 1970s; J. Welshman, 'Ideology, Social Science and Public Policy: The Debate over Transmitted Deprivation', *Twentieth Century British History,* 16(3)(2005), 306–41.

[15] Quoted in P. Gummett, *Scientists in Whitehall* (Manchester: Manchester University Press, 1980), 52.

[16] M. Kogan and M. Henkel, *Government and Research. The Rothschild Experiment in a Government Department* (London: Heinemann Educational Books, 1983).

[17] B. Croxson, 'From Private Club to Professional Network: An Economic History of the Health Economists' Study Group, 1971–1997', *Health Economics,* 7 (Suppl. 1), S9–S45.

psychological models also became important as health behaviour became central to public health—these will be discussed in Chapter 6 on the rise of health activism.

It was during the 1970s, too, that changes in the mechanisms linking science–research government and the medical profession were put in place. A network of governmental advisory committees on specific subject areas, with a research and policy brief, largely supplanted the influence of the old National Health Service (NHS) central committee machinery. The Advisory Council on the Misuse of Drugs, originally set up as the Advisory Committee on Drug Dependence in the late 1960s, and the Advisory Committee on Alcoholism (1978) were examples of these new arenas for the interaction between research, clinicians, scientists, and policy.[18] The story of policy on smoking in the early 1970s provides an early example of these technocratic approaches to policy making. So far as smoking was concerned this was a tale of four committees. Two of these are the subject of this chapter: the Royal College of Physicians' second report of 1971 and the cross-government enquiry into the impact of a decline in smoking, which also reported in 1971. The two other committees, the Standing Scientific Liaison committee and its successor the Independent Scientific Committee on Smoking and Health, will be considered in Chapter 5.

The second report of the Royal College of Physicians (RCP) on smoking in 1971 and the establishment of a cross-governmental enquiry into smoking policy by the Conservative Secretary of State, Sir Keith Joseph, was illustrative of new relationships between government and the medical profession on health issues, but also of the new emphasis on rational approaches to policy making and on the role of evidence within government. The enquiry, although it remained unimplemented, and indeed unknown until revealed in a series of articles in the *Guardian* in the early 1980s, demonstrated that government was taking on more responsibility for the smoking issue and was beginning to focus on the implications for taxation and wider economic issues. The rise of this economic perspective was important in differentiating British from American public responses on the issue. Britain began to use taxation as a tool of smoking policy and health policy more generally,

---

[18] V. Berridge, 'Doctors and the State: The Changing Role of Medical Expertise in Policy-Making', *Contemporary British History*, 11 (4) (1997), 66–85; B. Thom, *Dealing with Drink. Alcohol and Social Policy: From Treatment to Management* (London: Free Association Books, 1999).

while the United States took a different route. However, it was not until the latter half of the 1970s under the Labour Chancellor, Denis Healey, that these early moves were translated into practical taxation policies.

THE 1971 RCP REPORT, *SMOKING AND HEALTH NOW*

The publication of the second Royal College of Physicians report *Smoking and Health Now* on 5 January 1971 was the immediate catalyst for the setting up of a cross-government enquiry. The Royal College had maintained its interests in smoking and in air pollution after the publication of its first report on smoking in 1962. The College had continued with its air pollution committee, but its work had not proceeded with the same urgency as that of the smoking committee. The report on air pollution was not finally published until 1970 and its focus was rather different from that on smoking.[19] At a meeting in February 1965 it was recorded that the report would present scientific arguments more complex than those for smoking 'in which action by experts rather than by individuals was required for prevention'; so the report was to be presented in a style different to the smoking one, although still with sections of explanation for the lay public.[20] As the decade progressed, the work of the air pollution committee was paralleled by new work to produce a second smoking report: Charles Fletcher was again the secretary for both exercises. The membership of the committee was similar to the 1962 one, with the addition of air pollution specialists like Patrick Lawther of the newly established Air Pollution Unit at Bart's. The two reports were often considered together at meetings and the slow progress on the air pollution publication seems also to have held up work on the smoking report. Although consideration of a new smoking report first started in the mid-1960s, it did not appear until 1971. The report updated the latest research on lung cancer and the relationship of smoking to other diseases; it also had, for the first time, a strong emphasis on coronary heart disease and its relationship with smoking, based on research emanating from the US Framingham study and

---

[19] Royal College of Physicians, *Air Pollution and Health* (London: Pitman, 1970).
[20] London, Royal College of Physicians archive, Minutes of air pollution committee, 24 February 1965.

elsewhere.[21] It was during this committee's work that it was consulted by the tobacco manufacturers, represented by Todd, about the results of their work on nicotine, as discussed in the previous chapter.

The Royal College's work was a further example of that 'pressure from without' which the medical presentation of science provided. But this time in the new rational mode the issue was taken up within government. The motive force was Sir Keith Joseph, then Secretary of State for Social Services. Joseph was a reforming minister whose interest in poverty and the 'problem family' marked his time in office and who also initiated a period of interest in policy on alcohol.[22] He was a militant anti-smoker who chewed his handkerchief rather than give way to the urge to smoke.[23] The 'big issue' raised by the Royal College's report was the economic aspects of smoking. The 1971 report remarked that not much more was to be expected from small rises in taxation.[24] Larger increases might be effective, but would be undesirable in other respects in that they would bear on small incomes and might lead to crime. The report therefore, as had the 1962 one, favoured differential taxation, taxation which would be differentially applied dependent on the risk of the tobacco substance smoked. This could be used to encourage switching from cigarettes to less harmful pipes and cigars. But the report also called for a full economic enquiry and a balance sheet of benefit and loss from a fall in smoking.

The differential taxation issue will be considered in the following chapter. The cost–benefit call gave Joseph in government something 'modern' he could respond to. Here was an opportunity to look at costs and benefits over a larger canvas, and to apply business models to the health field. Discussion of the wider economic field up until this point had been limited and sporadic. The Royal College's 1971 report had an appendix on the economic consequences, but its referencing showed the limited state of the economic analysis field in the early 1970s. There were only two references in the report—to a chapter contributed by Harvey Cole, a financial journalist from the *Economist* Intelligence Unit, to Charles Fletcher's 1963 Penguin special on smoking; and to some work

[21] Royal College of Physicians, *Smoking and Health Now* (London: Pitman, 1971).

[22] See Thom, *Dealing with Drink*; R. Baggott, *Alcohol, Politics and Social Policy* (Aldershot: Avebury, 1990).

[23] Mentioned in A. Denham and M. Garnett, *Keith Joseph* (Chesham: Acumen, 2001), 218.

[24] Royal College of Physicians, *Smoking and Health Now,* 135 ff.

by Jerry Morris, in preparation. These were the routes—social medicine enquiry and journalistic—whereby wider economic issues were being discussed at this stage. There had been another route—through the insurance industry, as the Government Actuary's work in the early 1950s had demonstrated. This actuarial channel had been explored again after the publication of the first RCP report in 1962. But the insurance industry's calculations then had showed that the risk of shortening life due to smoking was not great. Representatives of the insurance industry had told government that they only contemplated imposing higher premiums when applicants for policies were already found to be suffering from defects like chronic bronchitis and were heavy smokers. But this was because the defect was already present. Future risk was more uncertain. Most companies had taken note of the RCP report and accepted that the risk of disease was higher among heavy smokers than nonsmokers. But 'actuarially the risks are not really significant and do not warrant special treatment'. In their opinion, the future risks were no greater than for other practices like eating fatty foods.[25]

The earlier political discussions within the Cabinet committee in the 1960s had focused almost entirely on the more immediate issue of differential taxation and what it might achieve, rather than on forward projections across a wider field of enquiry. In June 1962, for example, its view was that

there might ... be scope for a calculated discrimination against cigarette smokers, which, when coupled with the other anti smoking measures which were contemplated, might well produce a desirable marginal effect on the level of consumption. It would, moreover, produce additional revenue for the Exchequer.[26]

But the Treasury had produced arguments against the differential, or indeed the taxation route. It would bear more hardly on the poor and on women smokers; it would be unpopular and would be thought to be a wrong use of the taxation system. In the end the Cabinet committee could not agree on the issue. It rumbled on through the 1960s, ultimately feeding into the relationships with industry over safer smoking, which are discussed in Chapter 5.

[25] National Archives, Cabinet Office papers, CAB 21/4648, 3 April 1962, Notes of a meeting with representatives of the insurance companies.
[26] Ibid., CAB 134/2518, Ministerial committee on smoking and health, Minutes of second meeting, 1 June 1962.

The technical ability to discuss wider issues of economic analysis and projections of future mortality and morbidity patterns was limited. Again the industry scientists, as in other areas, filled some of the gaps. As part of the Tobacco Advisory Committee's (TAC) response to the draft 1971 report, the statistician Geoffrey Todd produced a twenty-page critique of the committee's estimate of smoking-related deaths from coronary heart disease. He summed up,

> The conclusion that there is a sub-group of cigarette smokers who died from coronary heart disease to which smoking did not contribute and whose death rate exceeded the death rate of non-smokers from this disease is therefore not unreasonable. But if it is a valid conclusion, the basis on which the RCP Committee estimated that in 1968 some 60,000 deaths of cigarette smokers were attributable to cigarette smoking is not valid.[27]

THE CROSS-GOVERNMENT ENQUIRY

However, the RCP had thrown down a challenge to government. The College proposed to take action after the report by coordinating the voluntary sector round smoking: this led ultimately to the formation of Action on Smoking and Health (ASH) and a new style of health activism, as discussed in Chapter 6. It argued that there was need for a standing government committee which could do the same within government, coordinating all the government departments with an interest in smoking. At the launch of the report, Lord Rosenheim, president of the College, said that this official enquiry was the most urgent single measure among those proposed. Matters were underway within government. In December 1970, in a brief for the Home Affairs committee, just before the RCP report was published, Joseph had argued strongly for measures which could influence the rising generation against cigarette smoking. He was prepared to use legislation if the manufacturers would not agree to his package of measures voluntarily (warning notices; details of the tar and nicotine content; and a requirement for the industry to notify government of changes in the composition of cigarettes). Government action could maintain this

---

[27] Royal College of Physicians archive, Papers of the committee on smoking and air pollution, Comments from Tobacco Advisory Committee on the draft 1971 report, 1970. Todd's paper, *Estimates of the Number of Deaths Attributable to Cigarette Smoking.*

position while a study of the economic effects of a reduction in smoking took place.[28] He was given three months to secure voluntary agreement. That agreement was reached by the following March. In a letter on 11 January 1971 to John Davies, Secretary of State for Trade and Industry, Joseph commented that the study was 'a proposal I regard as important presentationally as well as in substance'. He went on,

I am very anxious not only that these discussions should start without delay, in order to assess the pros and cons of antismoking measures more far reaching than those I have so far broached with the industry, but also that I shall be able to announce that they are taking place. The Government can be expected to derive credit for an early response to this point and be strongly criticised for refusing to carry out the study recommended.[29]

Moves to set up the officials coordinating committee were already in train. The enquiry was located at the centre of government in the Cabinet Office under the chairmanship of Paul Odgers, the head of the Social Services Coordinating unit, a unit which had been set up by Crossman in 1968. It lasted only from 1968 to 1971, although its research unit lasted longer. Odgers was not keen to take on the enquiry, in part because he already had too much to do, in part because if the enquiry was announced, the government would have to publish the report. But Ministers wanted a study of the effects of a substantial reduction in the sale of cigarettes, not of whether such a reduction would be justified on health grounds: Cabinet Office chairmanship was considered more appropriate than Department of Health and Social Security (DHSS) leadership. The committee had a membership drawn from the Central Statistical Office, Customs, DHSS, the Department of Trade and Industry, the Scottish Home and Health Department (SHHD), and the Treasury. Its work was to be in two parts—the economic and other implications of a substantial fall in cigarette smoking; and possible measures which might contribute to that fall.

The work of the committee was structured by two papers, one from the DHSS, which arrived early on in its life, and another from the

[28] National Archives, Cabinet Office papers, CAB 165/925, Home Affairs committee briefs, 8 December 1970, HA (70) 63, Cigarette Smoking and Health.
[29] Ibid., CAB 152/16/10/pt1, 11 January 1971, letter from Sir Keith Joseph to J. E. H. Davies, Secretary of State for Trade and Industry.

Treasury. In the 'received view' of the history of smoking policy, the final report of this committee has been presented as demonstrating the disbenefits for government of reducing smoking and the way in which health interests within government could lose out to fiscal ones.[30] However, the papers and discussion in the committee and the advice which came from the Treasury do not support these conclusions in their entirety. They show that, for the Treasury, the issue was rather more complex fiscally. The economic side of the committee's work was initially structured by a paper from the DHSS which arrived on 12 February 1971. The assumptions in the paper were that a fall in cigarette smoking of 20 or 40% would occur. The reductions would be a fall in the number of smokers rather than a reduction by people who continued to smoke. These falls would occur evenly over five years and then stability would be reached; and they would occur in equal proportions in all social classes in all age groups and in both sexes. The Cabinet Office found these assumptions rather one-dimensional. R. G. Watts, a Cabinet Office civil servant and secretary of the steering group, commented to Odgers that the DHSS had only made one set of assumptions and had left out a possible switch to less dangerous smoking habits:

Ministers, hopefully, might find it easier to introduce now the strong measures needed to bring about a substantial reduction in tobacco cigarette smoking if they thought that some of the awkward financial and other economic consequences would probably be diminished by the introduction of a new non tobacco cigarette.[31]

At the second meeting of the steering group on 17 February, it was agreed to use the DHSS predictions of 20 and 40% but to introduce switching smoking habits and non-tobacco cigarettes into the discussion as well. The DHSS was also to consider further whether it was correct to assume that any fall would affect all social classes equally.

Watts suggested that the departments represented on the steering group should consider three levels of action against smoking. Measure A consisted of large-scale, comprehensive, and continuing anti-smoking propaganda, the core being sustained TV advertisements. Measure B was the prohibition of, or alternatively, restrictions of varying degrees

---

[30] For example, Sir Richard Doll's comments in an interview in *The Observer*, 24 April 2005.

[31] National Archives, Cabinet Office papers, CAB 152/16/10/pt1, 15 February 1971, R. G. Watts to P. Odgers.

of severity on cigarette advertisements and cigarette promotion. And Measure C, the most wide ranging, was a package of compulsory practical measures, such as a ban or restrictions on smoking in public places; removal of vending machines from public places; the imposition of a statutory upper limit on tar and nicotine content; strengthened regulations forbidding sale to young people; and measures to help people to give up, including discrimination in taxation in favour of less dangerous smoking products. This would ensure coordination of activity rather than isolated initiatives such as the Home Office's consideration of raising the age of sale. [32] Eleven studies in all were carried out; study number one involved the DTI (Department of Trade and Industry), the Chancellor of the Exchequer, and the DHSS examining the likelihood of the cigarette industry producing a less dangerous cigarette and study number two the DHSS and the SHHD examining the beneficial effects on mortality and morbidity of a reduction in cigarette smoking.

The economic enquiry was structured at two levels. On 1 March James Collier, an undersecretary in the DHSS, told Bavin of the DHSS how he saw the shape of things. The report would look at the economic effect of the two proportionate reductions over five years; and then at the economic and social effects, advantageous to health and financially, over a generation. 'And we shall ask Ministers to decide whether the immediate cost is worth the long term gain.' The DTI, he reported, were cooperating very happily with the whole exercise. They thought the study would not tell against them and would undoubtedly question the validity of the conclusions on mortality. The note was copied to Odgers with a comment indicative of the administrative civil servants' attitude. 'I think you will be glad to see that I am seeking to protect our flanks from Ministers and George Godber!' [33]

At the start, political events intruded as some areas of the work— measures which might lead to these falls in smoking—were acted on in the political arena. Warning notices on cigarette packets had been adopted in the United States as a response to the Surgeon General's report in 1964. Both Labour and Conservative MPs of the anti-smoking persuasion wanted to see these and tar and nicotine tables introduced in the UK. Bills were introduced first by the Labour MP Laurie Pavitt,

[32] Ibid., 1 March 1971, Watts to Odgers, Notes for the meeting on 4 March.
[33] Ibid., 1 March 1971, J. Collier to Mr Bavin (both DHSS), copied to Odgers, Note by Collier.

chair of the Labour health committee, and then by the Conservative Gerald Nabarro. Nabarro had introduced a private members bill in the previous parliament, in 1970, which had fallen because of the general election. In December 1970 he had introduced his Tobacco and Snuff (Health Hazards) Bill, which proposed a warning notice, the 'poison content' of tar and nicotine, and an advertising ban. Initially Joseph worked with Nabarro, a strategic alliance so that he could exert pressure on the tobacco industry to agree to a voluntary deal. The government whips agreed not to oppose the Nabarro bill's second reading and it would then come to committee stage. If no voluntary agreement was signed with the industry then the committee stage would be delayed by two or three weeks. If there was still no voluntary agreement, then it was proposed that Nabarro's Bill would be used as the basis for legislation.[34] In an interview with the journalist William Norman some years later, Laurie Pavitt recalled that 'Nabarro thought he'd done a deal with Joseph as minister for social services—that it would go through—but he was sold down the river and the whole thing fell.'[35] As a result of the bill, the Department of Health was able to come to an agreement with the tobacco companies about their acceptance voluntarily of a warning on the side of the tobacco packet. Joseph also entered into negotiation over the second thing anti-tobacco forces were after—league tables of tar and nicotine—and there was agreement for the establishment of the Standing Scientific Liaison Committee, which is discussed in the following chapter. Nabarro, undeterred, continued with his Bill which was finally 'talked out' in May 1971.[36]

The civil servants on the steering group took note of these developments. On 23 March after Nabarro had decided to fight on despite the announcement of the voluntary agreement, Watts commented to Odgers there were only two strategies in the parliamentary discussions not already being considered by the officials group. Pavitt had proposed that ITV and the other commercial television companies make available to the Health Education Council the same amount of time as was spent on tobacco advertising; and also that the producers and wholesalers of tobacco products should make payments into a tobacco sales promotion

[34] National Archives, Cabinet Office papers, CAB 152/16/10/pt1, 18 February 1971, Note from Watts to Odgers re the Tobacco and Snuff (Health Hazards) Bill.
[35] Wellcome Library for the History and Understanding of Medicine, ASH archive, SA/ASH William Norman papers, Box 79, R.26, Interview with Laurie Pavitt.
[36] G. Nabarro, *Exploits of a Politician* (London: Arthur Barker, 1973), 174–91.

levy fund for use by the Health Education Council. The DHSS, commented Watts, was minded to oppose these measures—the first was seen as punitive and unfair to TV; and the second would founder on the Treasury's dislike of hypothecated taxes.[37]

The committee continued its work. It was noticeable how the civil servants at the centre took a balancing view of their role. This was apparent as the reports from the individual departments started to come in. The DTI prepared a paper on the pros and cons of the prohibition of advertising. The Home Office was already looking at raising the age of purchase to 18, the DHSS was to look at campaigns with the SHHD and at other measures, while the Treasury and the DTI took up differential taxation, and the DHSS looked at the switch to other forms of smoking. The DoE and the Home Office examined environmental measures like smoking on public transport and elsewhere. The DTI's paper on the prohibition of advertising was presented on 31 March; it stressed the lack of evidence that banning advertising would have a significant effect on consumption. But this did not find favour with the Cabinet Office team. Watts commented to Odgers on 2 April that they might agree with these conclusions. But at the last steering group meeting, the DTI had said that they saw themselves as the watchdog and spokesman for the tobacco industry. So the Cabinet Office should try to balance out the conclusions by stimulating the DHSS to produce a paper arguing in favour of the ban. However, the DHSS might not regard a ban as politically feasible at the present time and so might not bother.[38] The DTI also produced a paper on its allocated topic of safer smoking which summarized the current developments. It expected no significant effect from safer smoking materials over the next five years, but there might be significant and growing benefits over the following five. There was clearly also support for safer smoking within the DHSS. Collier commented to Odgers on 26 April 1971, after Joseph had spoken in the Commons in a debate on smoking, that the speech had been aimed at measures which would reduce the suffering caused by smoking:

These words were chosen very carefully, and you will note that they do not imply a Government decision to reduce substantially the amount of cigarette

---

[37] National Archives, Cabinet Office papers, CAB 152/16/10/pt1, 23 March 1971, Watts to Odgers.
[38] Ibid., CAB 152/16/10/pt2, Cigarette Smoking and Health, 2 April 1971, Note from Watts to Odgers.

smoking itself ... was designed deliberately as a way of working towards a policy of less dangerous forms of smoking, including switching to pipes and cigars.[39]

However, optimism in the committee about the likely impact of safer smoking was modified after a report was forwarded in May 1971 from two MRC conferences held the previous year on smoking and tobacco substitutes. The report stated that the comparative safety of such products could only be assessed by long-term epidemiological methods. These discussions at the MRC had involved representatives of the tobacco industry and a MRC committee chaired by the pharmacologist William Paton with a membership of Doll, Fletcher, Donald Reid of LSHTM, Guy Scadding, and Dr Julia Dawkins, the newly appointed (1970) medical civil servant in the Department of Health responsible for smoking policy. They were part of the manoeuvres which preceded the appointment of the Standing Scientific Liaison Committee in 1971 and the Independent Scientific Committee on Smoking and Health in 1973. The report concluded, in line with the general ethos of collaboration with industry, that the manufacturers should collaborate with appropriate independent research workers in the development and evaluation of experimental test systems. In 1971, the DTI modified its optimism about safer smoking materials after receiving a copy of this report. The prospects now seemed 'rather remote'.[40]

It was at this stage that the DHSS produced its promised paper on the health and economic consequences of the proposed falls in tobacco smoking. This provided some interesting figures which were not quite what any of the officials had been expecting. A paper produced by the government actuaries department on 12 May on the effect of a reduction of cigarette smoking on the future population of Great Britain had concluded that the effect on the population of both projected percentage falls, even over 35 years, would be small (see Table 4.1). Population would only increase by 3.5 per thousand for males and 0.5 per thousand for females in the case of the 20% reduction. There would also be a relatively small impact on expectation of life. There was only a two-year gain in life expectancy for men aged forty. If all smokers ceased to smoke—for 20 and 40% reduction—the gains

[39] National Archives, Cabinet Office papers, CAB 152/16/10/pt1, 26 April 1971, Note from James Collier, undersecretary in DHSS, to Odgers.

[40] Ibid., Report of the MRC conference on smoking and tobacco substitutes and the DTI response, 17 May 1971.

Table 4.1. Effects of a Reduction of Cigarette Smoking on the Future Population of the UK

	20% reduction			40% reduction		
	Fewer deaths	Net change in health care costs (£m)	Net change in security payments (£m)	Fewer deaths	Net change in health care costs (£m)	Net change in security payments (£m)
1981	3,000	−5	−2	15,000	−9	−5
1991	5,000	−6	+70	15,000	−8	+13
2001	9,000	−4	+20	18,000	−6	+39

would be even less.[41] However, the projected effects on welfare costs were considerable. These figures were considered by the steering group at its fourth meeting on 10 June 1971. The effect of such reductions was in fact substantial in terms of absolute numbers of lives saved and it was decided to emphasize this in the steering groups report to Ministers.

In the middle of June, Collier reported to Odgers that papers on health education and vending machines would come to the next meeting on 25 June, and he also had on the stocks the health arguments for and against differential taxation; anti-smoking clinics; smoking, alcohol, and drugs; and smoking in public places.[42] The DHSS favoured what he called the 'sophisticated' line on the taxation question—in the present state of knowledge it would be unwise to encourage pipes and cigars but they would go along with a negative discussion involved in raising the tax on cigarettes ('in fact our line on the latter will be influenced much more by the regressive effect on income distribution, special burden on the poorest families etc.').[43]

[41] National Archives, Ministry of Health papers, MH 148/1469, Cigarette smoking and health: medical commercial and policy aspects, 1971–79, 12 May 1971, Paper from Government Actuary's Department, Effect of a reduction in cigarette smoking on the future population of Great Britain.
[42] The attempt to look across the substances was a feature of this period, related to the MRC's growing interest in illicit drugs and the heightened policy attention to alcohol. See Chapter 9 for some discussion of this.
[43] National Archives, Cabinet Office papers, CAB 152/16/10/pt2, Cigarette Smoking and Health, 16 June 1971, Collier to Odgers.

It was after the next meeting that a memorandum arrived from the Treasury and Customs which demonstrated the complexities of the fiscal argument. Marked Secret, the memorandum dealt with the effect of increasing the duty on cigarettes. It considered the implications for tax revenue and demand management in the economy if the assumed falls in numbers smoking were achieved by increases in duty on cigarettes. It was as the Treasury civil servants commented, 'inevitably a sensitive document. The appraisal in it could be widely contested, and it could be used as a means of pressurising the Government, and it could cause considerable alarm in some circles.'[44] The document showed that the economic arguments were not as straightforward as they seemed and the implications for the economy were complex. Firstly the consequences of joining the European Economic Community (EEC) had to be considered. Indirect taxation would be harmonized and UK taxation was already at a rate higher than that in other EEC countries. Harmonized taxation would be at a level lower than the current UK level. But the major difficulty of the whole exercise was to quantify consumers' reactions to an increase in the price of tobacco; a firmly based estimate of price elasticity of demand was needed, but no academic studies existed. The Treasury conclusion was that it was not possible to bring about a controlled reduction in cigarette smoking. Duty changes were a blunt instrument: with an increase of five pence on a packet of twenty, and with other measures of a non-fiscal nature, the price elasticity of demand would approach minus two. This would result in an overall fall in consumption of around 30%, with a net loss of tobacco revenue of around £120 million. Consumer expenditure would switch to other taxed goods so the net loss would be less than this. Compensating revenue from pipes and cigars would not be that great and there would be an increase in imported cigars because the UK industry would not be able to adjust at short notice. An increase in tobacco duty would increase demand and would lead to an excessive level of demand in the economy, which would have to be offset by higher taxation. It would have a strange effect, in that it would lead to an increase and not a reduction in taxation. There was a reason for this—the high price elasticity of demand for these products. A large proportionate increase in price would be followed by larger proportionate falls in

    [44] National Archives, Cabinet Office papers, CAB 152/16/10/pt2, Cigarette Smoking and Health, 12 July 1971, Steering group on cigarette smoking, The Effect of Increasing the Duty on Cigarettes, Note by the Treasury and Customs.

consumption; duty accounted for a very large proportion (around 70%) of the retail price. Some individuals would be worse off by the fall in consumption because of fiscal action than by the fall through non-fiscal action. Some, for example the elderly and the poor, would lose out anyway—they would continue to smoke and they would be made even worse off by the increase in other rates of tax. The others made worse off would be those who did not smoke in the first place but who would be affected by overall higher taxation. The increase in duty would have the greatest effect on those on incomes of £1,000 a year, those below that limit slightly less and those above affected least. The increase in tax rates would affect the high income groups most. Collier commented to Odgers that the financial arguments for an increase in duty were not strong. This was the 'promised cockshy with some annotations'.[45] There was a case for looking at the economic and financial implications, but 'The case for reducing the damage done by cigarette smoking must rest on the State's duty to the health of its citizens.' The Treasury withdrew this paper ten days later on 22 July and copies were destroyed. A shorter paper was sent, which the Cabinet Office noted had dropped a lot of detail and did not assess the effect on revenue, balance of payments, and demand management. But the civil servants wanted their final report to note that the increase in demand because of the increase in taxation had to be mopped up by increases in other taxes. Watts' guess, he confided to Odgers in June, was that the Treasury regarded the size of the problem as manageable. They were not dismayed by the possible changes: the demand increase factor might offset the adverse effects on tax revenue and balance of payments.[46]

The first draft of the report was ready soon after on 26 July, but the final version was not presented until October 1971. The committee began to look at developments in Canada and in the United States. In the States advertising on TV and radio had been banned since January 1971 and the Canadian government had recently introduced a bill covering warning notices, an advertising ban, and statutory limits on tar and nicotine. But it was the economic effects which were most unpredictable. With the coming of entry to the EEC the tobacco industry faced a potential tax revolution and the officials also wrestled with the demand

---

[45] Ibid., Draft, Implications of a reduction in cigarette smoking, Note to Odgers from Collier.
[46] Ibid., 7 June 1971, Watts to Odgers, Notes for meeting on 10 June 1971.

implications of an increase in duty and taxation.[47] There were also the implications of the coming of VAT in 1973. A meeting of the group on August 19 led to the comment that a 15 to 30% impact on consumption might lead, together with health education, to a 10 to 20% reduction in the longer term. This would increase the Retail Price Index by 1 1/4% and the effect of the increase on pensioners would be even more marked. But the impact on demand management was unpredictable. If cigarette consumption fell by a proportion smaller than the retail price was increased, there would be a small reduction in the level of demand in the economy. If consumption fell by a greater proportion, the effect would be substantially to increase the level of demand. Tobacco duty was the most regressive of all the Exchequer duties and so any increase in duty would affect poor households more. But if demand increased and was therefore mopped up by a higher increase in tax, these households would do better and people paying tax worse. A DHSS memo on 9 September considered the impact on low income families earning under thirty pounds a week and spending more than two pounds on tobacco. The fiscal increase would be to increase their tobacco expenditure between twenty pence and one pound and to displace expenditure on food, clothing, and travel.[48]

To the uncertainties about demand management were added negotiations in the committee about statistics of mortality and morbidity. Collier wrote to Odgers in September 1971,

One of the difficulties with which Ministers will be faced when they come to make their policy announcements on smoking will be about statistics, and in particular the assumptions of mortality and morbidity arising from smoking. There is a wide range of assumptions upon which estimates of the number of premature deaths due to smoking can be based and hence a wide range of results.[49]

There were negotiations 'backstage' around the figures considered suitable for public presentation.[50] The report, it was decided, was to

[47] National Archives, Cabinet Office papers, CAB 152/16/10/pt3. The file contains a report: S. Aris, 'UK Tobacco Faces Tax Revolution', *Sunday Times*, 15 August 1971.

[48] Ibid., 9 September 1971, Miss M. E. Stuart at DHSS to Watts.

[49] Ibid., 17 September 1971, A. J. Collier to Odgers.

[50] D. F. Smith, 'The Social Construction of Dietary Standards: The British Medical Association–Ministry of Health Advisory Committee on Nutrition Report of 1934', in D. Maurer and J. Sobal (eds.), *Eating Agendas: Food and Nutrition as Social Problems* (New York: Aldine De Gruyter, 1995), 279–303; S. Hilgartner, *Science on Stage. Expert Advice as Public Drama* (Stanford: Stanford University Press, 2000).

take a figure of 52,000 deaths a year and they must stick by this as an absolute minimum and not allow sliding around. But there was also a need for other 'compelling figures' to make ministers realize the significance of the matter. At the eighth meeting on 23 September, it was decided that the report would go with the figure of 52,000 and not the higher 80,000 used in the CMO's annual report. [51]

After twelve meetings in all, the report was finally ready for Ministers on 14 October 1971. It was decided that around three hundred copies would be printed and it would go to the Home Affairs committee not to the Secretary of State for Social Services as the original discussion had been in that committee. The report struck a balance. It made clear the health issue—even without taking the CMO's preferred higher figures—and the potential duty of the government to its citizens on health grounds in terms of lives lost through smoking. It marked the formal assumption of government responsibility for the negotiation and management of health risk. But the economic arguments for that stance were by no means clear-cut. The report did not include the complexities of demand management which had been outlined in detail in the Treasury's secret memorandum. It argued that the effects on employment in the cigarette industry were manageable. Although there would be pockets of high unemployment in particular areas, the industry overall was not a large employer. It was in the revenue, balance of payments, and demand management fields where, as the memos presented to the committee had discussed, there was the most uncertainty. In the event the published report simply mentioned the increase in the retail price index (RPI) as the result of an increase in duty and the way in which this would bear on pensioners and the poor. The Treasury view of increased overall taxation to reduce demand in the economy, bearing on those with higher incomes and who did not smoke—a nightmare political scenario—was not presented to ministers. The report outlined the twin-track strategy which was to underpin both government and public health responses to smoking throughout the 1970s. The officials had examined the possibilities of making smoking less dangerous and of getting people to smoke less. 'The two approaches are not incompatible and neither can be guaranteed to produce substantial results; and, in the context of a major effort to reduce the ill effects of cigarette smoking, it would be desirable

[51] National Archives, Cabinet Office papers, CAB 152/16/10/pt3, 23 September 1971, Minutes of eighth meeting.

to pursue both.'[52] The strategy for the less dangerous cigarette was outlined in some detail as the tar and nicotine work had been referred to the newly established Standing Scientific Liaison Committee (SSLC). There was no mention in detail of the industry's moves to modify cigarettes apart from this. In order to achieve the drop in smoking, the report significantly placed most emphasis on health education and on advertising. The mediatization of health matters started after 1962 was amplified. The committee thought three million pounds a year would need to be committed to health education to make a difference. But there was no real evidence that health education would make any difference at all—so first a pilot study needed to be commissioned and evaluated. The focus would be on the young, but the real need was to change the attitudes of the adult world. Here the attitude to an advertising ban was equivocal. Evidence of the effect of advertising on consumption was inconclusive, but there was an argument that the continuation of advertising and gift coupon schemes 'might be held to hinder the decisive change in the climate of opinion which it would be the object of a health education campaign to bring about'.[53] In other words, the advertising ban had a symbolic importance, an argument which came to be widely used in public health circles. The report was not enthusiastic about measures which imposed environmental restrictions such as regulation of public space, or restrictions on vending machines or on the age of minimum sale.

Although there was some parliamentary questioning about the report during the autumn, it was never officially published. It was initially held back after its presentation to the Home Affairs committee on 17 November 1971 because Joseph intended to circulate policy proposals. When his memorandum was discussed in that committee on 22 December, he did not receive the support he had hoped for. Banning advertising and coupon gift schemes was seen as out of the question, so Joseph had put forward a package of other measures. He would seek voluntary industry agreement to ban vending machines, include safer smoking advice in cigarette packets, and also ban poster advertising and restrict overall advertising to its present level. Legislation would be held in reserve and Joseph also held out the possibility of the total abolition of advertising over a five- to ten-year period. But the committee did

---

[52] Cabinet Office, *Cigarette Smoking and Health. Report by an Interdepartmental Group of Officials, October 1971*, 7.
[53] Ibid., 8.

not support his tactics and insisted that voluntary agreement was to be sought, not backed up by such threats. The report and the legislative push fell flat.[54] Melanie Phillips, social services correspondent of the *Guardian*, 'discovered' the report in 1980 and published an exposé in the paper which presented its non-publication as a victory for smoking rather than health. 'Why smoking, not health, wins the day'.[55] Her reporting presented the non-publication as an example of how powerful economic interests within government could neutralize the Department of Health. This was to some extent true, but Phillips' characterization of the report tended to tread a well-worn path rather than look at the range of issues for politicians. The key issue as presented by officials was not the protection of the tobacco industry, although obviously industry-related strategies like less dangerous smoking were important. They stressed the effect which restricting advertising would have on the press and the popularity of coupon schemes with women voters. It was the economic and political implications for elected politicians. The report also appeared at a time when the harm reduction strategy within government was beginning to gather force. The voluntary agreement with the manufacturers and the establishment of the SSLC appeared to offer the way forward. This was the strategy favoured by the Conservative government for the rest of its duration even though the non-smoking prime minister, Edward Heath, also made Cabinet meetings non-smoking in 1973.

THE RISE OF HEALTH ECONOMICS IN PUBLIC HEALTH

The report was also significant because it made the wider economic argument central to discussion of the new public health. The economic arguments behind public health had a history which went back to the nineteenth century with the discussion of the 'human capital' elements of public health in the 1840s. The 1971 officials' report

---

[54] National Archives, Cabinet Office papers, CAB 134/3403, 17 November 1971, HS(71) 61, Cigarette smoking and health, Note by the secretaries; 9 December 1971, HS(71) 68 Smoking, Memorandum by the Secretary of State for Social Services. CAB 143/3402, Home and Social Affairs committee, 15th meeting, 22 December 1971, item 6 smoking. Denham and Garnett, *Keith Joseph*, 218, state that Joseph was reluctant to legislate against the industry. This does not appear to have been the case.

[55] M. Phillips, ' "Curb smoking" Call Unheeded', *Guardian*, 6 May 1980.

marked the beginning of that discussion in relation to smoking; but also the beginning of research-based investigation which focused on the economics of the issue. Health economics, as an emergent speciality, was the beneficiary of these discussions; and health economics was to become a central investigative tool for health in the technocratic era of the 1970s and beyond. The way in which this research developed in the rest of the decade began to challenge the arguments within government about the impact of a decline in smoking or of higher taxation on the poor. The political arguments began to change because of the argument from health economics.

Research capacity in this area had been severely limited at the outset of the committee of official's work. It had been recognized that economic assistance was needed, but there was little on offer. Maurice Peston's name came up and Collier had written to Odgers, 'Peston is not of course the only cost benefit practitioner; and we have had a proposal from the Metra Group to do something on the same lines.'[56] But in the end because of time constraints, the work was done in-house. In the early 1970s the interest in smoking was a major impetus for the economic perspective in public health. Peston (later Lord), Professor of Economics at Queen Mary College, spoke at the second world conference on smoking in London in 1971, along with George Teeling Smith, director of the pharmaceutical industry-funded Office of Health Economics, which had begun its work in 1962.[57] There was American influence, too. Weisbrod's *The Economics of Public Health* had been published in 1962 and there was American work on the costs of mental illness in the 1950s, with earlier work on tobacco as a commodity. In the UK, a classic early economic study on prevention was Reynolds' 'The Costs of Road Accidents' published in 1956 with further work after that commissioned by the Road Research Laboratory. This was an attempt to justify prevention of road accidents by indicating the benefits in terms of hospital costs and productivity which could be recouped if accidents were reduced.[58] As with the rise of mass media health education it was

[56] National Archives, Cabinet Office papers, CAB 152/16/10/pt1, 28 January 1971, James Collier, DHSS, to Paul Odgers, CO.

[57] M. H. Peston, 'Economics of Cigarette Smoking', in R. G. Richardson, *The Second World Conference on Smoking and Health* (London: HEC/Pitman Medical, 1971),100–10; G. Teeling Smith, 'An Argument for Swingeing Taxation', in Richardson (ed.), *Second World Conference on Smoking and Health*, 111–13.

[58] J. Roberts, 'Economic Evaluation of Health Care: A Survey', *British Journal of Social and Preventive Medicine*, 28 (1974), 210–16.

road safety which provided the initial model for prevention. Again there was 'policy seepage' from one area to another.

Peston's lecture at the world conference began to address some of the issues on which the government analysts had found little information. Estimating total economic costs was difficult. 'We do not as yet have all the evidence we need to produce a definitively accurate estimate of the economic costs of smoking. An elaborate and expensive research programme needs to be mounted.'[59] Price and income elasticities of demand was what had interested economists. Tobacco was an inelastic commodity and so it was not easy to reduce cigarette consumption by taxation alone. He began to address the poor consumers question. '[If] tax policy is used to reduce cigarette consumption, adjustments must be made in other taxes and benefits that affect poorer people in order not to lower their total real purchasing power.'[60] Teeling Smith argued for swingeing taxation. He pointed out that anti-smoking propaganda based on number of deaths and even life expectancy was rejected by the general public; the younger the audience, the greater the rejection. The only solution was really heavy taxation. A heavy smoker would spend between £200 and £250 a year; if this were trebled through taxation it would impose a very real deterrent.[61]

The interest in smoking came at a time when health economics research in relation to health services in general was expanding as government went down the route of technocratic and evidence-based approaches. The Health Economists Study Group was formed in 1972 and leading economists like Alan Williams and Tony Culyer at York linked with Norman Glass in the Department of Health, with the rise of cost effectiveness studies.[62] The first sustained smoking work came from a joint project in the early 1970s on the economic consequences of smoking organized between the MRC/DHSS Epidemiology and Medical Care Unit at Northwick Park Hospital and the Department of Economics at the University of Essex. There were personal connections as well as the institutional ones in terms of links established between MRC and DHSS research funding. Tony Atkinson, Professor of Economics at Essex, had been a pupil of the economist James Meade at Cambridge. Meade was the father of Tom Meade, Director of Northwick Park. The research officer was Joy Skegg, later Townsend,

[59] Peston, 'Economics of Cigarette Smoking', 104.   [60] Ibid., 110.
[61] Teeling Smith, 'An Argument for Swingeing Taxation', 111–13.
[62] Croxson, 'From Private Club to Professional Network'.

who came from a background of development economics.[63] The Atkinson–Townsend work impacted on a field which was small and in the course of development. One of the earliest publications in the 'new' health economics of public health was a paper by Michael Russell, a psychiatrist at the newly formed (1967) Addiction Research Unit at the Institute of Psychiatry. Russell, basing his argument on what had happened to cigarette consumption since 1946 with increases both in price and in duty, argued for a 10% increase in the price of cigarettes each year as an essential ingredient in smoking control.[64] Atkinson and Skegg's early work downplayed the effect of taxation in favour of that of health education, which had a greater (albeit temporary) effect.[65] Julian Peto, based at the MRC TB and Chest Diseases Unit, and previously a researcher at the Addiction Research Unit with Russell, joined in the debate with a defence of taxation:

[It] seems likely that systematic tax increases would have an immediate and progressive effect on consumption and recruitment, particularly among young people, who are less wealthy and less addicted. Although health education has some impact, there seems to be no other way of reducing smoking on the scale demanded by the still mounting evidence of associated morbidity and mortality.[66]

It was this work and its impact later in the 1970s which helped turn public health in a different direction—towards high taxation policies aimed at abstention from smoking. Townsend recalled that they were interested 'in building a model to look at economic effects on behaviour and the behaviour change effect on mortality. This was new work.'[67] In a paper published in the *Lancet* in 1977, she and Atkinson looked at the effects of a ban on advertising and at other policy developments, but also at what a 40% decrease in smoking would do to the government's budget. They argued that the effect on lower income groups would be greater, but could be mitigated by a sustained programme of health education. Smoking was a 'waste of working class, working age life'.[68] The same arguments were presented to a wider public in the pages

[63] Interview with Joy Townsend by Virginia Berridge, 7 March 2003.

[64] M. A. H. Russell, 'Changes in Cigarette Price and Consumption by Men in Britain 1946–71: A Preliminary Analysis', *British Journal of Social and Preventive Medicine*, 27 (1973), 1–7.

[65] A. B. Atkinson and J. L. Skegg, 'Control of Smoking and Price of Cigarettes—A Comment', *British Journal of Social and Preventive Medicine*, 28 (1974), 45–8.

[66] J. Peto, 'Price and Consumption of Cigarettes; a Case for Intervention?', *British Journal of Social and Preventive Medicine*, 28 (1974), 241–5.

of *New Society*.[69] This was the new view of inequalities and of public health by the end of the 1970s. Public health combined economics and psychology in an attack on tobacco consumption overall.

It was significant that much of the work in the early 1970s appeared in the *British Journal of Preventive and Social Medicine*. The economic perspective was emergent through the lens of social medicine and its changing focus. In the early 1970s there was still a twin-track approach to smoking within public health as outlined in the officials' report; to make smoking less dangerous and to make people smoke less. The former implied working with industry to secure a modified product. It is to this strategy and its implications for conceptualizing the health of the public which we now turn.

[67] Interview with Joy Townsend by Virginia Berridge, 7 March 2003.

[68] A. B. Atkinson and J. Townsend, 'Economic Aspects of Reduced Smoking', *Lancet*, 3 (1977), 492–4.

[69] J. Townsend, 'Smoking and Class', *New Society*, 30 March 1978, 709–10.

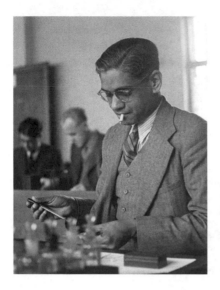

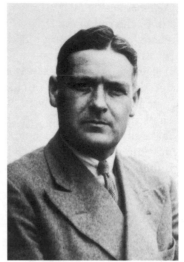

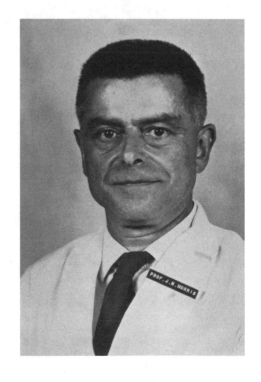

1. (*above left*) The culture of smoking. A student smokes at the laboratory bench, London School of Hygiene and Tropical Medicine, 1948.

Published in *Sport and Country*.

2. (*above right*) Sir Austin Bradford Hill.

Reproduced with permission of the London School of Hygiene and Tropical Medicine.

3. (*right*) Jerry Morris.

Reproduced with permission of the London School of Hygiene and Tropical Medicine.

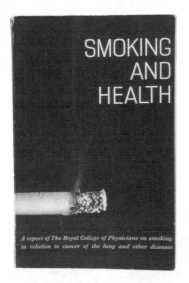

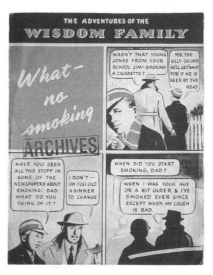

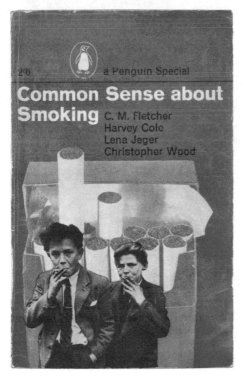

4. (*above left*)
Smoking and Health, the first
Report of the Royal
College of Physicians on
smoking, published in 1962.

Reproduced with permission of the
Royal College of Physicians.

5. (*above right*)
The Wisdom family,
a Central Council of Health
Education leaflet.

Reproduced with permission under
the terms of PSI licence
C2006010511.

6. (*left*) *Common Sense
about Smoking* by Charles
Fletcher shows the boy
delinquent view of
smokers in the 1960s.

Reproduced with permission
of Penguin books.

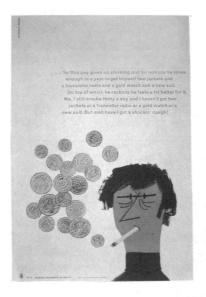

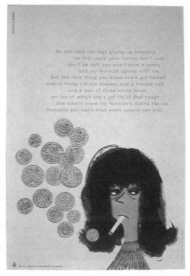

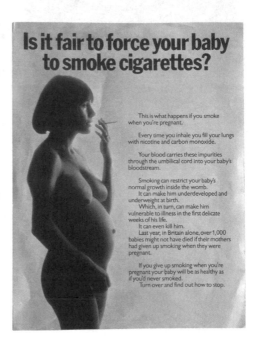

7. (*above left*) A young
man smoking, with
financial worries.

Reproduced with Crown copyright
permission and Wellcome Trust,
London.

8. (*above right*) A young
woman smoking, both
by Reginald Mount for
the Central Office of
Information, c.196?

Reproduced with Crown copyright
permission and Wellcome Trust,
London.

9. (*right*) The naked
smoking mother from the
Saatchi Health Education
Council campaign, 1973.

Reproduced with permission
under the terms of PSI licence
C2006010511.

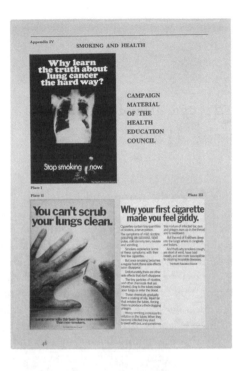

10. (*left*) The Saatchi influence on health education: You cant scrub your lungs clean.

Reproduced with permission under the terms of PSI licence c2006010511.

11. (*below left*) Women enter the picture: *The Ladykillers* by Bobbie Jacobson.

Reproduced with permission of Dr Jacobson OBE.

12. (*below right*) The female addict: Royal College of Physicians report on *Nicotine Addiction*.

Reproduced with permission of the Royal College of Physicians.

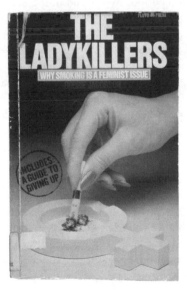

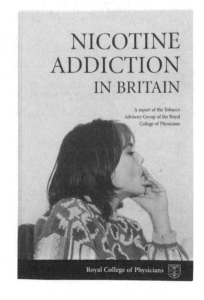

5

Expert Committees and Regulation in the 1970s

The 1970s were a crucial decade for the nature and focus of public health and also for the direction of smoking policy. The strategies of 'systematic gradualism' and 'coercive permissiveness' within public health strategies were increasingly polarized. 'Systematic gradualism' continued to operate throughout the 1970s as the major joint public health–industry–government initiative but it was under increasing strain. By the end of the decade that alliance fragmented: a new and more militant public health, which had been emergent since the early 1970s, came centre stage. These changes exemplified the direction which prevention and public health was taking overall by the end of the 1970s, and were reflected in government policy documents. The 1970s marked an important transition period. By the end of the decade a new public health creed had emerged with an agenda which became common to the discussion of a range of health issues. Drawing on chronic disease epidemiology and increasingly on mass psychology, it emphasized economic factors, and the role of higher taxation as a regulatory mechanism. The role of the mass media through mass advertising was central; advertising was either to be restricted or to be used as a public health tactic. It was part of a public health agenda which stressed both individual responsibility and the culpability of industrial interests. This template was to be applied in many areas—diet and heart disease was another—and smoking provided the blueprint.

But first the gradual approach was tried. By the 1970s that strategy appeared to have failed, although as we will see from Chapter 9 on the rise of addiction and nicotine-based strategies, failure of the strategy overall was far from the case. This chapter will examine the operation of systematic gradualism in the 1970s. It is a tale of two committees, the Standing Scientific Liaison Committee of 1971 and the Independent Scientific Committee on Smoking and Health (ISCSH), which replaced it in 1973. The operation of those two committees was illustrative also of a second strand of our analysis: the rise of the rational expertise-based model within government and specifically within health policy. This chapter examines the changing relationship between expertise and the state as expressed through the rise of a new style of expert committee in the 1970s. The operation of those committees in the 1970s also brought tobacco temporarily within the ambit of a whole set of further emergent government relationships with science. These were the mechanisms set up in the late 1960s and early 1970s to deal with the regulation of both licit and illicit medicines and drugs. Here is the third thrust of this chapter: the changing definition of tobacco as a substance during these years and the tensions between its regulation as a drug or as a medicine. Tobacco's positioning as a 'boundary substance' was also highlighted during these years.

THE RISE OF THE NEW EXPERT COMMITTEE

The reorganization of the National Health Service (NHS) in the early 1970s led to a reassessment of the central health advisory machinery. In 1969 it was calculated that more than a hundred central committees were in existence, the main statutory ones being the Central Health Services Council and its attendant Standing Advisory Committees (SACs), through which the smoking issue had wended its way in the early 1950s. These committees had been less than dynamic and were slimmed down to five in the course of the reorganization.[1] The most radical change came in the mental health area where the old Mental Health SAC was divided into three committees, one of which, the Advisory Committee on Alcoholism, chaired by Professor Neil Kessel, operated from 1975 to 1978. It produced three reports of crucial importance for alcohol policy in that decade.[2] This model of a committee of scientists or medical people in a much closer working relationship with government was also adopted in the area of illicit drugs when the Advisory Committee on Drug Dependence was set up in the late 1960s after the second Brain report had been published. This was replaced by the statutory Advisory

[1] C. Webster, *The Health Services since the War, vol. ii, Government and Health Care: The British National Health Service 1958–1979* (London: HMSO, 1996), 543–4.
[2] B. Thom, *Dealing with Drink. Alcohol and Social Policy: From Treatment to Management* (London: Free Association Books, 1999), 120–5.

Council on the Misuse of Drugs in 1972 under the terms of the 1971 Misuse of Drugs Act.[3] These committees have been characterized as part of the polite and gentlemanly relationships, out of public view, which characterized government–medical interactions in health policy.[4] They were certainly 'behind the scenes' in operation, with little public visibility, but there was also a significant change in the nature of governmental advisory mechanisms in the late 1960s and early 1970s. Doctors were moving from influence through 'outside' organizations (like the Royal College of Physicians (RCP) committee in the case of smoking) into positions of scientific influence which operated at the boundaries between government and the professions. The new expert committees were more clearly organizations which linked expertise within and outside government and which were founded on ideas of technical expertise and of the role of research.[5] It was significant that part of the reorientation of government–research relationships at this time also involved the establishment of a joint working party between the Medical Research Council (MRC) and the Social Science Research Council (SSRC) on smoking research. It achieved little but the 'rational' model which animated its formation was part of the ethos of these years.[6]

The expert committees which impacted more directly on smoking policy were the short-lived Standing Scientific Liaison Committee and the Independent Scientific Committee on Smoking and Health. Let us turn to their history in the 1970s. In June 1971 Joseph had announced the first of the voluntary agreements with industry with the labelling of cigarette packets and warnings on advertisements. The Consumers Association had published its own table of tar and nicotine in cigarettes in a report published in 1971, and so the Secretary of State referred the labeling issue to a new expert committee, a Standing Scientific Liaison

---

[3] M. Ashton, 'The Power of Persuasion', special supplement on the role of the ACMD, *Druglink,* 9(5), no pagination.

[4] G. V. Stimson and R. Lart, 'The Relationship between the State and Local Practice in the Development of National Policy on Drugs between 1920 and1990', in J. Strang and M. Gossop (eds.), *Heroin Addiction and the British System. Treatment and Policy Responses, vol. ii* (Abingdon: Routledge, 2005), 177–86.

[5] V. Berridge, 'Doctors and the State: The Changing Role of Medical Expertise in Policy Making', *Contemporary British History,* 11 (1997), 66–85.

[6] It did propose research into attitudes to smoking. See R. J. Merriman, *Attitudes towards Smoking: Indications for Further Research: Report of the Panel on Attitudes towards Smoking (Sub-committee of the Joint MRC/SSRC Committee on Research into Smoking)* (London: SSRC, 1981).

committee.[7] Chaired by Dr Dick Cohen, the Deputy Chief Medical Officer, the standing committee brought together scientists and industry representatives: it included Dr Herbert Bentley of Imperial Tobacco, Dr Colin Dollery, a clinical pharmacologist, and Geoffrey Rose of the London School of Hygiene and Tropical Medicine (LSHTM). Its civil servant was Frank Fairweather. Its first, and only, report was on tar and nicotine tables, whose publication it urged.[8] A participant in the committee remembered,

The RCP report in 1971 had made the point that there is a dose response relationship to tar and nicotine going into the lungs. Which way forward? At that time packets had no labels and we didn't know the significance of tar and nicotine ... The manufacturers gave us a tar and nicotine list and wanted to ensure it was available to the public. The Department was saying we don't want your figures—we'll ensure that all your cigarettes are looked at by the Laboratory of the Government Chemist (LGC). The LGC was acceptable to industry and the public would be happy. For new drugs the testing was done by industry, but industry put it out to contract houses and they could be inspected by the Department of Health. This was a different model. We needed independent assessment and a consumer model.[9]

When the Department of Health, acting on this advice, published its first tables in 1973, which gave three levels of tar in cigarettes—low, medium, and high—there were ten brands whose tar and nicotine content was lower than the brand which had headed the Consumers Association table. Ten new lower tar brands had been initiated within eighteen months. Clearly the industry could operate quickly when it had to.[10]

But the committee was plagued by problems. Cohen outlined them in an interview some years later.[11] The independent scientists were

[7] National Archives Ministry/Department of Health papers, MH 154/1013 contains a resumé of this history, 1972–7, Health hazards of carbon monoxide from cigarettes.

[8] Department of Health and Social Security (DHSS), *Report of the Standing Scientific Liaison Committee (on the Scientific Aspects of Smoking and Health) to the Secretary of State for Social Services on the Publication of Tar and Nicotine Yields of Packeted Cigarettes* (London: DHSS, 1972).

[9] Interview with civil servant by Virginia Berridge, 7 April 1997.

[10] National Archives, Department of Health papers, MH 154/1013, contains a copy of a letter from Michael Russell of the Institute of Psychiatry in the *British Medical Journal* which makes this point.

[11] Wellcome Library for the History and Understanding of Medicine, ASH archive, SA/ASH Box 77/13, William Norman papers, Notes of a meeting with Cohen, 6 August 1976.

a problem because they did not believe they should recommend any level of smoking since all levels were dangerous—but Cohen won them round. The problem was not the industry scientists' unwillingness to acknowledge the risks of smoking. They wanted to be treated as independent scientists and agreed to the draft report because they wished to show their scientific integrity. Herbert Bentley was the best of the group because he was a member of the Imperial Board and knew what the Board wanted. The other real problem was the disunity of the tobacco industry—a point which often emerges in the first two decades after the smoking–lung cancer debate began. Imperial was about to make a major investment in safer smoking products and so wanted the tar and nicotine issue out of the way. It was pressing strongly for publication of the tables and had been doing so since the late 1960s. But the attitude of the other companies was different and was a portent of changing relationships in the future. Gallahers reneged on publication because of pressure from the US brands and British American Tobacco (BAT) was also opposed and saw Joseph to press for non-publication. This made Joseph all the more determined to publish. An informant who was involved in the committee remembered how the relationships worked. The tobacco industry was disunited and wary about commercial confidentiality with its competitors.

It was sometimes unbelievable to go to meetings and they wouldn't speak. They were cooperative alone but not together—they had trade secrets and they were not going to give them away. But they would ring up after the meeting and offer the information. You always got the information, but not in the meetings.[12]

This wrangling over publication convinced Cohen that a totally independent committee was necessary. The MRC committee which had reported in 1971 on smoking and tobacco substitutes (see above) had advised that the manufacturers should collaborate with the appropriate independent research workers in the development and evaluation of experimental test systems. This group's report was to be considered by the Standing Scientific Liaison Committee, one of whose tasks was to seek to identify acceptable methods of determining whether new smoking materials were in fact less dangerous. However, the problems encountered on that committee meant that it was decided to establish an entirely new committee. The wider remit became the responsibility of

---

[12] Interview with civil servant by Virginia Berridge, 7 April 1997.

the Independent Scientific Committee on Smoking and Health, which was set up in 1973.

THE WORK OF THE INDEPENDENT SCIENTIFIC COMMITTEE ON SMOKING AND HEALTH

The ISCSH was composed not, as before, of a mixture of industry representatives and scientists, but of scientists alone. Its brief was 'safer smoking', the modification rather than the elimination of tobacco smoking. It reported direct to ministers, not to the Chief Medical Officer (CMO). Godber, who as CMO had taken such a strong line against modification of harm from smoking, retired in the same year and the Department's attitude seems to have softened under his replacement Henry Yellowlees. The committee's terms of reference were to advise on the scientific aspects of matters concerning smoking and health, in particular: to receive in confidence full data about the constituents of cigarettes and other smoking materials and their smoke and changes in these; to release to bona fide research workers for approved projects such of the above materials as agreed by the suppliers; to review research into less dangerous smoking and to consider whether further research, including clinical trials and epidemiological studies, needed to be carried out; and to advise on the validity of research results and of systems of testing the health effects of tobacco and tobacco substitutes and on their predictive value to human health.[13] The committee had a heavyweight chair, Dr Robert Hunter, vice-chancellor of Birmingham University who had recently chaired the Hunter enquiry into community medicine. Other members came from the public health, medical, and scientific community—the statistician Peter Armitage of the London School of Hygiene and Tropical Medicine; the public health–health services researcher Walter Holland from St Thomas' Medical School; Sir Theo Crawford, Professor of Pathology at St George's Medical School; Professor P. N. Magee, Professor of Experimental Biochemistry at the Middlesex; Professor A. Neuberger of St Mary's; and Professor David Poswillo from the Royal College of Surgeons among them. This membership

[13] Independent Scientific Committee on Smoking and Health (ISCSH), *First Report. Tobacco Substitutes and Additives in Tobacco Products: Their Testing and Marketing in the United Kingdom* (London: HMSO, 1975), Appendix.

symbolized the public health adherence to the gradualist agenda at this time.

The ISCSH was part of the trend of incorporating expertise through the new expert committee, as discussed previously. But it also formed part, both potentially and actually, of a whole set of other government–science relationships, those set up in the late 1960s and early 1970s to deal with the regulation of licit as well as illicit medicines. The period of the tobacco expert committees was also a time when the regulation of both licit and illicit substances was in flux: debates on tobacco formed part of the changes in the regulatory apparatus for medicines. Tobacco did not go down the 'treatment' route which characterized the policy responses to illicit drugs and which developed a strong specialist, psychiatric dimension at the end of the 1960s (we will return to this point in discussing addiction in Chapter 9). Its own expert committee, the ISCSH looked in the direction of regulation, of controlled public access, rather than maintenance or abstinence via doctors which were the primary aims of illicit drug treatment policy. These divergences were important for the emergence of addiction as a significant concept in the tobacco field in the 1990s.[14] Experts in the late 1960s and early 1970s did sometimes seek to draw the two areas—of tobacco and illicit drugs—together, but not with much success. In general, they remained separate and tobacco, as a licit substance, looked much more towards the arena of the regulation of licit medicines, which was also in flux during this period. The negotiations over the positioning of tobacco within that framework in the 1970s showed the indeterminate nature of tobacco as a substance. Was it food, medicine, or drug? Tobacco was a 'borderline substance' in both practical and conceptual terms.

The regulatory situation was complex. There were regulatory mechanisms for medicines, poisons, radioactive substances, and therapeutic substances.[15] By the end of the 1950s the focus of control had been on supply and sale and considerations of the cost of drugs was paramount. A series of Acts in that decade had dealt with substances which did not come under the earlier poisons legislation. The 1956 Therapeutic Substances Act, for example, covered vaccines and sera. But the key area relevant to tobacco was the new machinery set up to regulate new

---

[14] Discussed in Chapter 9.

[15] S. Anderson, 'Drug Regulation and the Welfare State. Government, the Pharmaceutical Industry and the Health Professions in Great Britain, 1940–80', in V. Berridge and K. Loughlin (eds.), *Medicine, the Market and the Mass Media: Producing Health in the Twentieth Century* (Abingdon: Routledge, 2005), 192–217.

drugs for safety. Here the thalidomide tragedy of 1961 had brought in its train moves for government regulation of the testing of new drugs. Government worked with the Association of the British Pharmaceutical Industry (ABPI) to set up drug testing machinery. It was decided early on that responsibility for testing should rest with the industry, but that a permanent expert body on safety should be set up. The Committee on the Safety of Drugs, set up in 1964 with Sir Derrick Dunlop as chair, had four subcommittees, on toxicity, clinical trials, therapeutic efficacy, and adverse reactions. Government work on the safety of drugs led to the Medicines Act of 1968, which consolidated the legislation relating to the safety, quality, and efficacy of medicinal products and the regulation of their sale and promotion. The Act confirmed the establishment of a Medicines Commission, which was set up in 1969 and which operated the licensing system for new drugs. Dunlop moved to chair the Medicines Commission, and the Committee on the Safety of Drugs became the Committee on the Safety of Medicines. The structures relied on the cooperation of industry and the relationships between Dunlop and Wheeler, the leader of the ABPI, were close. When Boots took a drug off the market after reports of adverse reactions, one member of the committee thought the decision should have been publicized to show general practitioners that the committee was doing something. But Dunlop disagreed because it would have antagonized the industry.[16]

The personal connections between this drug safety world and the new tobacco committee machinery were also close. Robert Hunter chaired the clinical trials subcommittee of the Committee on the Safety of Drugs and this was the model behind the operation of the ISCSH. Frank Fairweather, a toxicologist who became the scientific adviser first to the SSL Committee and then to the ISCSH, had worked in Carshalton for the British Industrial Biological Research Association (BIBRA), an independent research institute which provided information to government and industry on chemical toxicology issues. Dunlop, who

---

[16] E. M. Tansey, P. P. Catterall, D. A. Christie, S. V. Willhoft, and L. A. Reynolds (eds.), *Technology Transfer in Britain: The Case of Monoclonal Antibodies; Self and Non-Self: A History of Autoimmunity; Endogenous Opiates; The Committee on Safety of Drugs*, Wellcome Witnesses to Twentieth Century Medicine, vol. i (London: Wellcome Trust Centre for the History of Medicine at UCL, 1997). J. Abraham, *Science, Politics and the Pharmaceutical Industry: Controversy and Bias in Drug Regulation* (London: UCL Press, 1995). For drug regulation in different national contexts, see A. Daemmrich, *Pharmacopolitics: Drug Regulation in the United States and Germany* (Chapel Hill and London: University of North Carolina Press, 2004).

attended a lecture he gave, invited him to the Department of Health to
work as medical assessor to the Committee on the Safety of Medicines
(CSM). Reorganization brought a move first to the Standing Scientific
Liaison committee and then to the new ISCSH.

Godber wanted food, the environment and chemicals under one man ... I
didn't want to leave the Committee on the Safety of Medicines, but I did
and then they added smoking ... Cohen (deputy CMO) was concerned that he
needed someone who knew about chemicals in the environment—these were
similar issues to the CSM.[17]

Another scientist, who was not a member of the committee, but was
closely involved in tobacco related research, remembered,

Frank was suddenly asked to set up the ISCSH ... I invited him to lunch at the
Chanticleer restaurant ... I wanted to discuss who should be on the committee.
I said, Frank I don't know how you do it—here's me involved in tobacco
and can't keep up and you've got drugs, chemicals, food and smoking ... He
said ... I'll tell you what ... X asked me to discuss a problem and brought a
pile of papers and I asked him to write it on a single sheet—that's how I deal
with it.[18]

Soon Fairweather had plenty more paper to deal with. Hunter reflected
on the nature of the committee in a speech he gave in the mid-1970s,
and its difference from the SSLC. It had been considered important
that there should be a source of independent assessment to advise both
government and the tobacco industry about smoking and health. 'The
new purpose in setting up the committee was to give a manufacturer
contemplating the use of new materials the benefit of the advice of
independent experts in saying what testing was desirable.'[19] First it had
to establish its authority and a test case early on, in 1973, effectively
did this. The test case was not with the tobacco industry but with
textiles. The problem came not from the tobacco companies but from
the other industries moving into the 'safer smoking' area. There were
only a handful of tobacco companies. But with the advent of substitutes
as a possibility other companies entered the field—Celanese Fibres
Marketing in the United States, Courtaulds and Imperial Chemical
Industry (ICI) in the UK—because of the general industrial interest in

[17] Interview with civil servant by Virginia Berridge, 7 April 1997.
[18] Interview with industry scientist 1 by Virginia Berridge, 23 February 1998.
[19] R. B. Hunter, *Smoking and Health. The Philosophy of the Committee. Paper presented to the Royal College of Physicians, Edinburgh 21 April 1976*, and reprinted as a pamphlet.

these textile firms in synthetic materials.[20] In November 1973, Sir Keith Joseph rebuked Courtaulds for their decision to market their tobacco substitute, Planet, before it was cleared by the Hunter committee. Tests had been carried out at the Huntingdon Research Centre and Courtaulds claimed that the ISCSH's delay had held up their marketing. Although the committee had been set up in March 1973, it had only met for the first time in September. ASH (Action on Smoking and Health) attacked the decision to market and David McKie, writing in the *Lancet,* drew attention to the parallels with thalidomide and the issue of drug safety. Other companies like Imperial Tobacco had held back from marketing substitutes pending the committee's establishment and the operation of the new voluntary machinery.[21] Courtaulds' solicitors explained that they had cooperated fully with Frank Fairweather, sending him test results and data, but the ISCSH had not advised against going ahead until the end of October, despite correspondence with Joseph in March. The tests came to an end at the end of November and Courtaulds threatened libel action against ASH. This was a portent of things to come, but in the short term the incident served to establish the authority of the committee. Testing had to be reported to the committee before tobacco substitutes could be launched on to the market.

Tobacco substitutes were the major focus of the committee in the first stage of its work from 1973 to the mid-1970s. This was a period which members of the committee remembered as radical—when it was proposed that substitutes might replace tobacco and when changes in financial regulations made the use of such additives and substitutes more attractive. The ISCSH produced two reports in the 1970s which demonstrated the strength of this risk reduction initiative. In the first report, published in 1975, it stated that it had focused on the development of guidelines for the testing of cigarettes containing tobacco substitutes because a number of companies were planning to market these products and had undertaken smoke chemistry studies, animal tests, and human studies. It was also developing guidelines on the

---

[20] Courtaulds were also testing a meat substitute called KESP, which stood for Courtaulds Experimental Spun Protein. Information from Peter Hetherington, 1 August 2006. See also L. A. Reynolds and E. M. Tansey (eds.), *Cholesterol, Antherosclerosis and Coronary Disease in the UK, 1950–2000*, Wellcome Witnesses to Twentieth Century Medicine, vol. xxvii (London: Wellcome Trust Centre for the History of Medicine at UCL, 2006), where there is discussion of similar developments in food products, for example, the development of low fat margarine.

[21] Wellcome Library for the History and Understanding of Medicine, ASH archive, SA/ASH letter from solicitors acting for Courtaulds to Mike Daube.

testing and use of additives in tobacco products.[22] Prior to 1970, no additives had been allowed by Customs because of taxation issues. But the 1970 Finance Act had relaxed these restrictions. The report outlined the various stages of testing and also a future programme of work. There was hope that the remit of the committee would be expanded. It would need, so it reported, to continue to give attention to substitutes and to additives. It would be receiving submissions on tests and reports on tests from the companies for consideration and would be considering the form of long-term epidemiological studies. 'Nevertheless, the Committee hopes before making its next report to have been able to consider the wider range of problems on smoking and health that come within its terms of reference.'[23] The committee's terms of reference were widened after its first report had been published to make it clear that it advised both the government and the tobacco companies, although the industry representatives later claimed that they had never accepted this.[24]

THE DEVELOPMENT OF NEW SMOKING MATERIAL (NSM)

What was the response from the industry point of view? Two testing submissions were eventually made to the ISCSH: a consortium of Gallahers and Rothmans for a product called Cytrel 361 and from Imperial Tobacco for NSM14. BAT, which had little presence on the UK market, worked on a product called BATFLAKE.[25] This chapter will concentrate on Wills' work on the latter product—New Smoking Material (NSM).[26] In 1967 initial experiments into NSM were conducted at Wills no. 1 factory in Bedminster, Bristol. In the same year, Imperial Tobacco (ITG) joined forces with the ICI and

[22] Independent Scientific Committee on Smoking and Health, *First Report. Tobacco Substitutes and Additives in Tobacco Products: Their Testing and Marketing in the United Kingdom* (London: HMSO, 1975).

[23] Ibid.

[24] National Archives, Department of Health papers, MH 148/1473, Minutes of the Independent Scientific Committee on Smoking and Health, Thirtieth meeting, 16 November 1978.

[25] C. Proctor, *Sometimes a Cigarette is Just a Cigarette* (London: Sinclair-Stevenson, 2003), 84–5.

[26] The following section of the chapter is based on research conducted in the Bristol Record Office by Dr Penny Starns under the supervision of Virginia Berridge.

established a new offshoot company named Imperial Developments Limited (IDL). The sole purpose of IDL was to research, develop, and produce a safe and economically viable alternative to tobacco.

According to ITG, the smoking and health issue provided the strongest reason to develop NSM, but there were also economic considerations. If an alternative to tobacco could be found it would reduce the money the industry spent on import duty. Neither could it be argued that government concerns were entirely focused on the health aspects of NSM. From the government's standpoint the sale of NSM within the UK had the potential of saving foreign currency and sales of the material overseas held the possibility of improving the balance of payments. From the outset therefore, the development of NSM was not merely health orientated. But it was anticipated that NSM would replace between 10 and 20% of tobacco in cigarettes and that the substance would provide the consumer with a healthier alternative to conventional cigarettes. As Dr Herbert Bentley, ITG's research and development director, maintained,

While no-one is making health claims for NSM, it follows the government's view that if people do smoke they should smoke brands with low tar and nicotine yields. NSM is a neutral substance and is tasteless. It delivers only a quarter of the tar in an equal amount of tobacco. And tar from NSM is five times less biologically active than tobacco tar. It does not contain any nicotine. It is based on cellulose which is present in all natural vegetable matter, including tobacco. [27]

NSM was actually obtained from wood pulp which had been subjected to heat treatment. The material was condensed into black sheets and known in the industry as HTC or heat-treated cellulose. It was then mixed with water and six secret components which gave the material a variety of different properties such as moisture retention and ash cohesion. The HTC was transformed into liquid form by this process and then travelled down an air-heated steel band. Eventually the NSM appeared from this band as a film and was sliced and diced into a conventional blending silo. The usual tar yield and moisture tests were applied to NSM in much the same way as for tobacco, and the material contained no less than the 10% demanded by customs regulations. Laboratory tests and development procedures, however, also included

[27] Bristol Record Office, 38169/E/14/4, 'Now Public Gives Verdict on NSM', *Wills World*, 22 August 1974, 7.

other biological tests such as mouse skin painting. Research was stepped up as a result of the 1971 RCP report and by 1973 over three million pounds had been invested in the research and development of NSM. The director of IDL, Malcolm Anson, explained,

This is of course a commercial project, but it is expected that the new material could make a substantial contribution to mitigating the smoking and health problem. Whether it does so will ultimately depend on the medical authorities. The tobacco industry has always taken the view that however good they are at making cigarettes or however painstaking their research, the medical assessment must come from the doctors and that decisions concerning the nation's health must rest with the government.[28]

Members of the ISCSH quickly formed good working relationships with the directors of ITG and the latter felt confident in the future of NSM. They did not bother to wait for the official outcome of the Hunter committee's assessment of NSM before they invested a further thirteen million pounds in a new NSM production factory, based in Ardeer in Scotland. They had invested large sums of money into the development of low tar–nicotine cigarettes and continued to pour money into the research, development, and production of tobacco substitutes. By the time that NSM cigarettes were launched the sum had reached over twenty-six million pounds.

The first consumer tests of NSM were conducted 'in house' by Wills' own employees. Several had volunteered to take part in the testing of experimental cigarettes and volunteers were selected from a random cross section of the workforce, ranging from factory workers to laboratory chemists. This policy did not represent any radical departure from the practice of previous years, since Wills had traditionally tested new brands and blends of tobacco on its workforce. Initially no scientific protocols were followed. Usually Wills simply gave away free samples to employees and hoped for a straightforward reaction. Responses tended to be in the form of one-word answers which described cigarettes as 'wonderful' or 'disgusting'. However, from 1970 onwards the testing became more methodical and scientific in its approach. Volunteer cigarette tasters were trained along the same lines as food tasters and rigorously instructed as to how to taste cigarettes through the mouth and then through the nose. They were prevented from wearing any

---

[28] Bristol Record Office, 38169/E/14/4, 'NSM Stands on the Threshold', *Wills World*, 28 June 1973, 3.

deodorant, perfume, or aftershave which could possibly interfere with the aroma of the cigarette, and expected to complete standardized forms which included descriptions of all the components of the blend and to grade them accordingly. When Wills moved its workforce to its highly publicized and very expensive new forty-five-acre site in Hartcliffe in 1975, purpose-built smoking booths were constructed to accommodate the cigarette tasters. Furthermore the volunteers were not restricted to testing Wills brands. Many brands that 'the panel savour come from competitors and others are experimental cigarettes which cannot be sold on the open market because of present laws. These include cigarettes made with Imperial Tobacco's NSM, other substitutes such as Cytrel, and cigarettes made with additives or cased tobacco.'[29]

In 1974 the ISCSH committee permitted wider consumer tests and over five thousand people across the country began to sample forty different kinds of NSM cigarettes containing between 10 and 50% NSM. The cigarettes were produced by Wills and Players and consumers were asked to comment on flavour, aroma, and cigarette satisfaction. IDL was renamed NSM in the same year and new headquarters were established in Manchester. The tobacco substitute was seen as a major breakthrough for the British tobacco industry and the first to gain official recognition. Dr Bentley of Imperial Tobacco pointed out, 'We believe that NSM is the first substitute smoking material in the world to receive clearance from a government body.'[30] The level of investment into NSM, however, was beginning to take its toll and 1974 was one of the worst trading years for ITG since its formation. Group sales were actually higher than in previous years, but the increases in production costs, heavy duty, and inflation combined to depress profits. The chairman of ITG, Sir John Partridge, warned members of the group that future research might be curtailed,

We have invested heavily in recent years, mainly out of profits, in the equipment and housing of our businesses with a view to safeguarding their future and to reducing costs. We planned to invest over £50 million in this way in 1974. This expenditure, a great part of it contracted in 1973 will not be significantly reduced. But given our present artificially depressed level of profitability and consequently smaller cash flow, the further substantial investment programme which we had hoped to implement in 1975 is now gravely threatened.[31]

[29] Ibid., 'Course Is in Good Taste', *Wills World*, 20 November 1975, 3.
[30] Ibid., 'Now Public Gives Verdict on NSM', *Wills World*, 22 August 1974, 7.
[31] Ibid., 'Sir John Warns on Profits', *Wills World*, 25 July 1974, front page.

In reality most of the profit loss was due to Imperial's other interests such as food, packaging, and the brewery industry rather than tobacco sales. The group had diversified following the 1962 RCP report as a means of 'hedging its bets' over the smoking and health problem. The group even changed its name and dropped the word tobacco from its title in order to reflect this diversification. Imperial Tobacco Group Limited became Imperial Group Limited, and Imperial Tobacco Limited became the umbrella name for the tobacco division of the group. Imperial Group Limited (IGL), however, still retained its faith in the potential of NSM, and despite a subsequent severe recession in 1975 invested a further twenty-two million pounds in a new 'space age' factory at Ardeer, which was opened in 1977.

The Hunter committee had examined all the evidence with regard to tobacco substitutes and raised no objections to their use. Nevertheless, the committee did demand assurances from the tobacco manufacturers and retained some control over the use of NSM. Manufacturers were obliged to inform the committee of the exact proportion of substitutes and other cigarette specifications. The rationale behind this obligation centred on the fact that the scientific evidence which had been accepted by the committee was directly related to certain cigarette specifications: sales of NSM could therefore be withdrawn if manufacturers deviated from the original specification. The committee also wanted to have control over whether NSM was added to high tar and high nicotine cigarettes. A further condition was imposed whereby tobacco companies were required to agree on a date for the commencement of long-term health studies for NSM smokers.[32]

DAVID OWEN AND THE MEDICINES ACT INITIATIVE

This policy took a new turn under the Labour government of 1974 to 1979 and during David Owen's tenure as Minister of Health from 1974 to 1976. Owen, a doctor, was a keen non-smoker whose moves to do something about smoking were tolerated by the Secretary of State, the smoker Barbara Castle, whom he persuaded not to smoke in

---

[32] National Archives, Department of Health papers, MH 154/1013 has more on the testing of NSM. For example, see Minutes of ISCSH nineteenth meeting, 23 July 1976.

public.[33] Owen spoke at a joint ASH–Health Education Council (HEC) conference on smoking in 1974, 'Smoking—Whose Problem?'[34] He had plans to bring the tobacco substitutes being tested under the aegis of the ISCSH, under the regulatory provisions of the 1968 Medicines Act so they would be controlled like medicines. The implication was that tobacco would eventually go down that route, too. The ISCSH would be upgraded into the licensing body on the model of the Committee on the Safety of Medicines. In an interview in 1987 with Kenneth Harris Owen remarked that he became convinced that voluntary regulation was not the answer, and that there had to be statutory backup.[35] Part of the problem, as he recounted in a major speech in the Commons in January 1976, was that the home industry was prepared to cooperate but not the overseas one. He came up with the idea of changing the Medicines Act to bring tobacco products within its scope. That Act related primarily to the pharmaceutical industry, bringing scientific and medical expertise into a formalized relationship, providing for ministerial action and for appeals. Owen wanted to make the change by order rather than through an amendment to the Act to enable it to deal with tobacco products. The relevant Cabinet committee preferred a one-clause bill because they were worried that an order would be challenged by the statutory instruments committee. Owen got the agreement of the Home Affairs committee to his strategy but the chief whip, Michael Cocks, was a Bristol MP and reluctant to proceed too far on anti-smoking measures. Callaghan, the Prime Minister, was also opposed to intervention in areas of personal behaviour.

The minister operated cleverly to achieve his aim. The MP Robert Kilroy-Silk, a close friend of David Owen, had come top of the ballot for a ten-minute bill and asked Owen what he should do with the opportunity. Owen wanted action on tobacco, so Kilroy-Silk's motion, as eventually put to the House on 16 January 1976, proposed action under section 105 of the 1968 Medicines Act. If passed, this would bring 'tobacco and smoking substances which are not themselves medicinal products, but if used without proper safeguards are capable of causing

[33] B. Castle, *The Castle Diaries, 1964–1976* (London: Weidenfeld and Nicolson, 1980), entry for Tuesday, 5 August, 641. The department became Health and Social Security from 1968 (Crossman's tenure) until 1988.
[34] Wellcome Library for the History and Understanding of Medicine. ASH archive, Box 51, SA/AHS/M.1/6.
[35] D. Owen, *Personally Speaking to Kenneth Harris* (London: Weidenfeld and Nicolson, 1987), 58–9.

damage to the health of the community', under the regulatory provisions of the Act.[36] Tobacco and tobacco substitutes would be controlled just like medicines. In an interview conducted by William Norman at this time, Mike Daube, director of ASH, described how that organization was a vital conduit in the process. Owen could not offer Kilroy-Silk any direct departmental (Department of Health and Social Security, DHSS) help for his bill, but there was nothing to stop the minister asking his department to brief Daube and ASH on a hypothetical situation which related to its content. A 'very senior civil servant' discussed the terms with Daube, for reference to Kilroy-Silk. Kilroy-Silk's intervention, aided by ASH, brought matters to a head and secured Owen the leverage he needed to go ahead against the various competing interests. At the same time, ASH maintained its oppositional role, selectively leaking information to urge the minister on to more significant action.[37] Owen himself referred to this role (although not to the behind-the-scenes moves concerning Kilroy-Silk) in an interview at the time. He was 'orchestrating his moves' round the Medicines Act option — he used the Commons, ASH attacked him, and there were also informal contacts with sympathetic parts of industry.[38] Mike Daube remembered how Charles Fletcher, a diabetic, became hypoglaecaemic at one meeting and started spilling the beans about part of Owen's plans to Tory MPs who were sympathetic to the industry.[39]

Owen saw the Medicines Act strategy as the major option and was not enthused about taxation as a policy. This, he remarked, was not because of the revenue implications but because of the impact on the retail price index and also on wage bargaining. Godber thought that Owen was taking this route because 'it was safer politically.'[40] In his speech in the January 1976 debate, Owen did repeat the arguments on inequality which had also animated Labour politicians in the 1960s and which had electoral implications.

There are I know many people who believe that all cigarette advertising should be abolished. They believe and there is some evidence for this that advertising

[36] Hansard. House of Commons debates, 16 January 1976, vols. 93–4, cols. 785–871.

[37] Wellcome Library for the History and Understanding of Medicine, ASH archive, SA/ASH, William Norman collection, R.12, Box 77, Interview with Mike Daube, no date but *c*.1975–6.

[38] Ibid., R.24, Box 79, Interview with David Owen, 20 January 1976.

[39] Interview with Mike Daube by Virginia Berridge, 11 March 1999.

[40] Wellcome Library for the History and Understanding of Medicine, ASH archive, SA/ASH, William Norman collection, R.18 Box 77, Interview with Sir George Godber.

and promotions increase sales. On the other hand it would be absurd to pretend that abolishing advertising would mean that nineteen million people would stop smoking cigarettes and it would mean that brand switching to safer cigarettes would be more difficult to achieve. Some advocate stronger use of the price mechanism and there is clear evidence that price is a major factor. The Government has increased substantially the cost of cigarettes but pricing cigarettes off the market would have quite unacceptable social consequences in that the poor would suffer while the rich would continue to smoke. What is needed and needed desperately is a strategy for helping the nineteen million people who do smoke, and are heavily physically and psychologically dependent on cigarettes. The industry have made it clear that they will not support any measures which are designed even in the long term to abolish cigarette smoking whether by health education or other means. This is an area which will have to remain the Government's responsibility. The question is whether the industry can be involved in the long term strategy of safer smoking. Some believe that to even talk about safer smoking is to compromise one's stand against all smoking.[41]

Owen thought that was not realistic.

Owen recognized the divisions in the industry which he could exploit through these adroit parliamentary and extra-parliamentary manoeuvres. In an interview with Norman just after the January debate, he commented that Imperial, the main British company, were staffed by 'reasonably fair minded people' who did not like the adverse publicity and the image of being constantly at odds with government. However, the Tobacco Advisory Council (TAC), now the main industry representative body, was hopelessly split on the issue and could not deliver. 'There is a lot of competition between them, although they speak, seemingly, with one voice. It was quite interesting and quite helpful to ourselves that the TAC could not deliver. They had to admit to us that they were deeply split.'[42] So Owen astutely recognized that the most significant section of the industry in the British market—Imperial—had interests which potentially overlapped with those of the government and its independent committee of scientists.

Now what they have is a commercial interest which wants them to go down the Medicines Act. Because they know that we will not dare give them permission for additives and substitutes under the present provision. It is such a difficult

---

[41] Hansard. House of Commons debates, 16 January 1976, vols. 93–4.
[42] Wellcome Library for the History and Understanding of Medicine, ASH archive, SA/ASH, William Norman collection, R.24, Box 79 Interview with David Owen, 20 January 1976.

provision. And they also know that the Hunter Committee is very worried about being set up, as I think Professor Hunter has described it, as giving the 'good housekeeping seal' with no statutory authority and it all being done on a voluntary basis.

Those who want to go into the substitutes and additives market, which Imperial strongly wants to do, they can see that once this mechanism is going, first of all they get some sort of security from being given a licence. It doesn't protect them in a court of law, but they can be seen to have acted reasonably and taken all due care and precautions, so they have got some safeguard, which is quite important to them.[43]

The main British companies, Imperial in particular, had known prior to the debate what Owen was going to say in his speech: those who were opposed to the Medicines Act strategy had not been briefed.[44] Rothmans, Gallahers, Phillip Morris, and BAT, the latter company with no British market, had all been opposed to the strategy. These were influenced more by the precedent the legislation might be seen to offer to countries like the United States. The tobacco industry was fragmented and the interests of the British industry were different from those of the companies who were US-owned.[45] Owen was in part shadow boxing and flexing muscles which he was not sure he really had. He was sure that the tobacco industry would be aware that, if the strategy worked, the regulation of tobacco as a medicine would be next on the list.

I have always made it absolutely clear to them that I was prepared to do a 105 Order on a compromise basis, but that if they forced me into the position of going to substantive legislation in the next session, which I managed to convince them I would get the next session although I am extremely doubtful myself, I would not dream of doing a partial thing. I would do the whole lot.

And again, it can be a very short bill to put tobacco under the Medicines Act.[46]

In the event, the promised legislation did not happen. A draft bill was produced, but Owen's departure from the department for the Foreign Office in 1976 took the heat out of the issue. David Ennals, the

[43] Wellcome Library for the History and Understanding of Medicine, ASH archive, SA/ASH, William Norman collection, R.24, Box 79 Interview with David Owen, 20 January 1976.
[44] Ibid., R.7, Box 76, Interview and correspondence with G. C. Hargrove, Director of Public Relations for BAT.
[45] Gallahers had been nearly 80% owned by American Brands Inc since 1973. Information taken from detailed history on Gallahers website.
[46] Wellcome Library for the History and Understanding of Medicine, ASH archive, SA/ASH, William Norman collection, R.24, Box 79, Interview with David Owen, 20 January 1976.

successor to Barbara Castle, did not win Cabinet support for legislation and reached agreement in March 1977 for a voluntary monitoring role for the ISCSH.[47]

THE THIRD ROYAL COLLEGE OF PHYSICIANS REPORT, 1977

The years 1976 and 1977 were crucial for harm reduction as a central strategy for bringing together public health, government, and industry. But the strategy was under increasing strain from the public health side: this was demonstrated at meetings of the Royal College of Physicians committee between 1974 and 1977, which endeavoured to bring out a third report on smoking. Controversy about objectives marked the committee's work. There was disagreement between Jerry Morris and a new member of the committee, Michael Russell, the psychiatrist head of the smoking section of the Addiction Research Unit at the Institute of Psychiatry, a new unit bringing together smoking, alcohol, and drugs which had been set up with MRC funding in the late 1960s. Russell's re-draft of the chapter on the smoking habit was, Morris thought, 'too pessimistic and apocalyptic'. Morris thought it did not pay enough attention to the fact that smoking was a modern epidemic. The minutes recorded the basis of the disagreement. 'Dr. Russell did not agree that smoking was a modern epidemic and felt it would be more practical to make a much safer cigarette than to try to stop people from smoking.'[48] This divergence of opinion was unresolvable and later on, the minutes recorded that 'It was clear that there was disagreement in the committee as to whether the primary aim should be to urge people to stop smoking or whether the emphasis should be laid on safer methods of smoking. *It was agreed* that this dilemma should be discussed in the report as the kind of problem that doctors have to face in giving advice.'[49]

The work of the committee was also marked by a resurgence in statistical discussion of the controversy round the smoking and lung cancer connection. Papers and a book by Professor Peter Burch of Leeds University were published in 1974 and a subsequent paper was published

---

[47] Webster, *Health Services Since the War*, 666–7, describes the concessions on advertising and warning messages on packets which were obtained instead.
[48] Royal College of Physicians archive, Minutes of meeting of 7 April 1975.
[49] Ibid.

by the Royal Statistical Society in 1978. Although Bradford Hill had delineated his criteria for causal inference in 1965, Burch's publication briefly reignited interest in the issue. He noted the enormous impact of epidemiology since the original causal connection and the way in which it had come to underpin many aspects of everyday life. His complex calculations led to the conclusion that the secular trends for lung cancer did not support the idea that they were caused mainly by a change in smoking habits. The RCP committee was concerned about the possible public impact of such statements. Keith Ball went to visit Burch, representing ASH, but also as a member of the RCP committee.[50] The committee decided to have a review of the whole statistical question. Charles Fletcher reported at a meeting on 10 February 1975 that Dr Treasure, a friend of the College and chairman of the advertising agency J. Walter Thompson, had expressed doubt to him as to the validity of the statistical evidence on the effect of smoking on health. But statisticians were unwilling to publish criticisms for fear of being thought lackeys of the tobacco industry.[51] The statistician Harvey Goldstein produced an appendix for the committee on statistical controversy on smoking effects: this looked at work by Burch, Seltzer, and Yerushalmy, who had cast doubt in a paper in *Nature* on the connection between smoking and low birthweight. However, Goldstein's appendix did not find its way into the final report, much to his annoyance, although the birthweight controversy was mentioned in the chapter of the report on smoking and pregnancy.[52] The Hunter Committee also produced its own reply to Burch, which argued that his statements about smoking and lung cancer could not be proved or disproved. But the RCP clearly had no wish to reopen this area of statistical controversy.

The report itself, *Smoking or Health*, was published in 1977 and although it retained mention of the harm reduction option in policy, this strategy was more limited than it had been in the previous reports. Differential taxation for pipes and cigars was no longer favoured because people who smoked these continued to inhale. Less harmful smoking was still an option, but more research was needed and a new concept of 'high risk' smokers was introduced. Pregnant women and children figured

[50] Wellcome Library for the History and Understanding of Medicine, ASH archive, SA/ASH, Box 19 (old listing) Keith Ball's file, 29 September 1975, Keith Ball's account of his meeting with Burch in Leeds.

[51] Royal College of Physicians archive, Minutes of meeting, 10 February 1975.

[52] Royal College of Physicians archive, Papers of RCP committee on smoking, 23 June 1976, Letter from Goldstein to Ball.

more prominently and there was more discussion of the smoking habit. The economic dimension had also grown in importance. The economists had played a significant role in the work of the committee: Atkinson and Skegg had given evidence and the taxation option was favoured in the report. But its content was ultimately to be less significant than the circumstances of its publication, for it was overshadowed, public heath interests suspected perhaps deliberately, by the launch of New Smoking Material. This conjuncture and the fate of NSM finally sealed the fate of 'systematic gradualism' from the mainstream public health point of view.

THE FAILURE OF NSM

Meanwhile, Imperial had continued with its plans for the launch of NSM. The target date for the launch of NSM cigarettes was 1 July 1977: but the anti-smoking lobby was already pouring scorn on the whole concept of 'safer' smoking. Imperial Tobacco hit back by persuading eminent doctors to participate in a tribute film. The film was designed more for the company's employees than for the general public, but emphasized the long-standing responsible attitude of the tobacco industry, and Imperial in particular, towards the problem of smoking and health. The RCP report acknowledged the research efforts of tobacco manufacturers, and criticized the lack of government coordination in the area of research. Eventually NSM cigarettes left the warehouses on 28 July 1977. There were increasing tensions between the industry and government policy, however, particularly around the issues of price controls, smoking and health, and cigarette advertising. Members of the industry accused the government of not understanding the stress relief value of smoking. Speaking in 1976, John Pile, chairman of Imperial Group Limited, had stated that, 'For many of us smoking provides considerable solace and the realistic course is not to attempt a sudden radical reduction in the habit.'[53] Whereas there had been many who sympathized with John Pile's view in the mid-1960s, by the second half of the 1970s the context within which smoking policy was formed had changed. The launch of NSM in 1977 highlighted the new influences within smoking policy and the new players who had emerged.

[53] Bristol Record Office, 38169/E/14/4, 'Price Code Must Go', *Wills World* (supplement on trade), 25 March 1976, front page.

The new minister of Health, David Ennals, acknowledged in a House of Commons statement that 'calls to legislate smoking out of existence would not work,' and that 'it will not be banished quickly—but our long term aim must be its eventual disappearance.'[54] Ennals' speech was given a month before the Hunter committee gave the official go-ahead for the sale of NSM cigarettes and only four months before they were launched onto the open market.

The launch of NSM brought tensions to a head. There was a strong and organized lobby which opposed all smoking and the legitimacy of the industry. ASH, the new anti-smoking pressure group founded in 1971, took a more stringent position of opposition to safer smoking. The launch of NSM had upstaged, so anti-smoking campaigners argued, the launch of the third RCP report on smoking. Its title, *Smoking or Health*, epitomized the widening gulf over the issue of modified smoking.[55] The HEC, relaunched in 1973, was an anti-smoking ally of ASH's, and called smoking safer cigarettes the equivalent of jumping from the thirty-sixth instead of the thirty-ninth floor of a tall building.[56] The financial position on tobacco substitutes had changed too. In January 1978 the taxation system was revised and statutory controls over substitutes ceased.[57] Manufacturers gave voluntary undertakings rather than be subject to statutory controls.[58] The HEC had accused the tobacco industry of misleading the public and of making false health claims for its products. The directors at IGL were singularly unimpressed by what they believed to be an outright betrayal by the government. Indeed, such was the feeling of outrage that ITL chairman Tony Garrett took out a full-page press advertisement to vent his anger, and accused the government of failing to support its own policy on smoking and health.

By 1972 it had been established that a product could be used as a tobacco substitute in ways which showed every promise of reducing risks that had been associated by medical authorities with the smoking of cigarettes. Following its

[54] Bristol Record Office, 38169/E/14/4, 'Minister Outlines Strategy', *Wills World*, 24 March 1977, 8.
[55] Royal College of Physicians, *Smoking or Health* (London: Pitman Medical, 1977).
[56] Health Education Council, *Annual Report, 1977–78* (London), 11.
[57] These had been established under the Tobacco Substitutes regulations of 1970 after the 1970 Finance Act and had provided for tobacco duty to be charged on additives and substitutes used in the manufacture of smoking products.
[58] ISCSH, *Second Report of the Independent Scientific Committee of* [sic] *Smoking and Health: Developments in Tobacco Products and the Possibility of 'Lower Risk' Cigarettes* (London: HMSO, 1979).

consultation with scientific and medical authorities and of co-operation with the government, ITL started discussing the future of the product with the then Conservative government. The government without compromising its long term policy of discouraging smoking, agreed that this was an approach that should be pursued. The Hunter Committee was set up, and following ITL's research with ICI, product testing and the building of the NSM factory at Ardeer, it concluded there would be no objection to the making and selling of cigarettes containing NSM.

Accusations of misleading the public were sheer nonsense, Garrett declared. The ITL chairman pointed out that accusations were made on behalf of a body (the HEC) which had been appointed by the same government with whom the policy leading to the introduction of NSM was agreed.[59]

This sense of outrage continued as NSM cigarettes failed to gain acceptance in the marketplace. Wills had prided itself on being the peacemaker within the tobacco industry and along with ICI had funded all the research into NSM. Their competitors such as Rothmans meanwhile had relied on Cytrel, a tobacco substitute produced by the American Celanese Corporation. These competitors also experienced losses but since they had not made any huge investment these were minimal in comparison to Wills and the Imperial Group. Evidently the latter had expected some government support for their new products, yet despite the initial endorsement of the concept of 'safe' smoking none was forthcoming. Although the IGL chose to blame the government and the negative effects of the HEC's campaign, this was only one obstacle to the acceptance of tobacco substitutes. The issue of nicotine had been overlooked, and if smokers smoked to obtain nicotine they were not going to be enamoured of NSM. Since the Hunter committee had precluded manufacturers from adding NSM to cigarettes with a high nicotine content there was no incentive in terms of smoker satisfaction for consumers to buy the products. There was no financial incentive either, because the government had decided to tax NSM in exactly the same way as ordinary tobacco. The industrial policy of product modification and 'safer' smoking had fallen foul of a major shift in health policy.

There were attempts to build bridges between government and industry following the failure of NSM. In 1979 the outraged ITL

[59] Bristol Record Office, 38169/E/14/4, 'IMPS Accuse Government on NSM Policy', *Wills World*, 27 October 1977, 3.

chairman Tony Garrett was replaced by Andrew Reid. Reid defended the policy of product modification and the industry's responsible approach to the smoking and health controversy. He further stated,

Our relations with the government, its advisory committee and medical authorities are generally good. We have taken account of the judgments of medical authorities and have modified our products. Our quarrel is with the extremists who are running an hysterical propaganda campaign against the social acceptability of smoking. We believe that the adult citizen must be free to make his or her own choice and any measures that seek to limit that freedom should be resisted. Of course, some people dislike tobacco smoke and some smokers were discourteous, but the views of extremists in relation to the effect on non-smokers of smoking by others have not generally been supported by medical authorities.[60]

In 1981 Reid waxed lyrical about his faith in the future of Imperial Tobacco but the writing was already on the wall. A year later falling trade figures resulted in the closure of three factories at Bristol, Glasgow, and Stirling, and numerous job losses at Newcastle, Nottingham, Liverpool, Swindon, and Ipswich. On one level this situation arose because Wills and IGL had expanded furiously only to be caught out by unfavourable economic conditions. But changes in health policy and smoking had also played a role in the impending demise of Wills and IGL.[61]

THE SECOND REPORT FROM THE ISCSH: DIVISION IN PUBLIC HEALTH

Members and associates of the Hunter committee took different views of the failure of NSM. One saw it as a failure of marketing and distribution, not helped by the opposition from public health interests.[62] Another was still bitterly angry twenty years after the event.

You can't put your head in the sand, you couldn't ban smoking, what was the way forward? ... I was so angry when it came to nothing. It was the fault of the HEC ... The whole subject just went dead. You can't just grab people by

---

[60] Bristol Record Office, 38169/E/14/4, 'The Way I See It', *Wills World*, 27 September 1979, 3.
[61] A major reorganization began in 1981 because of losses on tobacco and Imperial was taken over by Hanson PLC in 1986, demerging ten years later.
[62] W. W. Holland and R. Wood, 'Policies on Prevention: The Hazards of Politics', *Proceedings of the Royal College of Physicians of Edinburgh*, 25 (1995), 189–203.

the neck and say stop smoking, it's an individual choice. Using substitutes is safer—but this was then cut off at the legs.[63]

The failure of NSM brought a change from radicalism to gradualism in the view of Peter Froggatt, who took over as chair of ISCSH in the 1980s. Tobacco substitutes were no longer important and the focus of the committee shifted to the role of additives and the reduction of tar.[64] Walter Holland had withdrawn from the ISCSH prior to the launch of NSM to advise the Tobacco Advisory Council through its research arm the Tobacco Research Council, in preparation for a major randomized controlled trial (RCT) on humans involving the material. The expense of such a trial was potentially so great that it had to be done by the tobacco companies, and it was 'too sensitive' for a government committee to be involved in it. But the lack of market share of such products made the trial impossible to run.[65] Holland remained the link with the Tobacco Advisory Council and was in attendance at the main meetings of ISCSH. This link was to lead to a RCT of low tar cigarettes in the early 1980s.

The second Hunter report, published in 1979, underlined the new policy situation. The report surveyed the work on tobacco substitutes and also the loss of financial incentives in relation to tobacco additives after 1978. It placed new hopes in lower risk cigarettes, in particular those with lower tar. It also raised the issue of nicotine and of carbon monoxide. In the longer term, since it was nicotine that the majority of dependent smokers seemed to require, it might be necessary for manufacturers to modify the nicotine delivery of cigarettes or alter the factors which could influence the rate of absorption from inhaled smoke into the body tissues. The reduction of carbon monoxide levels was also desirable. The main report was accompanied by a minority report from one of its members, the public health physician, Dr J. Donald Ball, brother of Keith Ball, one of the founders of ASH. Donald Ball took a different line from that of the main committee, insisting on a greater sense of urgency in reducing tar and carbon monoxide yields; he wanted to see maximum levels set. But the main thrust of his argument exemplified the increasingly dominant anti-smoking argument. His view was that consumption should be reduced as well as toxicity, and the emphasis had to be on prevention. It was important to stop people smoking or

63 Interview with civil servant by Virginia Berridge, 7 April 1997.
64 Interview with Robert Waller by Virginia Berridge, March 1995.
65 Interview with Walter Holland by Virginia Berridge, 6 March 1997.

prevent them starting, whereas the committee's main concern had been the health of persisting smokers.[66]

The discussion of Ball's proposed report which took place in the ISCSH shows that the difference was one of strategy. At the thirtieth meeting of the committee on 16 November 1978, Hunter said that the second report opened the way to a third one. 'In that Report the Committee would be able to set out its views on what was possible and desirable but its recommendations had to be based on science and he considered that it would be tactically unwise to set levels of noxious yields at this stage.'[67] Ball pointed out that industry had been able to get tar yields down quite quickly to avoid health tax on brands yielding 20 mg of tar or more. Professor Neuberger felt it was important to keep the industry in a cooperative frame of mind. The Committee's role was to act as an intermediary and a complete change of policy could prove harmful. Froggatt said that the committee could advise industry to reduce tar yields, but it could hardly advise it to reduce consumption. Hunter and other members of the committee were clearly envisaging a gradual two-stage process with a second and third report. These would fulfil different functions. The second report would give industry formal general guidance whereas the third report, already agreed with the minister of Health, would have specific recommendations on noxious yields based on the latest data. Dr Ball had misgivings about lack of progress—the industry could act quickly when it had to. Fairweather reminded the committee of the statement which Hunter had made to industry some while ago—that the cigarette of the future should not exceed 10 mg/tar, 1 mg/nicotine,and 10 mg/carbon monoxide—these were the long-term aims. Crawford considered 'that the industry had to be handled carefully and sympathetically if the Committee's intentions were to be implemented. If the Committee pushed the industry too hard it could prove counter-productive.'

Ball's stance was also founded on a change in smoking culture apparent by the end of the 1970s; for the first time, smoking was in decline, among both men and, to a lesser extent, women.[68] The voluntary agreement of 1977, signed after Owen's departure, had stated there

[66] ISCSH, *Second Report*; J. D. Ball, Minority report, 49–55.

[67] National Archives, Department of Health papers, MH 148/1473, Minutes of 30th meeting of ISCSH, Thursday, 16 November 1978, at Alexander Fleming House.

[68] V. Berridge, 'Constructing Women and Smoking as a Public Health Problem in Britain 1950–1990's', *Gender and History*, 13(2) (2001), 328–48.

would be no more high and middle tar brands, and a supplementary tax on cigarettes with a high tar yield had been imposed in September 1978.[69] But the second Hunter report, founded on this model of low tar, did not find favour with smoking researchers. Martin Jarvis and Michael Russell, writing in the *British Medical Journal* in 1980, lambasted the 'disappointing' record of the committee and criticized the report itself for the naïveté of its models of smoking behaviour. Low tar and nicotine cigarettes might actually lead smokers to take in more rather than less tar because of 'compensatory smoking'.[70] The report had failed to release information about carbon monoxide levels and the researchers implied that this was because of industry pressure. The leadership of the ISCSH changed in the early 1980s. Both Hunter and Andrew Nelmes, one of the civil servants working for it, went to work for the tobacco industry; however, it should be remembered that these relationships were normal in the world of drug safety at the time.

In some respects the end of the 1970s was also the end of a distinct stage in the scientific side of smoking policy and the beginning of a new stage for public health and its animating ideas. In fact, the alliance of the 1970s round harm reduction and involving public health with government and industry did continue into the 1980s and 1990s and this will be discussed in Chapter 9. However, from the end of the 1970s, for at least twenty years, harm reduction for tobacco was no longer a major strategy for mainstream public health. The work of the ISCSH can be seen in two ways. To some in the public health field, it was later seen as a waste of time, a diversionary activity by the tobacco industry and scientists which achieved little. However, in terms of the interplay between culture and regulation, the committee's role was significant. It may be argued it represented a stage in policy which was not without its achievements. Its search for alternative products looked forward to the later focus on nicotine replacement and the involvement of the pharmaceutical industry. The focus on lower risk cigarettes fitted with public attitudes and the general social support for smoking as a mainstream cultural activity.

By the end of the decade, that cultural centrality was showing signs of decline. A new public health alliance had been emergent since the

---

[69] Proctor, *Sometimes a Cigarette is Just a Cigarette*, 156.

[70] M. J. Jarvis and M. A. H. Russell, 'Comment on the Hunter Committee's Second Report', *British Medical Journal*, 280 (1980), 994–5.

early 1970s which took a very different attitude towards health risk and attendant factors. Its response to smoking typified a 'new absolutism' which aimed to eliminate risky habits rather than to modify them. The 1970s was also a crucial decade for this alliance and its ideology and it is to this we now turn.

6

The Rise of Health Activism in the 1970s: The Health Pressure Group

The 1970s was the era of the modernization of expertise and of 'systematic gradualism' but it was also, crucially, the era when a new style of public health activism emerged and became dominant. Formal public health as an occupation was in a state of disarray during the 1970s as public health doctors were relocated within health services and found their old contact with local communities removed. But the 1970s was a crucial decade when a new public health style and agenda emerged, separate from the organizational dislocation. As discussed in the Introduction, this was the decade when public health developed its twin-track emphasis on the evidence base and health services and on the lifestyle version of public health. Smoking was the crucial 'tracer issue' for the latter, the template for other public health issues subsequently. The previous chapter outlined some key components of the 'new public health' package of the 1970s. The next two chapters will analyse how this new public health consensus was established through a new style of health pressure group; through the rise of formalized state responsibility, at one remove, for health education; through the rise of the mass media as a tool for health and also as the object of public health campaigning; through a focus on women and children; through the role of research and rationality exemplified in 'evidence'; and through an emphasis on economics, on taxation as a tool, and, towards the end of the decade, on the role of inequalities in health.

All of these components were visible in the rise of anti-smoking activism in the 1970s. But they were apparent in other public health 'single issues' as well. They can be traced for the emergent public health interest in diet and heart disease; and for alcohol, to take two examples.[1] These were also part of an international movement in public health which saw the publication of the Canadian Lalonde report, *A New Perspective on the Health of Canadians*, in 1974 and the British prevention documents and enquiries at the end of the decade. Webster and French have related these broader changes to the influence of the radical critiques of medicine; the impact of concern about health in developing countries and the failures of health systems; concern about the growing costs of health care; and the dramatic impact of the oil price rises introduced by OPEC states in 1973.[2]

THE NEW HEALTH INTERNATIONALISM

Much of the impetus for these changes came from outside the UK and this new internationalism for health was also apparent in the smoking field. In the late 1940s Doll and Hill had been unaware of the research being carried out by Wynder and Graham but international networks developed apace after that. Health campaigners developed strong connections with their US counterparts and the American InterAgency Council became an important focus for overseas visitors. The First World Conference on Smoking and Health had been held in New York in 1967, at which Robert Kennedy had delivered the keynote address. The Second World Conference was held in London in September 1971; it was organized by the Health Education Council and the opening speech made by Sir Keith Joseph. Speakers came from the United States and Canada and the speech topics ranged from advertising to economics and pharmacology. Industry representatives were still welcome—Alan Armitage from the Harrogate laboratories and Dr Beattie, medical adviser to Gallahers in Belfast, were both

---

[1] M. W. Bufton, 'British Expert Advice on Diet and Heart Disease c1945–2000', in V. Berridge (ed.), *Making Health Policy. Networks in Research and Policy after 1945* (Amsterdam: Rodopi, 2005), 125–48; L. A. Reynolds and E. M. Tansey (eds.), *Cholesterol, Antheroselerosis and Coronary Disease in the UK, 1950–2000*, Wellcome Witnesses to Twentieth Century Medicine, vol. xxvii (London: Wellcome Trust Centre for the History of Medicine at UCL, 2006); B. Thom, *Dealing with Drink: Alcohol and Social Policy: From Treatment to Management* (London: Free Association Books, 1999), 105–33; R. Baggott, *Alcohol, Politics and Social Policy* (Aldershot: Avebury, 1990), 29–51.

[2] C. Webster and J. French, 'The Cycle of Conflict: The History of Public Health and Health Promotion Movements', in L. Adams, M. Amos, and J. Munro (eds.), *Promoting Health Politics and Practice* (London: Sage, 2002), 5–12.

there. But George Godber, who on his retirement as chief medical officer (CMO) had become chairman of the new Health Education Council, gave a ringing address, 'It Can Be Done', which was a portent of the absolutist agenda to come. Godber looked to the ways in which international networks would take forward the anti-smoking case. International manoeuvring was to be a significant tactic for new public health and activities after the First World Conference showed how these networks could be used to keep a health issue 'live' and secure an international body of support. After the First World Conference smoking became a serious issue within the World Health Organization (WHO). The European Regional Committee in Budapest had accepted a resolution from Sweden and the UK asking for no smoking in the rooms where it met. Dr Kaprio, the regional director, was asked to report on further action. The US regional committee met a fortnight later and Godber sent the Surgeon General the resolution from the European committee; the US committee followed suit. Both reported to the executive board of the WHO the following January, therefore making it possible for the WHO to pass similar resolutions for report to the World Health Assembly. Fletcher and Daniel Horn of the US Interagency council then produced a report for the Twenty-Second World Health Assembly, which was published and distributed to all doctors and medical students in the UK. This type of manoeuvring at the international level and through international organizations was to become commonplace over the following decades; but in the early 1970s it was something relatively new and a way of building a consensus and an alliance for action. Godber's view of the new stage public health was entering was prescient.

The old triumphs of preventive medicine were obtained first by doing things to the environment, simple though not inexpensive procedures which over a century have given most of the countries with sophisticated health services sanitary environments which with improved nutrition have been the main cause of better health and greater expectation of life. The second phase in public health was one of organising health care, and with that came the opportunity for specific prophylaxis against communicable disease; the sort of thing that has made possible the real prospect of success in eradication of smallpox from the world today. What we have to do here is not something that can be done to people or imposed on them by compulsion. It is a matter of education and persuasion that will lead the millions who now smoke, either from habit or addiction, to impose upon themselves a habit of self abnegation, of denying themselves the pleasure they undoubtedly get from cigarettes in a world that not only can still sell cigarettes to them but puts enormous effort and expense into persuading them to buy. We are asking for an almost infinite number of acts of self discipline.[3]

Godber hoped for a change in the social climate, a future in which it was accceptable only for the addicted to smoke in private with other consenting adults. The change in the tactics of public health in the 1970s was to bring this about.

THE NEW HEALTH PRESSURE GROUP

Key to this change of climate was the alliance which developed in the 1970s between centralized government campaigning on health and a new type of health pressure group. The rise of media conscious public health activist groups in the 1960s and 1970s dealing with single issues like smoking, diet, and heart disease or alcohol was a new development. This chapter will focus on the activities in the 1970s of one such activist group, ASH (Action on Smoking and Health), established in 1971; this was an exemplar of more general trends in public health. There, the 'health pressure group' largely replaced the formal public health occupation as a source of public pressure on health issues. The activities of such groups were at the national rather than the local level and they used the national media as the vehicle for their message rather than more localized campaigns. In that sense they were very much in the technocratic, marketing model outlined in the Cohen report on health education in 1964. However, their role went further than simply conveying health education. Their 'new radical/new social movement' style in fact masked close relationships with government, both strategic and through government funding. The groups, ASH in particular, were part of an essential policy-balancing act for government. These were government-funded pressure groups as well as new social movements and part of the 'policy community' which composed the network of influence.

[3] National Archives, Ministry of Health papers, MH 154/861, Second World Conference on Smoking and Health, 20–4 September 1971; background papers, notes and briefings; R. G. Richardson, *The Second World Conference on Smoking and Health. Conference Organized by the Health Education Council Held at Imperial College, 20–24 September 1971* (London: Pitman Medical HEC, 1971), Sir G. Godber, 'It Can Be Done', 141–7.

The creation of such campaigning groups was part of a wider trend. Between 1961 and 1971 the number of registered charities rose from 1,182 to 76,648. This dramatic increase can partly be accounted for by the introduction of more efficient methods for registering charities, but Johnson estimates that around 10,500 of these were entirely new organizations.[4] Just as significantly, these were different from many existing groups. Davis Smith asserts that the 1960s saw 'the appearance of a new generation of volunteers, who were entering existing organisations and creating new ones of their own'.[5] He attributes this to spillover from a renewed interest in the 'Third World' and overseas development, seen in the expansion of Oxfam which had begun with a European refugee focus, and the creation of Voluntary Service Overseas (VSO). They encouraged a re-evaluation of domestic welfare services which identified a series of startling deficiencies in certain areas, such as homelessness. Dramatized in a series of 'exposures' (consultancy reports, books, and television programmes) these issues became the focus of a new group of campaign organizations such as Gingerbread, Shelter (1965), the Child Poverty Action Group (CPAG, 1965), National Association for the Care and Resettlement of Offenders (NACRO, 1966), Radical Alternatives to Prison (1970), and the Disability Alliance.[6] In the health field, the new campaigning tradition was exemplified in organizations like the Patients Association established in 1963 and the rise of the human rights movement in mental health. There the National Association for Mental Health (NAMH) had its origins in 1940s notions of mental hygiene, but in the 1960s and 1970s, it became characterized by an opposition to psychiatry, culminating in a more radical and political organization which re-named itself MIND.[7]

The public health campaign groups were different from these new health campaigning groups in that their primary focus was not 'the

[4] J. Freeman and V. Johnson, *Waves of Protest: Social Movements since the Sixties* (Lanham, MD: Rowman and Littlefield, 1999), 89.

[5] J. Davis Smith, C. Rochester, and R. Hedley (eds.), *An Introduction to the Voluntary Sector* (London: Routledge, 1995), 49.

[6] Ibid., 49–50.

[7] N. Crossley, 'Transforming the Mental Health Field: The Early History of the National Association for Mental Health', *Sociology of Health and Illness*, 20(4) (1998), 458–88; G. Smith, 'The Rise of the "New Consumerism" in Health and Medicine in Britain, c.1948–1989', in J. Burr and P. Nicolson (eds.), *Researching Health Care Consumers* (Basingstoke: Palgrave/Macmillan, 2005), 13–38; R. Baggott, J. Allsop, and K. Jones, *Speaking for Patients and Carers: Health Consumer Groups and the Policy Process* (Basingstoke: Palgrave, 2005).

patient' or the provision or improvement of services. For smoking there were few health services and the treatment model was not dominant. But in one area, that of relationships with government, there was overlap. Voluntarism and charity had a long history in the provision of welfare; in particular the role of charity and voluntary relationships had been important within health services. Partnership between voluntary and statutory organizations had existed since the nineteenth century and had continued into the era of the National Health Service (NHS). Relationships with government also characterized the operation of the public health single-issue pressure group, although the image of such groups was one of independence from any interests and a robust campaigning stance. The role of ASH and of other health activist organizations shows how, from the 1970s, expertise and the pressure group were combining into a new media-centred approach to health risk.

ASH was by no means the first anti-tobacco organization. Such groupings came and went in the nineteenth century. Like the temperance, inebriety, anti-opium, and anti-alcohol movements, they drew on a crucial mix of medicine and morality. The issue of juvenile smoking saw more anti-smoking organizations established at the end of the nineteenth century.[8] ASH 's main predecessor in the twentieth century was the National Society of Non Smokers (NSNS), founded in 1926. Its secretary for much of its existence after the Second World War was Tom Hurst, an Edinburgh hospital administrator; the NSNS concentrated on the 'clean air' and environmentally harmful aspects of smoking, but its appeal was based on moral endeavour rather than on science. It argued that it was selfish to smoke near others. Of the initial 146 promoters of the society, only 38 were active scientists and the rest were moralists, evangelists, and social critics.[9] At its inception, the Society gained two thousand members in a few months, organized in local branches. The main aim was to protect the rights of non-smokers, not to stop all smoking, although the Society did oppose young people's smoking. Its

---

[8] R. B. Walker, 'Medical Aspects of Tobacco Smoking and the Anti Tobacco Movement in Britain in the Nineteenth Century', *Medical History*, 24 (1980), 391–402; M. Hilton and S. Nightingale, ' "A Microbe of the Devil's Own Make": Religion and Science in the British Anti-Tobacco Movement, 1853–1908', in S. Lock, L. Reynolds, and E. M. Tansey (eds.), *Ashes to Ashes: The History of Smoking and Health* (Amsterdam: Rodopi, 1998), 41–77; J. Welshman, 'Images of Youth: The Problem of Juvenile Smoking', *Addiction*, 91(9) (1996), 1379–86.

[9] M. Hilton, 'Constructing Tobacco: Perspectives on Consumer Culture in Britain, 1850–1950', PhD thesis University of Lancaster, 1996, 238.

campaign to secure premises with smoke-free areas had little success. The NSNS did not use science in its arguments at all and in general it regarded smoking as quite legitimate as long as it did not offend the sensibilities of others.

ASH's appeal was rather different. It was founded in 1971, at the time of the publication of the second Royal College of Physicians (RCP) report, *Smoking and Health Now*, but that was a catalyst; discussions of the need for an external pressure group had been going on for some time. It was significant, and a portent of ASH's later relationship with government, that the first mention of such an organization came from within the Ministry of Health. The need for some kind of external pressure group had been foreseen there long before ASH's foundation. Ten years previously, in the early 1960s, an exchange of views within the health department looked forward to pressure from without. During the discussions on what policy line should be followed in response to the first RCP report in 1962, various options—legal, fiscal, and publicity—were on the agenda. The central problem was the widespread social acceptability of the habit, and the perceived fluidity of the 'scientific facts' surrounding smoking risk. What could justify action? Enid Russell Smith of the Ministry of Health wrote perceptively

There is at present very little in the way of an anti smoking lobby and it may well be that at the present intermediate stage, when the nature of the connection between smoking and lung cancer has still not been fully established, the most effective measure to limit smoking would be the promotion of a voluntary anti-smoking movement. It would be much easier for the Government and the local authorities to take regulatory measures against smoking if there were a body of opinion pressing them to do so.[10]

The setting up of ASH, some nine years later, illustrated this interaction between anti-smoking sentiment among civil servants and public health activists outside. It was an example of the political science concept of the policy community, linking interests in and outside government.[11] The initial planned focus for the organization was on information dissemination. In 1969, after an internal departmental group had reviewed progress on smoking and health, the Central Health Services Council decided to advise the Secretary of State for Social Services

[10] National Archives, Ministry of Health papers, MH 55/2204, Minute from Enid Russell Smith, 5 February 1962.
[11] D. Marsh and R. A. W. Rhodes, *Policy Networks in British Government* (Oxford: Clarendon Press, 1992).

to encourage the establishment of a body comparable to the US InterAgency Council and to establish a section in the Department of Health and Social Security (DHSS) able to collate the large amount of information coming forward about smoking and health. After some delay, the internal section was set up under a senior medical officer, Dr Julia Dawkins, who had previously been in the Department of Education dealing with drugs and sex education. But the minister, presumably Crossman at this stage, was doubtful about the value of setting up a body comparable to the InterAgency Council and so the initiative did not come directly from government.[12]

Doctors with public health interests had been having similar discussions since the late 1960s. There was a need for a 'central information point', and also a body which, as a group of doctors independent of the Ministry, would be able to exert more pressure.[13] A meeting in March 1968 at which Godber was present, along with Holland, Fletcher, and others, concluded 'there was a need for a central point, either within the Ministry, or working closely with it, to coordinate information on the health aspects of smoking.'[14] The eventual initiative for the founding of ASH came from Dr Charles Fletcher, secretary of the first two RCP committees, and Dr Keith Ball, a doctor with a strong interest in public health. Ball worked at the Central Middlesex Hospital, a powerhouse of social medicine sentiment.[15] However, Dr Dawkins was also closely involved, emphasizing the close relationship with government.

ASH's foundation was central to moves by anti-smoking interests to secure government action and to publicize the risks of smoking to the public in the wake of the 1971 report. There was some discussion initially about what the new organization should be called. Names suggested at a steering committee in October 1970 included NCSH (National Council on Smoking and Health), BASH (British Association on Smoking and Health), CASH (Council or Commission for Action on Smoking and Health), and the subsequently adopted ASH.[16] The

[12] National Archives, Ministry of Health papers, MH 154/619, 1969–71, Royal College of Physicians, Working party proposals for a national council, Registration, membership and organisation of ASH (Action on Smoking and Health Ltd).

[13] Wellcome Library for the History and Understanding of Medicine, ASH archive, SA/ASH/C.8, Box 7, Letter from Keith Ball to Charles Fletcher, 5 February 1968.

[14] Ibid., Box 19 (old series), 7 March 1968, meeting on smoking and health.

[15] C. Webster, 'Tobacco Smoking Addiction: A Challenge to the National Health Service', *British Journal of Addition*, 79 (1984), 11.

[16] Wellcome Library for the History and Understanding of Medicine, ASH Archive, Box 70, SA/ASH/Q. 3/2/1, Meeting of steering committee, 19 October 1970.

form the organization might take was also fluid at this stage. Dawkins saw it as 'a group of members of the various professions, including industry, who were concerned with tobacco', while Fletcher and Max Rosenheim, president of the RCP, initially saw it as a 'very large group of people representing all sorts of organisations', which was to be sponsored by the College. The American model of an InterAgency Council was clearly influential, along with similar Australian organizations, although it was subsequently agreed that those models would not be applicable in the UK.

Sir George Godber, as chief medical officer, had already stimulated action through the RCP in the 1960s in order to goad government into action.[17] He saw ASH as fulfilling a similar ongoing irritant function, in alliance with the newly established (1968) Health Education Council (HEC). In a 1969 minute, he commented,

If the RCP will start it and the HEC also take part we would have something very different from the interdepartmental committee. A voluntary group may be a thorn in our flesh—but only if we are inert and deserve it. This is one of our biggest health problems. We made a start five years before the Americans and they are really doing something now while we are in the doldrums. We really must show we are in earnest.[18]

The launch of ASH in January 1971 was attended by between 150 and 200 people representing around seventy-five organizations. The Council of the new body was primarily medical, but with input from both new style (advertising and the media) organizations and traditional voluntary bodies: Lady Anglesea, past chair of the National Federation of Women's Institutes, represented women's interests. (She thought there should be pipes suitable for women.) The function of the new organization was not entirely clear and this caused some problems at the outset. Dr Keith Ball, one of the founders, saw its activities as a traditional research and education body. In a paper on 'what we have done and what we should do' he saw work for ASH in health education, regional groups, and research into the economics of smoking and ways of discouraging the habit. However, the dominant impetus was towards

---

[17] C. C. Booth, 'Smoking and the Gold Headed Cane', in C. C. Booth (ed.), *Balancing Act: Essays to Honour Stephen Lock* (London: Keynes Press, 1991), 49–55.

[18] National Archives, Ministry of Health papers, MH 154/169, Minute from George Godber, 18 June 1969.

changing public opinion.[19] Dr Robert Murray, medical adviser to the Trades Union Congress (TUC) who was also an early supporter, put this eloquently. The habit of giving and receiving cigarettes and the camaraderie of smoking and drinking was a 'kind of ritual' he noted in a letter in 1970.

The idea of disease arising as the result of repeated exposure to an environmental cause is of fairly recent origin. The generally accepted idea of disease is a dramatic attack as the result of accident, infection or 'Act of God'. Because the cause and effect relationship is so distant in time and so statistical in character the average individual does not see it, and is not convinced by argument. This I believe accounts for the failure of direct propaganda except among doctors who are trained to see the relationship.

Smoking was an individual not an industrial problem, in his view.

By all means make it obvious that smoking cigarettes is not 'with it'. Increase the number of 'non smoking' railway compartments and places of entertainment. Label cigarette packets as the Americans are doing. Build up a climate of opinion against smoking. It will be a long and discouraging job.'[20]

Dr John Dunwoody, a former junior minister in the Department of Health and ex-MP, was ASH's part-time secretary. In a letter enclosing a launch leaflet which he sent to Dawkins in 1971, he clearly envisaged a media and public opinion role for ASH:

ASH intends to examine the problem very thoroughly; it will not be just a clearing house for posters. ASH will sponsor research into why people smoke and into patterns of smoking. It will also act as a pressure group and as a centre for information on smoking and health ... the most important activity that ASH will undertake will be an advertising campaign to discourage people from smoking.

Dunwoody wanted to drop the 'Black Widow' approach of the road accident campaigns, which had aimed to shock drivers into responsible behaviour. Instead, he envisaged marketing social acceptability. Financial and material incentives were to be encouraged, with group therapy on the lines of Weight Watchers and a focus on children and young people. 'Primarily the campaign will attempt to take the social cachet

---

[19] Wellcome Library for the History and Understanding of Medicine, ASH Archive, Box 19 (old series) (Ball file), paper (undated) on 'What we have done and what we should do'.

[20] Ibid., Box 29 (old series), 14 September 1970, Robert Murray, medical adviser to the TUC.

that surrounds smoking and turn it on its head.'[21] But Dunwoody's proposals to start this ruffled feathers initially. Dawkins had seen ASH as a high-powered professional body, but these ideas infringed on the territory of the Health Education Council. The HEC was annoyed at the overlap with its role. Max Rosenheim apologized and ASH's launch leaflet was hastily withdrawn.

At its inception ASH endorsed the twin-track strategy of public health. The initial aims of the proposed national council were a mixture of risk reduction and risk elimination; to maintain pressure on government to bring in legislation; to increase efforts to discourage smoking among all sections of the population; but also to encourage less hazardous forms of smoking and to consider the economic problems related to a reduction of cigarette smoking.[22] Later drafts of ASH's aims dropped the explicit commitment to risk reduction and this was a portent of the future stance of the organization. At the outset, there were moves to involve friendly figures from industry. Fletcher wrote to Todd in December 1970 suggesting the industry might like to support the new organization:

Naturally, much of this organisation's activity must, in the present state of knowledge, be devoted to trying to persuade people not to smoke the sort of cigarettes which are sold today, but one of its objects is to stimulate research into less harmful forms of smoking ... I can conceive that the tobacco industry itself might like to have a voice in the affairs of this body.[23]

Two years later, when ASH was hoping to raise funds, Fletcher also approached Sir John Partridge, chairman of Imperial Tobacco. He wanted Imperial's assurance that they would not penalize companies who supported ASH financially.[24]

The stance was one of harm reduction at this initial stage. H. B. Wright of the Institute of Directors Medical Centre agreed to come on to the ASH committee 'provided I am allowed to go on smoking my pipe'. The acceptance list was annotated 'Yes and pipe'.[25] Murray, too, commented,' I am quite prepared to defend pipe smoking but I hold

---

[21] National Archives, Ministry of Health papers, MH 154/169, Letter from Dunwoody to Dawkins, 5 January 1971.

[22] Ibid., Aims of proposed national council, 2 June 1970.

[23] Wellcome Library for the History and Understanding of Medicine, ASH Archive, Box 19 (old series), 7 December 1970, Letter from Charles Fletcher to Geoffrey Todd, Director of the Tobacco Research Council.

[24] Ibid., 22 September 1972, Letter from Fletcher to Sir John Partridge.

[25] Ibid., Box 29 (old series), 1971–2, Papers relating to the setting up of ASH.

no brief for cigarette smoking.' He was told, 'Your pipe will certainly not be a disqualification for service on the committee and it is really cigarettes we are after!'[26] In 1973, the organization set up an expert group to look at the issue of the safety of pipes and cigars, about which it had received many enquiries. Switching to a pipe or cigar smoking instead of cigarettes was widely advocated as a harm/risk reduction strategy. The expert group came up with no clear answer, although it concluded that it was likely that risk was reduced. There was, however, a risk to others from so-called 'passive smoking'. But this risk was minute. This report was reproduced as a leaflet by the Health Education Council.[27]

For the first year or two ASH's activities were relatively low key. A group of supportive doctors wrote letters to the *Lancet* and it set up a research committee in 1973. Publicity activities had a rather amateurish air. 'Doctors weren't good at publicity', said one of the ASH pioneers.[28] In December 1971, ASH 'Christmas dolly birds' made their appearance in Camden High Street to publicize ASH's first public exhibition. 'Dressed as a mini skirted "Father Christmas", each girl will make her present to Camden's shoppers, an invitation to see the ASH display inside the centre and to take home a copy of the Health Education Council leaflet, "How to stop smoking".'[29]

Dunwoody's departure in 1973 and the arrival of Mike Daube as director brought a change of emphasis and style. Daube brought with him a campaigning stance from his previous work at the housing charity Shelter, which had pioneered a media and publicity conscious approach to social issues. He was strongly influenced by the new style of campaigning which the director of Shelter, Des Wilson, had introduced. He also had a background in student politics. He joined ASH because it was an interesting job, not because he was fanatically anti-smoking at the outset. Daube's arrival was significant in importing the human rights new social movement style of campaigning into the public health

[26] Wellcome Library for the History and Understanding of Medicine, ASH Archive, Exchange, 5 August 1970.

[27] 'Pipe and Cigar Smoking: Report of an Expert Group Appointed by ASH', reprinted from *The Practitioner,* 210 (1973). Health Education Council (later Authority) leaflet archive, 14 950.1.

[28] Interview with Keith Ball by Virginia Berridge, 5 December 1997.

[29] Wellcome Library for the History and Understanding of Medicine, ASH archive Box 36 (old series), Press release, 7 December 1971.

arena. A letter he wrote to Charles Fletcher in 1973 about a funding application gives a flavour of this style:

I have tried to define the areas of commitment fairly widely, while also conforming to the requirement that they be controversial. I suspect that one of the reasons for ASH's failure has been that it has been to a large extent a reacting organization, rather than one that has set out to create news ... so the suggestions that I have made in this application ... are concerned with creating news in a way that could have a fair impact on the anti smoking campaign.[30]

In an interview he gave to the Australian journalist William Norman, in the mid-1970s, he argued in a similar way. 'It seemed to me when I came into ASH that here was a pressure campaign that was ripe. It hadn't been properly used. You had your villain. You had your St. George and the dragon scenario, you had your growing ecology bandwagon, growing interest in consumerism. It seemed there were a lot of prospects of making something out of it.'[31] An indication of this new approach came shortly after Daube's appointment when he wrote a piece for the journal *Adweek*, attacking the textile firm Courtaulds for 'irresponsible action' in marketing Planet, a tobacco substitute, before it had been reviewed by the DHSS's Independent Scientific Committee on Smoking and Health (ISCSH). Courtaulds threatened a libel action, although this was never ultimately brought to court. In Daube's view, the furore was a good thing. 'The first thing it did was to show that we had teeth. I think if I were being a little honest and a little arrogant, I would say Courtaulds established ASH as a pressure group.'[32]

This was the tone of ASH's activities throughout the 1970s. It was intensely media conscious. The organization bought shares (or one share) in tobacco companies and would then turn up to ask awkward questions at the AGM. It collaborated on a Thames TV *This Week* programme. It also worked with journalists like Peter Taylor; the journalist's anti-smoking programmes in the 1970s, *Dying for a Fag, Licensed to Kill* (1974) and later on *Death in the West* (1977) were also part of this new media trend. ASH also cooperated in television programmes on stopping smoking and received funds to help with the enormous response. Over half a million people responded to one

[30] Ibid., SA/ASH/0.4/3, Box 71, Letter from Mike Daube to Charles Fletcher, 3 August 1973.
[31] Ibid., SA/ASH William Norman collection, R. 12, Box 77, Interview with Mike Daube.
[32] Ibid.

programme in the mid-1970s. Daube operated by the American activist text, *Rules for Radicals*, 'rule one is to personalize the problem—the people running the major companies are responsible for those deaths.'[33]

The medical and health correspondents, a newly emergent occupational group—Ronnie Bedford at the *Daily Mirror*, Nicholas Timmins at the Press Association, Oliver Gillie, and Christine Doyle—were vital allies. A major aim was to keep tobacco on the front pages; the story did not matter, but the media coverage did. Daube favoured ASH's move to new offices at the Family Planning Association in Mortimer Street mainly because the organization would be closer to the BBC in Portland Place. The organization did not just react to news, but also created it in a way which has become more familiar since. Daube described to Norman how he set up a media storm over the production of a low tar cigarette called Westminster Abbey. He got onto a journalist and suggested, ' "I wonder what Westminster Abbey think about that, why don't you ask them." She phoned up W. A. and they said, no, we don't know about it. Ten minutes later I phoned up as Mike Daube from ASH and they said, "Funny, we have just had a journalist on to us asking about this." I said, "Really, well it shows how wide the interest is." '[34] Then a piece appeared in *Adweek* and Westminster Abbey sent Daube a copy. He wrote to the Dean of the Abbey complaining, the Dean consulted lawyers, and he and the journalists were phoning up and keeping in touch. It was what Daube called the 'rapier and stiletto' approach—now better known as 'spin'.

Twenty years later, he was remembered by Keith Ball as 'a young man with long hair and a purple suit'; he made ASH important as a political force in the 1970s.[35] Daube helped to set up the Commons All Party group on smoking in 1976, which, although chaired by the Labour MP Laurie Pavitt, had active members from the Conservative Party, among them the MPs Lynda Chalker and Sir George Young. ASH's great strengths lay in its media skills—relatively new at the time—and its radical outsider image. But it was not too much of an outside organization. The Duke of Gloucester and Angus Ogilvy, husband of Princess Alexandra, visited the Royal College of Physicians

[33] Interview with Mike Daube by Virginia Berridge, 11 March 1999. Notes of interview.

[34] Wellcome Library for the History and Understanding of Medicine, ASH archive, SA/ASH William Norman collection, R. K, Box 77, Interview with Mike Daube.

[35] Comment at witness seminar at Ashes to Ashes conference on smoking at Wellcome Institute, 26–7 April 1995. Author's notes.

for ASH's anniversary celebrations in 1975 and the Council of ASH remained doctor-dominated with a sprinkling of radicals such as Joan Ruddock, the director of Oxford Housing Aid.

ASH was also an insider–outsider organization so far as government went. The relationship with government had been close from when ASH was first set up and Sir Keith Joseph was Secretary of State. ASH was primarily funded for much of its first two decades by the Health department. After initial unsuccessful attempts to mount a national appeal, most funding came from government. The organization had £25,000 of government money between 1971 and 1972, initially intended to be 'start up' funds.[36] But in 1974, it was granted £13,000 for 1975–6, together with money for alterations to its new premises.[37] Later attempts by government to reduce its financial responsibility and to involve the cancer charities in funding ASH were unsuccessful. Daube commented in the mid-1970s that more government funding had come just in time. '[If] the grant from the department stopped then we'd be in trouble. If the grant from the department did stop, however, I'd kick up such a fuss, that it would soon start again.'[38] An ASH development committee chaired by the comedian Brian Rix, with support from Clement Freud, Spike Milligan, and Norman Vaughan, launched a £200,000 appeal, but raised little.[39] Pump priming funding from government initially was replaced by an ongoing DHSS grant. By 1978, it was reported that 90% of ASH's income came from the DHSS. The organization expanded, with a deputy director, an information officer, and other posts. In 1977, the grant was £31,000 with donations standing at just over £5,000. In addition, there was a special government grant of £80,000 to enable ASH to deal with over half a million responses it had received to a television programme on stopping smoking. It has been argued that the policy changes of the 1980s and 1990s brought a government-funded voluntary sector, but the example of ASH shows that this relationship had an earlier history.[40]

[36] Wellcome Library for the History and Understanding of Medicine, ASH archive, Box 19 (old series), 22 November 1972, Letter from Dunwoody to Fletcher.

[37] Ibid., Box 36 (old series), 3 December 1974, David Owen to Daube; Royal College of Physicians, *Smoking or Health* (London: Pitman Medical, 1977), 27.

[38] Wellcome Library for the History and Understanding of Medicine, ASH archive, SA/ASH, R.12, Box 77, William Norman collection, Interview with Mike Daube, no date but *c.*1975–6.

[39] Ibid., R. 5.7.

[40] R. Whelan, *Involuntary Action. How Voluntary is the 'Voluntary' Sector?* (London: IEA, Institute of Economic Affairs, Health and Welfare Unit, 1999), 23.

The great advantage of ASH to the Labour government of the mid-1970s was the visible pressure it was able to put on government, on the lines of the model Enid Russell Smith had outlined earlier. ASH worked closely with David Owen over the Medicines Act initiative, as we have seen in Chapter 5. This was the function which ASH came to fulfil as part of the policy community round smoking. It was an external pressure group, urging government to greater activity, but at the same time part of the policy network, working with the DHSS while it was agitating outside. ASH was extremely useful, especially to those ministers who wished to follow a stronger anti-smoking line. In 1974, Owen as minister of Health, echoed Russell Smith at a joint ASH/HEC conference.

The facts of life are that Government in this area will respond to pressure, and I, instead of acting defensively on the pressure that you will put me under, am coming to you with a different message, which is to say, 'Put me under as much pressure as you like.'[41]

During the Medicines Act events, Kilroy-Silk's intervention, aided by ASH, brought matters to a head and secured Owen the leverage he needed to go ahead against the various competing interests. At the same time, ASH maintained its oppositional role, selectively leaking information to urge the Minister on to more significant action.[42] Daube's role was of a useful stalking horse. For example, he told Norman of an exchange where Charles Fletcher had called him and reported on a lunch with Robert Hunter, chairman of the ISCSH. Hunter had been at a meeting with Owen and the industry and had told Fletcher that Owen was proposing a pact with industry. Fletcher could not do anything with the story—but Daube could. He felt the pressure put on Owen by these sort of selective leaks was an important force, 'the best thing to happen for ten years'.[43]

A similar relationship operated over the answering of parliamentary questions (PQs), where Daube would be rung up from within government for help; and sometimes he encouraged the 'planting' of PQs. But there was always a limit to the overt opposition. 'With several

[41] RCP, *Smoking or Health*. The Third report from the Royal College of Physicians of London (London: Pitman Medical, 1977), 27.
[42] Wellcome Library for the History and Understanding of Medicine, ASH archive, SA/ASH, William Norman collection, R.12, Box 77, Interview with Mike Daube, no date but *c*.1975–6.
[43] Ibid.

PQs I have discussed with them what the terms of the PQ should be. Because I want to embarrass them, obviously, in some ways, but I don't want to ask the kind of really embarrassing question. It is not my job just to make life difficult.'[44] This was, indeed, as two ASH activists recalled in an interview in the 1990s, the 'golden age' so far as the organization was concerned.[45] ASH fulfilled an important facilitating role within the political process with networks between government and this outside organization. It achieved this role within politics while at the same time becoming a high-profile public presence. In fact, its media profile was part of its attraction to politicians because it made it appear a 'force to be reckoned with' and therefore useful as a counterweight to the stance of industry and of other government departments.

As the decade progressed ASH's stance became increasingly hard line. The harm reduction twin-track strategy of the early 1970s continued in organizations like ISCSH but, for ASH, this was increasingly untenable. It was opposed to the industry and the tactic of 'safer' smoking. The sections of the industry which opposed further regulation under the Medicines Act also took strong exception to Daube's line. In an off-the-record conversation, G. C. Hargrove, director of Public Relations at British American Tobacco (BAT) said that Daube was doing more harm than good because of his arrogance. He had only one share in BAT, but he had taken up two hours of the annual meeting's time.[46] ASH criticized the Hunter committee's first report. Daube was concerned that substitutes or additives might be used as a means of slowing up the trends in cigarette smoking in the 1970s which were beginning to move downwards. His organization was also concerned about the Hunter committee's plans for human trials of the new materials. A close working relationship with Jim Welch, a civil servant involved in smoking policy at the DHSS, brought in confidence a copy of Hunter's plans for the studies and their management. Welch's comment underlined the 'balancing act' relationship between ASH and the department, 'This is the text of a letter from Hunter re long term human health studies. Could we please discuss Press Notices before

[44] Ibid.

[45] Interview with Ann McNeill and Patti White by Virginia Berridge, 10 November 1997.

[46] Wellcome Library for the History and Understanding of Medicine, ASH archive, SA/ASH, William Norman collection R.8, Box 76, Correspondence with G. C. Hargrove, director of Public Relations BAT, 1975–6.

you go public (if you think that necessary).'[47] The overall consensus
for public health ended in the course of the 1970s.[48] The end of
Owen's strategy of regulation (abandoned after he moved to the Foreign
Office) and a feeling that ASH had 'marked time' while this strategy
was in play politically also contributed to the new hostile public health
stance.[49] ASH submitted evidence to the Royal Commission on Civil
Liability and Compensation in 1973–4 recommending that tobacco
manufacturers be liable for the harm caused by their cigarettes and for
the establishment of a compensation fund. It was this hostility which
was to develop further into a new agenda for public health by the end
of the decade.

Daube and ASH were key mediators of the new science of anti-
smoking in the public domain. The role of public health science, the
epidemiology of smoking, was of central importance in the organization.
The scientists, Doll and Hill, did not see themselves as campaigners.
Daube thought that, in a way, they were right. 'The researcher is
seen to lose his objectivity as soon as he becomes a campaigner.' He
was the pressure group tactical expert and this was his job within
the organization. Yet ASH set up a research committee and the role
of science was central to its mission. Daube was also instrumental in
changing the policy agenda which had been developed since the 1950s.
The new position was more anti-industry and aimed at the elimination
of the habit rather than its modification. There was already public health
support for this line. Sir Robert Platt, for example, the president of the
RCP who had encouraged the publication of its first report, and Dr
Keith Ball, one of ASH's founders, had always been opposed to industry
links. This became the dominant strategy within public health in the
course of the 1970s.[50]

ASH's key ally throughout the 1970s was the Health Education
Council, which was chaired by George Godber after his retirement as
chief medical officer and whose campaigning is discussed in more detail

[47] Wellcome Library for the History and Understanding of Medicine, ASH archive,
Box 36 (old series), 6 July 1977 and 2 August 1977, Letters from Daube to Jim Welch
and Welch to Daube.
[48] Although it continued as an objective in parts of the policy network. See Virginia
Berridge, 'Post-war Smoking Policy in the UK and the Redefinition of Public Health',
Twentieth Century British History, 14(1) (2003), 61–82.
[49] M. Daube, 'The Politics of Smoking: Thoughts on the Labour Record', *Community
Medicine* (1979), 306–14.
[50] Although it continued as an objective in parts of the policy network. See Berridge
'Post-war Smoking Policy'.

in the following chapter. A briefing note for a meeting with Owen in 1975 showed that the earlier confusion about their respective roles had been resolved. The HEC was to pursue research, education, and publicity activities; ASH was to act as a campaigning organization and a catalyst, operating as a pressure group. At the end of the decade, the two organizations took a notably antagonistic stance to the launch of tobacco substitutes like New Smoking Material (NSM). They were concerned that part-substitute brands like NSM and Cytrel still contained 75% tobacco and could be stronger than cigarettes already on the market.[51] The major press conference by Imperial Tobacco to launch its part-substitute brands, held the day after the launch of the RCP's third report, *Smoking or Health,* effectively upstaged the Royal College. ASH was concerned, as letters from Daube to Jim Welch, a civil servant at the DHSS make clear, that the publicity for substitutes would slow down the downward trend in smoking which was becoming apparent in the 1970s.[52] The aim, said the Council's report for 1978, was 'deterrence', a new terminology which epitomized the war between some public health interests and the industry.[53]

This new agenda for smoking was part of a larger agenda for public health and prevention epitomized in the government's prevention documents at the end of the 1970s and part of a wider international movement.[54] The Health Education Council itself, with its advertising campaigns formulated by the advertising agency Saatchi and Saatchi, also showed a distinctively different approach. The 'new public health' concentrated on relationships and on the responsibility of the individual. Self-discipline, central publicity, and habit-changing campaigns were central to its ethos. The height of this new approach was to come in the 1980s, so far as smoking was concerned, with the elaboration of the science of passive smoking. Already, at the end of the 1970s, ASH was moving its policy agenda in this direction. The issue of the non-smoker was initially a moral one, one of human rights, as some of the activities at the end of the decade demonstrate. Fletcher had not been in favour

[51] Wellcome Library for the History and Understanding of Medicine, ASH archive, SA/ASH/G.1, Box 23, Letter from Daube to David Ennals, 24 June 1977.

[52] Ibid., SA/ASH/G.3/1, Box 71, Letter from Daube to Jim Welch, DHSS, 6 July 1977.

[53] Health Education Council, *Annual Report, 1977–78* (London, 1978), 11.

[54] C. Webster. *The Health Services since the War, vol. ii: Government and Health Care. The British National Health Service, 1958–1979* (London: HMSO, 1996), 676–80; Webster and French, 'The Cycle of Conflict', 5–12.

of concentrating over much on the 'nuisance' aspects of smoking—he saw this as a moral issue rather than a scientific one. By the end of the 1970s Daube was moving ASH's focus towards the human rights issues involved in smoking. Important in this respect was a conference held at the Kings Fund (date probably about 1977–8) on The Rights of the Non Smoker.[55] The epidemiological case was to follow in the early 1980s.[56]

CENTRE AND PERIPHERY: LONDON AND SCOTLAND

ASH was new in its use of the media, and its organizational structure also made new departures for a pressure group. Its membership was around the 500 mark in the 1970s, but Daube did not wish to broaden it further. Such efforts would be pointless: a large membership, if it needed to be regularly serviced, would use up resources and be more of a hindrance than a help. ASH did develop some local branches in the 1970s, but these were few in number. The focus of the organization instead reflected its emphasis on London, the media, and political lobbying, as for example through its involvement in the Commons All Party Group on Smoking.

But there was an important centre of activity outside London. This was Scottish ASH in Edinburgh. Founded in 1972 in a corner of the Royal College of Physicians there, it was originally local authority funded, with the Scottish Office taking over after the 1975 local government reorganization. Its work was different from that of ASH in London. It carried out projects and had project funding for action research: a dominant theme was to do something about advertising. Sir John and Eileen Crofton were leading figures in the organization and Eileen Crofton was its first director, Their influence was considerable, also that of the subsequent director, Alison Hillhouse. They had close links into the Scottish health establishment and government. Scottish ASH did its own thing, but Eileen Crofton and Daube got on well, so the

---

[55] Wellcome Library for the History and Understanding of Medicine, ASH archive, Box 36 (old series), 18 February 1977, Letter from Daube to David Ennals.

[56] V. Berridge, 'Passive Smoking and its Pre-history in Britain: Policy Speaks to Science?', *Social Science and Medicine*, special historical issue, Science Speaks to Policy, 49(9) (1999), 1183–95.

combination worked. Their campaign initiated in 1985–6 against the chewing tobacco, Skoal Bandits, was highly successful and resulted in a ban.[57] The Scottish dimension to anti-smoking policy was an important one in many respects, and there were differences between Scottish and English activism on smoking, underlined by the differences between the two organizations. Scottish ASH ran community projects and also, through the work of Eileen Crofton and Alison Hillhouse, initiated work on children and smoking. It gave a lead to the growing interest in women and smoking in the anti-smoking field in the 1980s.[58] It, too, saw science as central and the Croftons set up a research committee for Scottish ASH.[59] The activities of the separate Scottish organization and its close links into Scottish public health policy emphasized the importance of the interest group in the Scottish as well as English policy community.

The later history of ASH will be discussed in Chapter 8. Under a Conservative government in the 1980s, it was less influential within policy. In that decade, the anti-tobacco alliance broadened and new players like the British Medical Association (BMA) joined in. ASH became one among several organizations and was no longer the dominant force on the UK anti-smoking scene. The movement became an international one, stretching out to networks in Australia and the Far East and it also developed local roots on a more extensive scale. ASH's activist agenda was founded on its interpretation of the science of smoking; it translated the connections between smoking, lung cancer, and heart disease, into the policy and public environment. Its appeal was in the way in which it made these 'scientific facts' media friendly and part of the everyday milieu of the discussion of smoking. They became 'common sense' which few could gainsay. Here was a change from the moral stance of the NSNS where there had been little reference to science. David Simpson, who took over as director after Daube's departure, recalled, 'We had the massive scientific evidence against smoking, which is the biggest single resource ASH has ever had.'[60] ASH's authority in part arose

---

[57] M. Raw, P. White, and A. McNeill, *Clearing the Air. A Guide for Action on Tobacco* (London: BMA/WHO, 1990), 100–12.

[58] Interview with Eileen and John Crofton by Virginia Berridge, 17 March 1999; E. Crofton, *Some Notes on the Women's Committee of ASH. A Personal Account by Eileen Crofton* (ms, 1999). Copy in author's possession.

[59] Sir John Crofton autobiography, ms copy.

[60] D. Simpson, 'ASH: Witness on Smoking', in Lock, Reynolds, and Tansey (eds.), *Ashes to Ashes,* 209.

from the translation of the moral agenda into one which was justified by the tenets of risk factor epidemiology. It was an organizational style which became the model for other health activist organizations. The Coronary Prevention Group was established by a similar group of public health activists at the end of the 1970s. The reference to science was similar. The Canterbury conference in 1983 and its report on heart disease published in 1984 displayed many of the tactics which ASH had pioneered, and some of the same people were involved.[61]

ASH was an important insider–outsider organization. It was part of the policy community linked into smoking in the health department, but its utility also lay in its overt opposition, its absolutist stance which would always urge the government to more action. Its image was of a charitable body appealing for funds, and a pressure group at the same time. But its main funding, for this period at least, was from the Department of Health. It was very closely a part of a 'policy community' round smoking which had its links into government. But government, of course, also had other interests in the formulation of policy on smoking and many different government departments were involved. So far as the health interests were concerned, the existence of a body like ASH had clear advantages. ASH was useful to ministers. As Simpson pointed out 'there was brinkmanship over the grant each year', but 'good ministers expected us to attack and knew how to use a campaigning charity… there was a lot of stuff behind the scenes.'[62] Simpson, said one observer, 'knew how to influence people.'[63] ASH was used by the DHSS as the bogeyman in its negotiations with the tobacco industry over voluntary agreements. It was thus the model of an outside campaigning group, but also linked inextricably to government, both financially and in strategic terms.

It was able to fulfil this role because of its policy line. ASH had an extraordinarily broad policy agenda, but its overall aim by the end of the 70s, as we have seen, was to stop smoking. This was an absolutist agenda rather than one of moderation. The changed emphasis

[61] *Coronary Heart Disease Prevention. Plans for Action* (London: Pitman, 1984), HEC collection.
[62] Comments from Simpson at witness seminar at Ashes to Ashes conference on smoking at Wellcome Institute, 26–7 April 1995.
[63] Interview with journalist by Virginia Berridge, 15 March 1992.

of anti-smoking activism in the 1970s was paralleled by a new more general government emphasis on individual responsibility for health after the 1976 policy report *Prevention and Health: Everybody's Business*. ASH and its ally, the HEC, were representative of this more prohibitionist anti-smoking coalition and of a new style and content for public health and prevention more generally. ASH never forgot that it had held fire during the initiatives round tobacco substitutes in the 1970s, and that the launch of the third RCP report in 1977 had been eclipsed by the much publicized launch of New Smoking Material. The battle lines were drawn—as Simpson put it, 'If there was such a thing as a safer cigarette, then there would be no need for ASH.' The style and agenda of the organization was bound up with its stance of opposition to reduction of risk and in favour of its elimination. To achieve this necessarily pitted it against industry interests, but also against sections of government which saw the way forward in cooperation and voluntary regulation.

But these were later developments, as were the troubles which beset the organization after Simpson's departure. For much of the 1970s and 1980s ASH represented a new type of health voluntarism which had its parallels with social justice organizations such as Amnesty and Shelter. This was a pressure group which took its authority from its ability to translate scientific facts into media sound bites, while, at the same time, forming part of the policy community linking into health interests within government. It was in contrast to an organization like the Consumers Association, which shared its interest in tobacco. That organization had avoided the idea of direct activism in exchange for a different form of appeal to science. But the stress on science was common to both organizations.[64] It could be argued that ASH also had much in common with earlier pressure groups combining activism with expertise, for example, the inebriety organizations founded in the last quarter of the nineteenth century. These too mingled medical and lay membership with an appeal to science.[65] There were recognizably elements of that earlier package in ASH. But there were also significant differences, not least the close funding relationships with government

[64] M. Hilton, *Consumerism in Twentieth Century Britain: The Search for a Historical Movement* (Cambridge: Cambridge University Press, 2003), 206, also makes the point about the Consumers Association and science.

[65] V. Berridge, 'The Society for the Study of Addiction, 1884–1988', *British Journal of Addiction,* special issue, 85(8) (1990), 983–1087.

and the appeal to the public through the mass media.[66] ASH was the first of the health pressure groups actively to market the science of public health to politicians and to the public.

[66] This chapter has not considered the US voluntary situation in the smoking field which was different. There the cancer charities, in particular the American Cancer Society, pressed the issue on government initially. GASP (founded in 1971) was the Group Against Smokers' Pollution. American ASH was a separate organization. See C. Nathanson, 'Social Movements as Catalysts for Policy Change: The Case of Smoking and Guns', *Journal of Health Politics, Policy and Law*, 24(3) (1999), 421–88.

7

The New Public Health Package

Action on Smoking and Health (ASH) was typical of the new style public health pressure group of the 1970s. Its agenda by the middle of the decade was an absolutist one which stressed stopping smoking and began to focus on the media—campaigns and banning advertising—and on fiscal moves to reduce smoking through higher taxation. It also began to develop a strong human rights emphasis in relation to the rights of the non-smoker. ASH was one component of a 'new public health' which emerged during the 1970s. The developments in focus, philosophy, and scientific underpinning were epitomized in a number of policy documents published during the 1970s. The new public health was an international movement, and documents such as the Canadian Lalonde report of 1974 were important. In the UK, the government consultative document *Prevention and Health: Everybody's Business* issued in 1976 was overshadowed by the resignation of Harold Wilson as prime minister. The White Paper, *Prevention and Health*, was published at the end of 1977. It was influenced by the pioneer 1977 report on prevention from the Social Services and Employment Subcommittee of the Expenditure committee.[1] That committee's evidence was important for another reason too. It gave a snapshot of the players in the public health field and their attitudes towards the end of a decade: it was indicative of the attitudes of some key players. In its report the Committee saw smoking as a greater evil than alcohol and was willing to promote stronger measures for its control. It recommended an advertising ban; an annual price increase; the abolition of coupons; the restriction of cigarette machines; stronger health warnings on packets; more non-smoking areas; targeted education; action on weight and smoking; and more research into the problem of physiological addiction.[2]

[1] C. Webster, *The Health Services since the War, vol. ii: Government and Health Care. The British National Health Service, 1958–1979* (London: HMSO, 1996), 676–8.
[2] *First Report from the Expenditure Committee 1976–77 Session. Preventive Medicine, vol. i: Report* (London: HMSO, 1977).

This was the standard public health agenda by the end of the decade. As Alistair Mackie of the Health Education Council commented, the key issue was smoking: 'the big Beelzebub, the big destroyer, the 50,000 deaths a year one, is smoking. It has a sort of fascination for me that thirty six million pounds was the parliamentary answer for treating smoking-related diseases. It has a sort of bell-wether capacity; it leads all the other health education.'[3] Jerry Morris, the doyen of social medicine, showed, in his evidence, how the precepts of the 1940s and 1950s had transmuted into a new style of public health by the end of the 1970s. The public, he said, had to be 'educated into probabilities'. The issue of class was redefined as the social class gradient in lifestyle behaviours. In this Morris saw 'the perpetuation of the diseases of poverty, because of differences in personal behaviour in relation to the same social class factors as we saw were important in tuberculosis, bronchitis and rickets and so forth. This is a real mass educational thing.'[4] Morris' comments summed up the transmutation which had taken place by the end of the 1970s. This had been a crucial decade for public health. This decade had seen a huge change in the ethos and style of public health issues, developments which had been almost totally divorced from public health practice on the ground. By the end of the 1970s public health had developed a new agenda, more radical in some respects in its attacks on industrial interests and its demands for higher taxation of the risky products, but also narrower than the social medicine vision of social class and occupation. The following chapter will examine how this modernization of public health was achieved in relation to smoking. It drew on a mix of new and old—a focus on the role of women as mothers which had a long history within public health, but also a new reliance on hard-hitting mass advertising informed by social science and social psychology in particular. It also saw a new role for economic arguments and a growing focus by the end of the decade on the more general issue of inequality.

The Health Education Council (HEC) was an important force in the modernization of public health. Formed as a central body in 1968 out of the old Central Council for Health Education (CCHE) in the wake of the recommendations in the Cohen report, it had, as a 'semi

---

[3] *First Report from the Expenditure Committee 1976–77 Session. Preventive Medicine, vol. ii: Minutes of Evidence* (London: HMSO, 1977), Evidence of Alexander Mackie, Director General, Health Education Council Q.542, 119.

[4] Ibid., Evidence from Professor J. N. Morris, 30.

independent Board', clear advantages to government in that it allowed government to intervene directly when necessary but also to distance itself from responsibility for the content of campaigns.[5] The Council was reconstituted in 1973 at the time of the reorganization of the National Health Service (NHS). Smoking was a central concern for the new Council and its tactics exemplified the use of commercial consumerist and market-driven strategies which, as we have seen in Chapter 3, had also begun to develop in the public health field from the publication of the 1962 Royal College of Physicians (RCP) report. The Council, like ASH, developed an absolutist agenda on smoking in the course of the 1970s. ASH and the HEC formed a formidable public health duo. One of the HEC's earliest perceived successes was its advertising campaign in 1973 which used a picture of a naked mother smoking: this was mounted for the Council by the new advertising agency Saatchi and Saatchi. 'Is it fair to force your baby to smoke cigarettes?', it asked. The campaign raised many issues, not least that of the role of women in the 'new public health' and it is to this aspect which we now turn.

WOMEN AND PUBLIC HEALTH: WOMEN AS MOTHERS

Women emerged in the 1970s as a problem for public health and specifically in relation to smoking. In the initial incarnation of the 'problem' in the 1970s, this had echoes of the earlier debates at the turn of the nineteenth and twentieth centuries, of 'women as mothers' and the future of the race.[6] But there were several redefinitions from the 1970s of the way in which the 'woman issue' was seen in public health. The role of women as mothers was the concern in the 1970s: towards the end of the decade feminist concern developed a view of women's smoking which uncoupled it from women's reproductive function and tied smoking to issues current within feminism and communications theory. Initially the foetus had been the 'innocent victim' of the mother's smoking but then the women themselves became 'innocent victims' of media manipulation. The early 1980s brought a further redefinition through the emergence of the concept of 'passive smoking' as a scientific fact: women were seen as the non-smoking victims of their

[5] Webster, *The Health Services since the War*, 137–8.
[6] J. Lewis, *The Politics of Motherhood* (London: Croom Helm, 1980).

husbands' smoke. Such formulations and redefinitions were related to the dominant tendencies within post-war public health and with health-related feminism, and to ideas also about class and inequality.

Although women's smoking had increased during the War, smoking was overwhelmingly a male habit when the Doll–Hill findings were first published. In the 1950s, men and boys were by far the largest group of smokers in the UK. The earliest anti-smoking campaigns had therefore stressed the role of males. The CCHE leaflet of 1957 detailing the adventures of the Wisdom family and their discussion of whether to give up smoking focused on men and boys, not women. The participants were Mr Wisdom and his son, taking advice from a male GP. Mrs Wisdom had only a walk-on part, restricted to throwing up her hands in horror at the money wasted by smoking—'£70 a year—the price of a wonderful summer holiday abroad'.[7] Part of the Ministry of Health's reluctance to carry out a health education campaign in the wake of the new research had been the fact that this was a male rather than a female habit and therefore would be unusual as a public health campaign. Mr Pater in the Ministry of Health was told 'Public health campaigns in the past have tended to concentrate on mothers and young children ... A campaign against smoking would have to be directed mainly to men.'[8] This was considered to be inappropriate.

The 1962 RCP report had nothing specifically about females although there was a separate table of statistics relating to men and boys.[9] Despite the rise in female smoking there was little that was woman specific. Numbers of male smokers were far larger; and investigation into the effects of inhalation encouraged a belief that women smokers, many of whom did not inhale, would be less susceptible to the harmful effects of smoking. Women's smoking seemed less of a problem; and the implication was that the real problem was male. In the 1960s the CCHE commented,

We are greatly concerned to keep our skins clean and few of us would willingly drink dirty or polluted water. But the air we breathe is often appallingly filthy and therefore unhealthy. There are two reasons for this—general atmospheric pollution caused by the burning of large amounts of coal for industrial and

---

[7] Health Education Authority leaflet archive, *The Adventures of the Wisdom Family: No. 2, 'What—no smoking?'* (London: CCHE, 1957).

[8] National Archive, Ministry of Health papers, MH55/2220 (4), 1 April, 1957, Minute to Mr Pater about Medical Research Council (MRC) statement about the connection between smoking and lung cancer.

[9] Royal College of Physicians, *Smoking and Health* (London: Pitman, 1962), 4.

domestic purposes, and voluntary pollution by the individual of the air *he* [my emphasis] breathes—brought about by smoking.[10]

The front cover of Charles Fletcher's Penguin Special *Commonsense about Smoking,* published in 1963 after the RCP report, featured two wizened working-class boys smoking, recalling the turn of the century concern about juvenile male smoking, national deterioration, and hooliganism.[11] In the 1960s women were not absent from campaigns but had no special prominence. Illustrator Reginald Mount produced posters for the Central Office of Information which featured a female smoker as well as a male.[12] The Central Council's van campaign in 1962–3, which disseminated anti-smoking propaganda, had no suggestion that women were needed to provide a female role model, and little of the material produced was directed at women. In 1964, the Ministry of Health had produced a strip cartoon which featured Bobby Moore, 'the soccer star who never runs out of puff'. This appeared in children's magazines and comics and was specifically aimed at boys. 'A jolt for Johnnie from Bobby Moore'. Of the other sports stars taking part in the campaign, only one was female.[13]

The late 1960s saw a change in this male-only emphasis and the emergence of women into the gaze of health education. The technique and rise of the social survey was important in this process. John Bynner's study of *The Young Smoker* published in 1969 was of young schoolboys. In 1966 5,601 boys between eleven and fifteen from sixty schools were surveyed. This stressed the accepted view of the young smoker—that he was a working-class boy of low educational attainment, who had started smoking because of family influence and because it was considered 'tough'. Smoking boys had more out-of-home activities while non-smokers were more home-based and preferred to spend their money on books, sweets, and bicycle spare parts.[14] But McKennell and Thomas'

[10] HEA leaflet archive, leaflet reprinted from the CCHE magazine *Better Health*, no date but 1960s.

[11] C. M. Fletcher, H. Cole, L. Jeger, and C. Wood, *Commonsense about Smoking* (Harmondsworth: Penguin, 1963). Illustration 6.

[12] Young woman smoking with silver coins representing the expense of buying cigarettes: colour lithograph after Reginald Mount (Central Office of Information issued by Ministry of Health, Wellcome Library collection, BRN 22670). Illustration 8.

[13] Wellcome Library for the History and Understanding of Medicine, ASH archive, SA/ASH, William Norman collection, R.19, cutting.

[14] J. M. Bynner, *The Young Smoker. A Study of Smoking among School Boys Carried out for the Ministry of Health. Government Social Survey,* 383 (London: HMSO, 1969).

study, published in 1967, of *Adults' and Adolescents' Smoking Habits and Attitudes*, a survey carried out under the auspices of the Government Social Survey for the Ministry of Health, found its most striking trends in the smoking behaviour of females. The youngest age groups were found to be smoking earlier and in greater numbers than older women and this trend had accelerated since the end of the War. The pattern of female smokers, the survey concluded, had transformed over the past twenty years to resemble that of males. The legacy of past social taboos had operated to prevent older women smoking, but there was now nothing to prevent the incidence of smoking among women rising until it equalled that of men.[15]

In the late 1960s and early 1970s, in particular through the work of the Health Education Council, this emergent concern crystallized in the issue of women as mothers. The context of the time was important. Armstrong, in her analysis of the scientific debates which surrounded the establishment of parallel concern about women's ingestion of alcohol and the rise or discovery of Foetal Alcohol Syndrome (FAS), has drawn attention to broader social forces which contributed to this period of concern in the early 1970s. Among these were a period of environmental risk; the thalidomide disaster of the 1960s and the fear of what ingesting drugs could do to the foetus; rubella; and the rise of technology whereby techniques such as ultrasound enabled observation of the foetus. This foetus became more visible and women became seen as 'foetal containers'. It was feared that women, in the era of the pill, were stepping beyond their traditional roles and gaining control of reproduction. There was a maternal–foetal conflict which led to a punitive response. The 'baby boom' was coming to an end in the 1970s followed by a period of baby 'bust', which in its turn led to an emphasis on the quality rather than quantity of the population.[16] There were strong parallels between the women and alcohol debates and those round women and smoking. In Britain, the role of the social survey and of epidemiology were important technologies of observation.

The way in which the smoking and pregnancy issue was redefined in the 1970s shows how science and the media interacted in the new public health. There had been interest in the relationship between women's

---

[15] A. C. McKennell and R. K. Thomas, *Adults' and Adolescents' Smoking Habits and Attitudes. Government Social Survey 353/B* (London: HMSO, 1967).

[16] E. A. Armstrong, 'Diagnosing Moral Disorder: The Discovery and Evolution of Fetal Alcohol Syndrome', *Social Science and Medicine*, 47(12) (1998), 2025–42.

smoking and its impact on pregnancy since before the Second World
War although then the interest was in the health of women tobacco
workers, building on the occupational health interest of the time. In
the 1950s some research had suggested that smoking might prevent
a successful outcome to pregnancy. Researchers began to show that
when smokers and non-smokers were compared, the former had the
smaller babies. This was not initially seen as particularly worrying. The
eminent obstetrician Josephine Barnes commented in a collection on
The Dangers of Smoking edited by Charles Fletcher in the early 1960s
that such babies were not unhealthy and not difficult to bring up.[17] The
main hardening of stance came through the British Perinatal Mortality
survey whose participants were followed up in the National Child
Development Study, funded by the National Birthday Trust Fund.
The results emanating from this study provided the main evidence of
the association which were taken up within health education circles,
although not without controversy. Harvey Goldstein, Neville Butler,
and E. M. Ross published a paper in the *British Medical Journal* in April
1972 which concluded from a survey of 17,000 births in one week in
1958 and 7,000 late foetal and neonatal deaths from a three-month
period in the same year, 'an estimate can be made of the potential saving
in new born lives per year if all these women [regular smokers] could
be persuaded to stop smoking during pregnancy. With the 1970 overall
foetal and neonatal mortality rates, this might amount to a saving of
approximately 1,500 babies each year.' Goldstein also wrote an article in
Concern, the journal of the National Children's Bureau, which opened
with the statement that smoking during pregnancy 'caused the deaths
of 1,500 babies in Britain last year'.[18] The follow-up to this research,
according to one researcher on the study, was funded by the tobacco
industry. 'We found the connection between smoking and low birth
weight and Butler wanted to do further research but felt the tobacco
industry wouldn't fund it. I suggested they tell them that smoking led
to easier births—and so they got the money!'[19] The publications led to
controversy round causality which involved the statistician Peter Burch
and the American statistician Jacob Yerushalmy, but also to discussion
of what the correct line to advise mothers would be. An editorial in

---

[17] J. Barnes, 'Smoking and Motherhood', in C. Fletcher (ed.), *The Dangers of Smoking*,
reprinted from CCHE magazine for parents *Better Health,* HEA leaflet collection.
[18] The *Concern* article is referred to in 'Smoking, Pregnancy and Publicity', *Nature,*
245 (1973), 61.
[19] Interview with Ann Dally by Virginia Berridge, 18 July 1995.

Nature was critical of the unscientific nature of the results: no proper randomized controlled trial (RCT) could be carried out and these were entirely self-selected people who had given up. 'Lack of control over the observations undoubtedly led to personality entering in as a variable. The woman who can give up smoking easily is a different type of person from the one who cannot, and for all we know may be less prone to perinatal fatality and light babies.'[20] The question was what was to be done about this? Mothers, thought *Nature,* should be encouraged to stop, but not put under undue pressure. 'This study has not shown that the 1,500 babies could be saved because it has not shown that compulsory abstention produces the same sort of statistics as voluntary abstention. In fact, the later stages of pregnancy seem no time to try to break the habit, with all the well-known tensions that usually implies.'

The implications of the research were seen differently in the public health field than they were a decade earlier. The research led to a groundbreaking campaign mounted for the Health Education Council in 1973 by the new advertising agency Saatchi and Saatchi. There had been a few earlier women-focused materials which had concentrated on the links between smoking and losing sexual attractiveness—a HEC commercial based on 'Fag Ash Lil' in the early 1970s and a British Medical Association (BMA) Family Doctor leaflet which emphasized the connection with wrinkles. In 1973, the striking image of the naked mother smoking was the main image in a campaign which cost £160,000 and took up nearly two-thirds of the HEC's anti-smoking budget for the year. Two further campaigns were planned and over 20% of the HEC's anti-smoking budget was to go on smoking in pregnancy. There was a clothed version of the naked mother but evaluation concluded that it was less effective as a campaigning tool.[21] Some critics disputed the campaign's effect. Surveys commissioned by the HEC before and after the first campaign showed that the proportion of pregnant women among smokers had fallen from 39 to 20%. This seemed significant, but the research was flawed because it had not compared a group of pregnant women who watched the advertisements with a group of pregnant women who did not. HEC research into later campaigns showed no overall impact and also that

[20] 'Smoking, Pregnancy and Publicity'.
[21] *First Report from the Expenditure Committee 1976–77 Session*, vol. ii, Evidence from Department of Health witnesses, Q. 2137–8. Illustration 9.

15% of women who smoked stopped smoking anyway when they were pregnant.[22]

The Council's main preparatory work for the campaign had been based on a clothed model and had not used the nude option. Alistair Mackie, the director of the HEC, later explained that the nude emerged out of a conversation he had with his chief medical officer. 'I can remember thinking in a crude way what a tremendous topic this was for public relations work.'[23] There was no doubt however that the foetus at risk was male. The HEC press release for the second campaign said, 'Mums-to-be will be told that smoking can restrict the baby's growth, make *him* underdeveloped and underweight at birth and even kill *him*' (my emphasis).[24]

The problem was thus defined in the 1970s as women in their reproductive role, although there was little epidemiological evidence that this was the major issue. Smoking was rising and then, later in the decade, failing to decrease as swiftly as among men. But this was among women and young girls in general rather than specifically among pregnant women. But this way of seeing the issue was increasingly common in policy documents. The RCP reports on smoking had separate chapters on smoking and pregnancy from 1971 onwards. The Select Committee on Preventive Medicine, which sat in 1976 to 1977 and spent much time on smoking as emblematic of the new preventive medicine, also focused on pregnant women smoking. Dr Macara of the BMA stressed that stopping smoking was a family matter. 'One has to make one's attack simultaneously on parents and children, particularly on those who are most susceptible to good advice, such as the pregnant mothers, who can be shown that they are more likely to lose their babies and to have smaller babies who find it more difficult to survive when they are born (if at all) if they smoke.'[25] David Owen, as minister of Health at the time, was also strongly in favour of the approach which linked smoking and pregnancy.

[22] Wellcome Library for the History and Understanding of Medicine, ASH archive, William Norman collection, Box 77, R. 14, A. Mackie file, *Anti-smoking in Pregnancy Campaign: Pre and Post campaign Study* (Communication Research Ltd., May 1974); ditto (June, 1975). Also cited in B. Jacobson, *The Ladykillers: Why Smoking is a Feminist Issue* (London: Pluto Press, 1981).

[23] Jacobson, *Ladykillers*, 72.

[24] Wellcome Library for the History and Understanding of Medicine, ASH archive, William Norman collection, Box 77, R.19, A. Mackie file.

[25] *First Report from the Expenditure Committee 1976–77 Session, vol. ii*, Evidence from Dr Macara, Q.1715.

Not everyone accepted this definition of the problem. Certainly the mothers themselves were only minimally consulted. In 1976 an article appeared in *Social Science and Medicine* by the sociologist Hilary Graham, who reported on a research project which had taken account of the views of mothers who smoked. Graham pointed out that the health education agenda stressed the mothers' 'selfishness' or their reliance on 'old wives' tales' or on advertisements on television and in the media. She analysed the view of expectant mothers and showed that they were aware of the arguments, but differed in their assessment of the validity of the scientific case. Medical evidence was seen as a 'tale' and assessed against 'proof' which came from experience and through lay systems of referral. The 'wrong' sort of proof would not be accepted and there was antipathy to pre-packaged standardized information. Women, Graham concluded, assessed family needs rather than simply reproduction.[26] The women as mothers argument was coming under fire; ultimately this critique linked with the feminist arguments of the early 1980s. It also brought into the debate the 'view from below' and the arguments round inequalities which were to revive at the end of the decade.

THE NEW HEALTH EDUCATION

Women as mothers and the Saatchi campaign drew on some old turn of the century trends in public health remodelled in the advertising speak and style of the 1970s. That campaign and the new and enhanced role of the HEC was also symbolic of the role of the mass media and advertising within public health as it redefined itself in this decade. We have already seen in Chapter 3 how the Cohen committee of 1964 and the formation of the HEC in 1968 carried through a new centralized and technocratic agenda for health education which began to make greater use of the techniques of mass persuasion. The 1960s had begun to bring a change in tempo—towards a mass media focused, slicker, pre-tested by market research, advertising agency product. At the same time, the nature and content of the message changed—away from neutral information presentation, away from reduction of risk, towards more direct advice and an absolutist line. The Cohen report presented the advertising

---

[26] H. Graham, 'Smoking in Pregnancy: The Attitudes of Expectant Mothers', *Social Science and Medicine*, 10 (1976), 371–82.

and the PR sections of commercial organizations as models of effective action and expenditure. The image was one of up-to-date, media savvy professionals who knew their market. The 1960s were a boom time for advertising and market research in the UK. Membership of the Market Research Society grew from 23 to 2000 in the years between 1947 and 1972.[27]

Expenditure almost doubled on the HEC's smoking campaign in the early 1970s, after the further RCP report in 1971, and a reconstitution of the HEC itself. TV campaigns and press advertising were areas of growth: £413,899 was spent in 1972–3; £702,292 in 1973–4.[28] Research also became more important in the design of campaigns and their evaluation. The quantitative sociologist Ann Cartwright had evaluated a campaign carried out in Edinburgh in 1959. There had been another evaluation by the sociologist Margot Jeffreys in Hertfordshire in the early 1960s. In the 1960s, this style of research expanded. There was OPCS (Office of Population Censuses and Surveys) research on smoking; research surveys by the educationalist John Bynner on boys smoking; and research surveys by the public health researcher Walter Holland on the impact of health education on schoolchildren.[29] The social survey found a role in health through the smoking issue.

The new style of advertising campaign was mounted for the HEC by the advertising agency Saatchi and Saatchi. Saatchi's emerged originally out of the reconfiguration of advertising in the UK in the 1960s, under the influence of developments in the United States. Vance Packard's *The Hidden Persuaders* was published in 1957, and Charles Saatchi visited the United States in the early 1960s.[30] He recalled how the press advertising people dominated the UK advertising scene, with little knowledge of the possibility of TV. The new style agencies changed the image of advertising and started calling in academics to help—here was a more

[27] K. Williams, *Get Me a Murder a Day!: History of Mass Communication in Britain* (London: Hodder Arnold, 1997), 217.

[28] HEC Smoking and Health Campaign Activities *c*.1975. Typescript document in HEA (now HDA) information centre collection.

[29] Walter Holland, Interview by Michael Ashley Miller, Oxford Brookes University/Royal College of Physicians video interviews, May–December 1996. Interview with Walter Holland by Virginia Berridge, March 1997. J. M. Bynner, *Medical Students' Attitudes towards Smoking. A Report on a Survey Carried out for the Ministry of Health* (London: HMSO, 1967). Bynner, *The Young Smoker.*

[30] V. Packard, *The Hidden Persuaders* (London: Longmans, Green, 1957); A. Fendley, *Commercial Break. The Inside Story of Saatchi and Saatchi* (London: Hamish Hamilton, 1995).

professional scientific approach, also using typically a combination of humour and hard sell. Cigarette advertisements were among the first to use it, as for example in the Gold Box Benson and Hedges advertisements created by the agency Collett Dickinson and Pearce. The HEC account was Saatchi's first big break and marked the importation of the new advertising style into the ranks of the public health opposition. At first the work was confined to posters and brochures, but later came full-scale advertising. Saatchi produced a number of advertisements early in 1970 with the lines 'The tar and discharge that collect in the lungs of the average smoker' and 'You can't scrub your lungs clean' (Illustration 10). Images like these generated an anti-aesthetic around smoking; visible effects, such as the unsightly nicotine stains on fingers, provided a visual cue to deeper more significant damage. The rest of the media started to become interested. The *Sun* newspaper wrote about the anti-smoking campaign, noting how dynamic and brutally effective the copywriting was. Earlier hesitations about generating public fears concerning cancer were swept aside. Graphic images of diseased lungs were featured in posters asking, 'Why learn the truth about lung cancer the hard way?' In 1970, the Saatchi brothers formed the agency Saatchi and Saatchi and Charles Saatchi brought the HEC account with him. For the first time the anti-smoking campaign was extended to TV. Advertisements in 1971 showed smokers crossing London's Waterloo Bridge intercut with film of lemmings throwing themselves off a cliff. A voice-over said, 'There's a strange Arctic rodent called a lemming which every year throws itself off a cliff. It's as though it wanted to die. Every year in Britain thousands of men and women smoke cigarettes. It's as though they want to die.'[31]

This was the advertising style which developed into the women as mothers campaign and which was paralleled by the doleful pregnant man campaign 'Would you be more careful if it was you that got pregnant?' In early 1976 the HEC ran its third smoking in pregnancy campaign and also, for the first time in the world, so it maintained, a campaign aimed specifically at teenagers. By the mid-1970s the Council had spent around two million pounds on smoking alone since its formation in 1968. It was spending just over one hundred thousand pounds a year in the late 1960s but over £413,000 in 1972–3 and over £700,000 in 1973–4. The Scots also mounted a smoking and health campaign in

---

[31] Quoted in A. Fendley, *Commercial Break. The Inside Story of Saatchi and Saatchi* (London: Hamish Hamilton, 1995), 35.

1973–4 with four TV films and large advertisements. The advent of local commercial broadcasting offered health education opportunities.

EVIDENCE-BASED PUBLIC HEALTH: THE ROLE OF SOCIAL PSYCHOLOGY

In Chapter 3 we have seen how social medicine and emergent medical sociology were closely connected in the 1950s. The social medicine focus on class had begun to mutate to an emphasis on behaviour. Sociology was joined in the 1960s and 1970s by other social science disciplines, most notably social psychology and health economics. There were the technical tools of the new public health, the scientific package which underpinned chronic disease epidemiology. This reliance on the social sciences seems to have been a development common across other industrialized countries in Western Europe, after its inception in the United States earlier on. Certainly in France, health education campaigns on smoking began to use the mass media in the 1970s and to draw on social psychology and market research.[32] Luc Berlivet has drawn attention to the role of motivation research developed in the United States in the aftermath of the Second World War and used in French health education from the late 1970s.

This was a different role for psychology, less studied than its better-known role in the treatment and health service world from the 1960s. There, psychology emerged as part of the redefinition of treatment for substances like alcohol and illicit drugs and as a new development within primary care. Historians and sociologists have discussed the rise of psychology in general practice in the 1970s and also in new directions in alcohol treatment.[33] Developmental psychology became important in the post-war discussions of 'bonding' between mother and child.[34] Treatment was not important for smoking at this time nor

[32] L. Berlivet, 'Uneasy Prevention. The Problematic Modernisation of Health Education in France after 1975', in V. Berridge and K. Loughlin (eds.), *Medicine, the Market and the Mass Media: Producing Health in the Twentieth Century* (Abingdon: Routledge, 2005), 95–122.

[33] See, for example, D. Armstrong, *Political Anatomy of the Body. Medical Knowledge in Britain in the Twentieth Century* (Cambridge: Cambridge University Press, 1983), 113–14; B. Thom, *Dealing with Drink. Alcohol and Social Policy: From Treatment to Management* (London: Free Association Books, 1999), 140–2.

[34] D. Riley, *War in the Nursery: Theories of the Child and Mother* (London: Virago, 1983).

for public health in general. But there were areas of overlap in terms of the significance of psychology for the promotion of a general ethos of individual responsibility within society. Miller and Rose in a study of the Tavistock Clinic and the Tavistock Institute of Human Relations outline the links between psychological models and government strategy. Ideals drawn from psychological and psychoanalytic models of human relations and development spread into the social and public domain. A programme at the Clinic aimed at preventive mental health through family and group management and policies were implemented at the Institute aiming to promote these ideals within the workplace. These techniques became indiscernible from government techniques aimed at regulating subjectivity through the promotion of individual ideals.[35] Here was a congruence with the notions of individual responsibility which also came to animate public health.

However, historical research on psychology in the twentieth century has strangely neglected the importance of the discipline as part of the evidence-based paradigm in public health. [36] Psychological research in public health initially focused on attitudes and the modification of behaviour. Smoking, as one leading researcher commented, 'was run by the social psychologists in the early 1970s'.[37] Social psychology moved into public health through two routes: via the social survey and through commercially funded research, initially funded by the tobacco industry and later through the commercial research used to develop and evaluate mass media campaigns. Subsequent controversies over industry funding have detracted from the more general significance of those developments for the role of social science and public health. Here was a further stage in the focus on behaviour rather than class which had marked the social medicine publications of the 1950s. Tobacco industry-funded research was important but so, too was a more general interaction between academic and commercial forms of research which marked the field, in particular the links with market research.

In terms of the mass communication and health education side of public health, the emergence of psychology as a technical tool came

---

[35] P. Miller and N. Rose, 'The Tavistock Programme: The Government of Subjectivity', *Sociology*, 22 (1988), 171–92.

[36] The most recent publication, M. Thomson, *Psychological Subjects. Identity, Culture and Health in Twentieth Century Britain* (Oxford: Oxford University Press, 2006), makes no mention of the role of psychology within public health and addiction research and conceptualization.

[37] Interview with Michael Russell by Virginia Berridge, 16 February 1995.

initially via industry-funded research on motivation and through the work of the government social survey. Let us turn to see how this came about. Even in the earliest discussions of appropriate research into the smoking question, there had been pressure from health education interests for more social science research. The tenor of health education advice in the 1950s—that people should make up their own minds—also brought in its train the question of how to motivate that decision. In July 1957, Dr John Burton, medical director of the CCHE, had written to Sir John Charles, the chief medical officer, about the lack of social science research. He wanted a research project undertaken via CCHE or the MRC into epidemiological, motivational, and educational factors. 'While many hundreds of thousands of pounds are being spent on laboratory research it is being assumed that the educational aspects—on which, as far as I can see, the whole preventive policy now rests—are to operate with no accurate data and as yet no indication of any capital investment.'[38] The question was referred to the MRC, whose secretary Harold Himsworth, was unsupportive.

My own feeling is that problems of this kind, while of considerable interest, are fraught with great difficulties for the investigator. The trouble is that they lie in that uncharted territory between medicine, sociology and psychology, and few techniques have been devised for their investigation. It would be very easy to expend a great deal of effort merely to find out that one had found out what one knew anyway.[39]

Despite Himsworth's cynicism, out of this discussion did come the suggestion, later acted on, that the social survey section of the Central Office of Information should be asked to conduct a survey into the attitudes of smokers.

At the same time, the tobacco industry was taking on the psychological question. In the 1950s and 1960s the earliest contribution to the smoking field had come from psychologists trained in the psychoanalytic tradition. Smoking was not a rational activity but was linked to other forms of compulsive orality such as eating, drinking, and sex. The cigarette had obvious phallic associations for this literature.[40] This psychoanalytic school was criticized by the psychologist Hans Eysenck

[38] National Archives, Ministry of Health papers, MH 55/2224, 12 July 1957, Dr John Burton to Sir John Charles.
[39] Ibid., 30 August 1957, Himsworth to Charles.
[40] A. Marsh, *The Dying of the Light. Smoke Free Europe: 7* (WHO Euro and BMA, n.d. but *c.* late 1980s), discusses the earlier history of psychology for smoking.

in the 1960s. Eysenck argued that smoking itself was probably not the cause of disease but that the habit and the disease shared a common origin. He promoted the idea of a genetic predisposition to cancer: people who developed cancer were also predisposed to smoke. Eysenck's work was funded by the Tobacco Manufacturers Standing Committee. In its report for 1960, it listed research on the physiological and psychological aspects of smoking being carried out by Mass Observation Ltd in conjunction with Eysenck.[41] In an interview in 1996, Eysenck looked back on this period. 'In the 1950s I was interested in individual differences, personality differences—I was interested in the social consequences of individual differences. I wanted to derive a prediction from the theory which could be applied.'[42] Eysenck worked with an oncologist on the relationship between personality and cancer and whether repression of emotions influenced the development of cancer. 'Those who scored highly in emotional repression were six times as likely to have lung cancer.' There was also a synergistic relationship—and some repressed people needed fewer cigarettes to get lung cancer. Eysenck published papers on this in the 1960s.[43] Such theories were not 'mainstream' for smoking at the time, although personality theories were strongly supported in the addictions field, and Eysenck's reputation has suffered since because of the large sums he was paid from industry sources.[44] In the 1996 interview, he expressed the hostility of an outsider whose criticisms of epidemiology had been ignored. The epidemiology of smoking was

very primitive and unscientific. They take lung cancer patients and controls and how many smoke. That's fine on paper, but people who don't smoke are also different—through diet and alcohol. Social class is the most important in any disease. The expression 'kill' is used in quite a different way—the relationship to a death thirty years later is purely a statistical one ... It's only a correlation and badly confounded with other correlations. There's a relationship with personality, especially ... You cannot rationally look at smoking alone—it has differential effects on different types of person.[45]

---

[41] National Archives, Ministry of Health papers, MH55/2222, Report for the year ended 31 May 1960 of the Tobacco Manufacturers Standing Committee.

[42] Interview with Hans Eysenck by Virginia Berridge, 22 July 1996.

[43] H. J. Eysenck, *Smoking, Health and Personality* (London: Weidenfeld and Nicolson, [1965]).

[44] See list of special projects funded by the Tobacco Industry Research Committee, the Council for Tobacco Research, USA, and the Council for Tobacco Research, USA, Inc.: <http://tobaccodocuments.org/bliley-pm/26463.html>, accessed 31 July 2006.

[45] Interview with Hans Eysenck by Virginia Berridge, 22 July 1996.

Although Eysenck presented himself as an outsider in terms of public health epidemiology, personality theories were important in the emergent field of research studies across the substances in the 1970s—they were important for drugs and alcohol. But personality tests on smokers and non-smokers showed minute differences. As the psychologist Alan Marsh commented in a review of psychological theories, it was

not plausible that the tendency for half the population to become dependent on a life threatening habit is the outcome of some abiding personality syndrome. We would then be forced to accept that one fifth of smokers in advanced industrial countries have undergone a revision of personalities in order to stop ... By the end of the 1970s it was recognized that this line had run into the sand.[46]

Such theories were influential at the time; the tobacco industry began to use psychological theories derived from commissioned social surveys. Government also developed psychological work through the social survey. In 1966 the then Tobacco Research Council published Geoffrey Todd's *Reliability of Statements about Smoking Habits*, which took forward previous work which had been published at the end of the 1950s. D. H. Besse and G. W. Hoinville of Research Services Ltd were thanked for the research work.[47] Men had been interviewed at intervals since the late 1940s, with the latest interviews being carried out in 1964. Such work married market social survey work and psychology. It was overlapped with the psychological input into the government social survey work on smoking. Work was carried out in conjunction with McKennell and Thomas' research on adolescent smoking; the role of psychology was important and links with universities were developed on the new rational model of research funding. Bram Oppenheim, a psychologist at the London School of Economics, reported on discussion groups set up for 11–16 year olds.[48] McKennell's resultant report was strongly influenced by psychology with its talk of 'dissonant' and 'consonant' smokers. Dissonant smokers were those trapped by smoking

---

[46] Marsh, *Dying of the Light*, 13.
[47] G. F. Todd and J. T. Laws, *The Reliability of Statements about Smoking Habits, Tobacco Manufacturers Standing Committee, Research Report no. 2* (London: TMSC, 1958); G. F. Todd, *Reliability of Statements about Smoking Habits, Supplementary Report Tobacco Research Committee, 2A* (London: Tobacco Research Committee, 1966).
[48] National Archives, Ministry of Health papers, MH 151/27, Smoking and health; social surveys, 18 February 1965, A. N. Oppenheim, Children and smoking. Hypotheses derived from John Downing's report on ten discussion groups.

against their will, while consonant ones had no wish to give up smoking and rejected anti-smoking arguments. Here the idea of addiction started to emerge—dissonants were said to be more highly addicted than consonants. But social influence was the principle factor in making consonant smokers into ex-smokers. The research identified subgroups among the population—the middle class, better educated, religious or non-alcohol drinking all had a high proportion of non-smokers. It might be worth focusing anti-smoking campaigns on them to reduce numbers. McKennell used a model based on the social psychologists experiments on the effects of persuasive communications. Communication could produce a 'boomerang' effect if it was too far from the initial standpoint of the person receiving the message. In a marked change from the 1950s position of information giving and civic responsibility, the report pointed out that everyone knew about smoking and lung cancer so there was no point in efforts simply to inform the public. 'Effective communications have to be designed to counter the more sceptical defences of smokers.' It was important that communications built on the belief that the habit was helpful—'there seems little need to fear that a communication which recognizes that smoking can be helpful and pleasant will lower receptivity to negative themes.'[49] This research and the tobacco industry-funded research pursued similar lines. Emery, Hilgendorf, and Irving of the Human Resources Centre at the Tavistock Institute of Human Relations published a Tobacco Research Council paper in 1968 on *The Psychological Dynamics of Smoking*; McKennell also expanded his work on smoking typologies in a Tobacco Research Council paper in 1973.[50]

Government and industry interest in the insights of psychology ran parallel and often overlapped. In the 1970s, government funding of this type of research continued and psychology research became part of the developing research remit of the research councils. Part of the elaboration of the 'rational' model of research outlined by Rothschild was the negotiation between the research councils and government departments about who was responsible for areas of relevant research. The Medical Research Council (MRC) continued to be reluctant, as

[49] A. C. McKennell and R. Thomas, *Adults' and Adolescents' Smoking Habits and Attitudes*, Government Social Survey 353B (London: Ministry of Health, 1967), 5–6.
[50] F. E. Emery, E. L. Hilgendorf, and B. L. Irving, *The Psychological Dynamics of Smoking*, Tobacco Research Council Research Paper no. 10 (London: TRC, 1968); A. C. McKennell, *A Comparison of Two Smoking Typologies*, Tobacco Research Council research paper no. 12 (London: TRC, 1973).

it had been in the 1950s, to be involved in the communications and attitudinal side of psychological research. In 1971 a joint MRC/SSRC working party on smoking research was set up at the suggestion of the MRC's committee on epidemiology, chaired by Doll. The joint working party recommended that the SSRC fund work on attitudes to smoking, while research on biological aspects was remitted to the MRC's committee on the biological aspects of drug dependence, chaired by Sir William Paton. It was through the latter initiative that work on the psychopharmacology of smoking was funded in the 1970s and which was important for the establishment of concepts of addiction later on.[51] Most research on the psychological attitudes of smokers came through the DHSS and the SSRC. The GHS (General Household Survey) inserted a question on smoking in 1972 but then, according to one psychologist, 'it all went to sleep'. In the mid-1970s, things began to wake up again. Psychologists began to move away from the earlier personality theories towards new intellectual influences within the discipline. Fishbein and Ajzen's theory of 'reasoned action' brought cognitive psychology into the equation—this was the idea that people work out their behaviour for themselves. Research on this strategy began initially in a SSRC survey unit and then a large-scale Office of Population Consuses and Surveys (OPCS) study was funded designed to examine how attitudes could be changed by information and persuasion. This brought out publications in the 1980s.[52] By then, psychology as a public health technique and tool was no longer anything to question. Its rise was also closely linked to a new type of commercial model, the use of market research and evaluation of campaigns by the Health Education Council and the focus on children's smoking in the research carried out by people like Beulah Bewley and Walter Holland.

EVIDENCE-BASED PUBLIC HEALTH: ECONOMICS, TAXATION, AND INEQUALITIES

The new health paradigm—public health and health services research—being established in the 1970s also had a strong economic agenda. The rise of economics had come, as we have seen, through social medicine and its changes in the 1950s; the RCP reports and the subsequent

---

[51] Medical Research Council, *Annual Report 1972–73* (London: MRC, 1973), 30–1.
[52] Interview with Alan Marsh by Virginia Berridge, 3 November, 1997.

discussion of differential taxation; and the economic balance sheet of lives lost and gained provided for the Joseph cross-government enquiry. This emphasis on taxation as a public health tool and on an economic dimension to the public health argument was to become characteristic of the new public health in other areas as well. Health economics was coalescing as a separate specialty in this decade.[53] It was certainly the case for alcohol, where, during the 1970s, an internationally based group of public health researchers put the case for a set of population-focused public health policies for alcohol with a central role for taxation.[54] During the 1970s the economic arguments made about smoking began to change as the demography of smoking changed: governments began to use taxation for public health purposes. The period when Denis Healey was Chancellor of the Exchequer between 1974 and 1979 was important for this change. Alcohol and tobacco taxes became linked to the management of the economy during a period of crisis and the issue of the effect of taxation on people with different incomes was addressed. The 1974 Budget introduced the notion of essential and less essential goods, with wine, spirits, and tobacco being seen as less essential goods. The health case for taxation started to be accepted. Although it was not accepted in 1974, by 1976 the health case had gained economic weight. In 1977 a voluntary agreement agreed to drop advertising of high tar brands and in 1978 Healey raised taxation on higher tar cigarettes, specifically to alter consumption habits; this was the start of the differential taxation which had been discussed for so long.[55] Increased duty on cigarettes clearly had a considerable impact on consumption. Company reports showed that the tobacco companies themselves thought that increased taxation had been the major cause of a drop in sales. Changes in the excise tax had exceeded inflation in

[53] B. Croxson, 'From Private Club to Professional Network: An Economic History of the Health Economists' Study Group, 1971–1997', *Health Economics*, 7 (Suppl. 1), 59–545.

[54] K. Bruun, M. Lumio, K. Makela, L. Pan, R. Popham, R. Room, W. Schmidt, O. Skog, P. Sulkunnen, and E. Osterberg, *Alcohol Control Policies in Public Health Perspective* (Helsinki: Finnish Foundation for Alcohol Studies, WHO Regional office for Europe, Addiction Research Foundation of Ontario, 1975).

[55] W. Leedham and C. Godfrey, 'Tax Policy and Budget Decisions', in A. Maynard and P. Tether (eds.), *Preventing Alcohol and Tobacco Problems, vol. i: The Addictions Market* (Aldershot: Avebury, 1990), 96–132. M. J. Daunton, *Just Taxes. The Politics of Taxation in Britain, 1914–1979* (Cambridge: Cambridge University Press, 2002), 302–38 makes the point that the Labour government in the 1970s was rethinking the basis of its taxation policy and that it was no longer so easy for it to use taxation to extract money from the rich to give to the working class.

1974, 1975, and 1977 and this trend continued into the 1980s.[56] There was also competition from imports and unemployment. The tobacco industry began to diversify into other markets.

This economic cause became a central plank of the new public health stance. ASH had been involved in pressing the Chancellor for action on taxation for public health purposes. It had also consistently pressed an economic case before various official enquiries in the 1970s. Its evidence to the Royal Commission on Civil Liability in the early 1970s had pressed the case for the industry to be made liable for the damage its products caused. Again it gave evidence to the Royal Commission on the NHS in 1977 calling for a health levy on cigarettes. Five pence a pack would raise £350 million to pay for the cost of treating smoking-related diseases. Even Daube was moved to comment that the taxation policies of the Labour government had been quite successful.[57] In the late 1970s these arguments became powerfully connected with a revived political interest in inequalities and, for the first time, with a new generation of public health doctors. The arguments from health economics began to challenge the politicians' case round inequality at a time when health inequality was back on the political agenda. Inequality was rediscovered through the work of Titmuss and others in the 1960s when it had been thought that it would wither away with the coming of the NHS and of the post war welfare state.[58] The abrupt end of welfare state expansion after the 1973 oil crisis brought it further to the forefront and the 1970s saw a concentrated burst of research into inequalities in access to health care. In the 1970s under the aegis of Michael Young and the Institute of Community Studies, annual *Poverty Reports* contained updates of earlier Fabian essays on inequality. The Castle–Owen partnership at the Department of Health and Social Security set up the Resource Allocation Working Party, which reported in 1976. In 1977 their successors appointed the committee chaired by Sir Douglas Black to look at the more general questions in inequalities in health. Inequalities in health were back on the government agenda.

[56] M. Booth, K. Hartley, and M. Powell, 'Industry: Structure, Performance and Policy', in Maynard and Tether (eds.), *Preventing Alcohol and Tobacco Problems, vol. i: The Additions Market*, 151–78.

[57] M. Daube, 'The Politics of Smoking: Thoughts on the Labour Record', *Community Medicine* (1979), 306–14.

[58] C. Webster, 'Investigating Inequalities in Health before Black', in V. Berridge and S. Blume (eds.) *Poor Health. Social Inequality before and after the Black Report* (London: Frank Cass, 2003), 81–103.

This revival of inequalities was also apparent for smoking and the impact of media discussion was important for both areas. One impetus for action on inequalities had been a *New Society* article headed 'Dear David Ennals', written by Richard Wilkinson, a former Nottingham MSc student whose dissertation had been on the widening social class differential in death rates. Wilkinson had won a prize in an essay competition run by the food company Van den Bergh (Tony van den Bergh was an early supporter of ASH). He had thrown down a challenge to Ennals to do something. 'As Labour Secretary of State for Social Services you have the misfortune to be confronted by the largest social class differences in death rates since accurate figures were first collected.' The personal interaction with the Department of Health and Ennals' office after this article showed the power of the media to define such issues to ministers.[59]

A similar sequence of events developed for smoking. Atkinson and Skegg (later Townsend) had continued their work on taxation as a public health strategy. In March 1978, after the publication of the government's White Paper on prevention and health, Joy Townsend published an attack on the failure to commit to various anti-smoking initiatives, including an annual increase in the price of cigarettes. Recognizing the important advances which had been made, including a reduction by half in the tar content of cigarettes which could reduce the risk of lung cancer by a half, she drew attention to the disturbing class gradient in smoking which was developing. In the early 1960s, smoking had been a cross-class activity. By the end of the 1970s trends which showed sharp social class differences for lung cancer and bronchitis and also for heart disease and the rapid rise on women's mortality for all three diseases were visible. This 'waste of working class, working age life' called for a major three-part programme. Duty could be raised to increase the real prices of cigarettes by 56% over ten years, and so reduce demand by about 20%; advertising campaigns and sports promotions by tobacco companies could be greatly reduced; and health education could be raised to a major sustained programme costing about ten million pounds a year. This would save 8,500 lives rising subsequently to 22,000 lives a year. Townsend saw the results of such a coordinated programme as reducing the cost of living for the poorest rather than raising it. She placed faith in the power of health education to make a contribution to the public will

[59] V. Berridge, 'The Origin of the Black Report: A Conversation with Richard Wilkinson', in Berridge and Blume (eds.), *Poor Health*, 120–2.

to succeed. A recent Granada programme, *Report in Action*, had resulted in an overwhelming response from people wanting to quit—'mainly from the worse-off. People do need help. Only the government can act on the scale required.'[60]

Townsend's argument was part of the new public health consensus. More stringent measures like tax increases, hard-hitting health education informed by social psychology and communications theory, and an anti-industry line were becoming the norm for public health by the end of the decade. Inequalities as an issue was becoming the watchword for a new young public health profession emergent from the ashes of the 1973 reorganization. The ideology of public health had undergone a radical change in the 1970s: in the 1980s this knowledge base began to be assimilated by a profession in search of a new role.[61] Smoking had epitomized this transformation in public health, and its essential duality. There was the focus it offered on lifestyle issues and the role of individual behaviour, especially, as we have seen, the behaviour of females. But there was also the role it offered for 'evidence' and the social sciences.

[60] J. Townsend, 'Smoking and Class', *New Society*, 30 March 1978, 709–10.
[61] M. Bartley, *Authorities and Partisans* (Edinburgh: Edinburgh University Press, 1992).

8

Environment and Infectious Disease in the 1980s: From Passive Smoking to AIDS

The policy and scientific climates changed in the late 1970s and early 1980s. Concerns about the environment re-emerged as part of public health rather than separate from it. Epidemic disease, previously consigned to the 'dustbin of history', suddenly made a reappearance. New alliances emerged within the science of public health; epidemiology was no longer proof enough and gained greater legitimacy through support from biomedicine and the science of psychopharmacology. Occupational health revived as a public health matter. In Britain, the decade was marked at its start by the emergence of 'passive smoking' as a scientific fact and later by the irruption of HIV/AIDS as a central policy issue. The two appeared to be totally different, but as we will see, they were linked in the new public health discourse of environmentalism and infection. This discourse was an international one; and internationalism in public health was a defining feature of this decade.

The environment had been almost entirely absent from the redefined public health ideology which had emerged during the 1970s. Government policy documents placed responsibility on the individual and behavioural modification of individual lifestyle. New concerns about occupational health or about environmental pollution had no particular connections with public health. Rather they had emerged as separate 'single issues' through organizations which had little to do with formal public health. Greenpeace and Friends of the Earth had both been founded in 1971. They were part of the rise of pressure group activism exemplified by Action on Smoking and Health (ASH) in the health field, but the 'environmentalism' of the 1970s had few connections with public health concerns.[1] Infectious diseases were also remote from 'modern' public health, although in a different way. They were a feature of the past, associated with pre-war diphtheria or the even more distant environmentally induced diseases, like cholera, or typhoid, in the nineteenth century. The revolution in high-tech medicine of the 1950s had removed the need to worry about such epidemic incursions: penicillin, the antibiotics would deal with it all. The rise of the chronic diseases as central to population health had removed the centrality of epidemic disease. Or so it was thought. The 1980s were to witness a revival of environmentalism and also a revival of epidemic disease but within a different form within public health. The environment and the individual reached a new accommodation.

Epidemics and the environment were interconnected: a key issue which came to symbolize this interconnection was the irruption of 'passive smoking' as a scientific fact onto the public health scene. Passive smoking symbolized the redefinition of public health in the 1980s: it married the 1970s 'population health' emphasis on the behaviour of the individual as part of the population with an environmental turn. It reintroduced the idea of infection within public health. For ETS (environmental tobacco smoke) was an infective agent for the population at large. Passive smoking also symbolized new scientific alliances within the public health fold. The 1970s had been the decade when the social sciences came to be used as technical tools. In the 1980s the legitimacy of passive smoking was predicated on an emergent alliance between epidemiology and pharmacology, disciplines which previously had been distant from each other in scientific terms. Such alliances and influences developed further with the advent of HIV/AIDS as a policy issue towards the end of the decade. HIV/AIDS represented the central re-emergence of epidemic infection on the public health stage.

The revival of environmentalism and infection was accompanied by a new militancy within public health both in the UK and at the increasingly important international level. Passive smoking both stimulated and represented a rupture with industrial interests. This was a strategy which some public health activists had worked towards in

[1] M. Jackson, 'Cleansing the Air and Promoting Health. The Politics of Pollution in Post War Britain', in V. Berridge and K. Loughlin (eds.), *Medicine, the Market and the Mass Media. Producing Health in the Twentieth Century* (Abingdon: Routledge, 2005), 221–43, surveys these developments but does not draw out the separation from health concerns.

the 1970s and which was also the aim of some industrial interests. The smoking issue became more 'heroes and villains' or 'them and us', more adversarial in general style. Industry, as Sir Peter Froggatt, the new chair of the Independent Scientific Committee on Smoking and Health (ISCSH), noted, focused on disproving the science rather than modifying it as previously. This scientific and policy advocacy and opposition was a mirror image of harsher attitudes towards many public health issues on the part of the new Conservative government which was elected in 1979.

POLITICAL RUPTURE

Let us look at the political rupture first. What was striking about the early years of the new government was just how many public health initiatives initiated by the previous Labour administration were abruptly overthrown. Smoking, alcohol, inequalities, diet, all saw political change. The stories are usually told separately but there were interconnections, in particular for the subsequent fate of smoking and health inequalities as policy issues. Such events also provided the context of the revival of public health as an occupation during the 1980s. This 'new public health' took on an oppositional stance initially in part because of its exclusion from the corridors of power.

The story of what happened to smoking is well known.[2] The arrival of Sir George Young in the new government as junior health minister with responsibility for prevention brought a stand-off with the industry over proposals to regulate or ban tobacco advertising. Discontent on the backbenches and industry pressure led to his removal in the autumn of 1981 and replacement by Geoffrey Finsberg, who was more sympathetic to industry interests. Patrick Jenkin, the Secretary of State, who had supported Young's stance, was promoted to the Department of Industry and replaced by Norman Fowler, who had long supported individual liberty arguments, as for example in his opposition to legislation on seat belts. Dr Gerard Vaughan, the only survivor at the Department of Health and Social Security (DHSS), was subsequently replaced as minister of Health by Kenneth Clarke, who had connections with the tobacco industry. The sequence of events was later used as the basis of

---

[2] See P. Taylor, *Smoke Ring: The Politics of Tobacco* (London: Bodley Head, 1984), Chapter 8, 'The Freedom Fighters'.

an episode in the popular TV series *Yes Minister*, for which Young acted as adviser (the programme was transmitted in 1986).

The events represented an attempted reordering of the balances which had operated within policy. The civil servants in the DHSS favoured moderate reform and 'holding the ring' between interests; Young, who was a member of the Commons All Party group on smoking and of ASH, represented the 'new public health'. Outside government, the industry was also changing: overseas US-dominated interests were more important than they had been in the period from the 1940s to the 1970s. The corporate relationships with Imperial were less important than they had been. Young used outside pressure groups like ASH (now under the directorship of David Simpson) much as David Owen had used ASH and Daube some years earlier.[3] A briefing written in the spring of 1979, before the change of government, summed up the attitudes of the civil servants in the negotiations leading up to the renewal of the voluntary agreement and threw light on the way in which the balancing act within government operated. A major speech on smoking by the minister, it suggested, would be appropriate as negotiations with the industry got under way. The object would be to soften up the industry and rally public opinion to the extent necessary to achieve the government's objectives. The civil servants noted that an advertising ban would be promoted strongly by anti-smoking interests; but they opposed 'anti smoking' in their document to 'lower risk smoking'. Relations with industry were

good, formally and informally ... The strained relations with one or two firms over substitutes have not left a permanent scar. If there is any scar it should largely disappear with the retirement at the end of this month of the Imperial Chairman (Mr Garrett). Industry are genuinely grateful for the Government's adherence to agreements. Informally, they expect to have substantial new proposals put to them during the next round of negotiations.

Other government departments were a problem—not the Treasury, however. 'Relations with the Treasury have been excellent; Treasury Ministers fought hard and successfully for the high tar tax and have publicly acknowledged the part which health factors must play in fiscal policy.' Not all departments took the same line. 'Relations with the DoI [Department of Industry] have come under some strain—on substitutes, loans to tobacco firms and awards to industry. Ministers

---

[3] Interview with David Simpson by Virginia Berridge, 8 July 2003.

have had to fight hard to maintain the health factor. Similarly with DoE [Department of the Environment] as regards sports sponsorship.'⁴

These established relationships were ruptured during negotiations. The industry wanted to maintain the focus on safer cigarettes and product modification while advertising was of greater interest to Sir George and the anti-smokers. In a speech on the role of government to a conference on smoking and smoking-related diseases at the National Health Service (NHS) training centre in Harrogate in December 1980, he stated this clearly.

I am bound to say this [lower risk smoking] has a relatively low priority in my book ... I cannot be as enthusiastic—all cigarettes are dangerous and there is always the risk that smokers will be confirmed in their habits by a belief that Low Tar cigarettes are somehow safe.

A greater priority was to get future generations to give up and to change attitudes to smoking in public places. 'In Alexander Fleming House [then the DHSS HQ] one is greeted by the sight of a hall porter chain smoking next to a 'No Smoking' sign.'⁵ Daube, in a speech to the same conference, noted that Sir George's arrival would disrupt the comfortable stance of civil servants in the DHSS who saw their job to 'hold the ring' between health interests and industry interests. But the situation was complicated by the transfer into the Health department's civil servant team of Ray Petch, who had had friendly relationships with the industry during many years in Customs and Excise, a department with close contacts with the tobacco industry. In January 1980 he pointed out that he brought to his new job the advantages of having been closely concerned with tobacco taxation and VAT between 1969 and 1972. He had then moved to the London Business School, and also had been a 'cigarette addict' for 25 years. 'Also that I had lunch with Sir James Wilson and Mr Grice on Friday' (Chairman and Director, respectively, of the Tobacco Advisory Council).⁶ Petch was to become

---

⁴ National Archives, Ministry of Health papers, MH 148/1469, 16 March 1979. Notes from B.A.R. Smith on smoking and health, circulated for discussion at Secretary of State's strategy meeting, 21 March 1979.

⁵ HEA collection (later HDA, now NICE), Smoking and Smoking-Related Diseases, Proceedings of a seminar held 3–5 December 1980, NHS Training and Studies Centre, Harrogate. Unit for Continuing Education Department of Community Medicine, University of Manchester.

⁶ National Archives, Department of Health papers, Cigarette smoking and health; medical, commercial and policy aspects, 1979–1981, memorandum from Ray Petch, 14 January 1980.

notorious to anti-smoking interests later in negotiations over the possible transfer of Mike Daube to the HEC.

This rupture of established relationships or 'policy communities' in health was also the case in other areas of policy. The fate of the Black report on inequalities in health was another cause célèbre. Commissioned by the Labour government, which had set up a working party to look at this issue in 1977, the report was presented to the incoming Conservative government nine months after the 1979 election victory. It was published on the August Bank Holiday 1980 by Patrick Jenkin but without any commitment to its proposals. One of the reasons for the delay and poor timing of the report's presentation was severe disagreement on the committee itself between two leading members, Professors Peter Townsend and Jerry Morris, who, as Morris stated in a seminar on the report in 1999, had a major difference of opinion, 'a sort of Isaiah Berlin view of two great values colliding which are incompatible and you can't do anything about it.' It was a clash between social medicine and sociology, as the scientific secretary to the committee, Stuart Blume, characterized it: it was about how the changes were to be funded and whether hospital services were to take second place to those in the community.[7] But the 'non-publication' form of publication led to greater interest being paid to the report than otherwise might have been the case; and the fate of the report led to more research on inequalities in the 1980s. This became a growth area of research.

This media furore underlined the changed attitude to health issues of the incoming government. The Central Policy Review Staff Report on alcohol, commissioned in 1977 and produced in March 1979, likewise fell foul of electoral timing. The report argued for the population theory of alcohol consumption which was part of the epidemiologically based 'new public health' case. It wanted a coordinated response across government departments with a range of measures, such as price and availability controls. Never officially published, it finally appeared in a 'pirated' edition in Stockholm in 1982, while the government published its own new document, *Drinking Sensibly*, in the same year.[8] A similar sequence of events marked the

---

[7] V. Berridge and S. Blume (eds.), *Poor Health. Social Inequality before and after the Black Report* (London: Frank Cass, 2003).

[8] K. Bruun (ed.), *Alcohol Policies in United Kingdom* (Stockholm: Studies in Swedish Alcohol Policies, 1982).

NACNE and COMA reports on diet and heart disease, where the latter's report, published in 1984, took a more circumspect attitude to the role of dietary fat.[9] Such events were part of the reordering of relationships around health issues which marked the new government.

The recommendations of the Black report did not lead to formal government policy initiatives, but its rejection did, as the 1999 seminar participants remembered, lead to a growth of research on the subject and an 'underground' interest. At least forty articles a year were published on inequalities throughout the 1980s; and the rerun of the 'government censorship' battle over the follow-up report, *The Health Divide*, in 1987 drew further public attention. For the new generation in public health, work on what came to be known as 'variations in health' was a key aspect of their work in public health. The health services researcher Nick Black, one of those public health 'Young Turks', remembered in 2004, 'samizdat publications ... in public health ... there was a very exciting period in the early 1980s when I think public health was much more political, and I can remember all sorts of exciting fringe events.'[10] The sociologist David Blane remembered a senior civil servant telling him,

it was absolutely naïve to expect someone like Peter Townsend would get funding for any further research in the area of health inequalities in the 1980s and most of the work that was done then was done by people like John Fox and Peter Goldblatt at City University, who were very much going against the grain, and whose careers, I mean they left academic work and went back into the civil service in a way to escape the fallout.[11]

This underground culture of interest in inequalities was important because it marked a generation of new entrants to public health who went on to have significant roles in health promotion and health services research and in the revived occupation from the late 1980s. It was also significant for the particular issue of smoking. This issue increasingly intersected with academic and policy discussions of inequalities as the social profile of smoking rapidly altered during the decade.

[9] M. W. Bufton, 'British Expert Advice on Diet and Heart Disease, c.1945–2000', in V. Berridge (ed.), *Making Health Policy. Networks in Research and Policy after 1945* (Amsterdam: Rodopi, 2005), 125–48.

[10] Nick Black speaking in the witness seminar on recent public health, in V. Berridge, D. Christie, and E. M. Tansey (eds.), *Public Health in the 1980s and 90s: Decline and Rise?* (London: Wellcome Trust, 2006).

[11] David Blane speaking in the witness seminar on recent public health, in Berridge, Christie, and Tansey (eds.), *Public Health in the 1980s and 90s*.

THE RISE OF PASSIVE SMOKING

It was in this changed political and public health situation that passive smoking arrived on the scene as a scientific fact, and, quite quickly, became a policy fact as well. Environmental tobacco smoke reintroduced the environment centrally into discussions of tobacco, into activist public health discussions, after some decades of absence. The policy significance of passive smoking was considerable. It was a 'science waiting to happen' in the sense that the policy objectives of the anti-smoking alliance had already begun to shift in the direction which the new science supported. ASH had been gathering international evidence on the rights of the non-smoker since 1975. As Peter Froggatt, chair of ISCSH during the 1980s later commented, 'The argument that smokers poison only themselves (or their unborn children?) can no longer be convincingly sustained. The conceptual framework within which government, industry, and the profession have worked, is fundamentally changed.'[12] The nature of its emergence as a scientific and a policy fact shows a symbiosis of political and scientific developments: the re-emergence of the environment as a health issue; the change from a rights-based activist discourse to a science-based one; a new role for technology and new scientific alliances within public health.

The connection between air pollution and the rise in lung cancer had, as we have seen, been dropped as a focus of scientific discussion in the 1960s. The Royal College of Physicians' (RCP) subsequent report on air pollution attracted none of the press coverage which had marked the earlier smoking report. The Medical Research Council (MRC) funded a unit at St Bartholomew's Hospital to look at air pollution after the 1952 great London smog; it was funded out of part of the MRC's tobacco benefaction. But Pat Lawther, later its director, remarked in an interview in 2003 that the research in that unit had gone down the wrong track. They 'got it wrong—they worked on small particles and it was large particles'. The MRC did not renew funding of the unit after the mid-1970s.[13] Environmental issues were not central to public health. Environmental activism took other routes in the 1960s

---

[12] P. Froggatt, 'Determinants of Policy on Smoking and Health', *International Journal of Epidemiology*, 18 (1)(1989), 1–9.
[13] Interview with Pat Lawther by Virginia Berridge and Suzanne Taylor, 3 February 2003.

and 1970s, in particular through the issues of car transport and of lead in petrol. This was in contrast to the early advent of environmentalism in the United States in the 1960s, where there was some input from traditional public health concerns about water purity and sanitation.[14]

The rise of asbestosis as an issue can, with hindsight, be seen as a marker of new developments which were to bring the environment back in to public health. The discovery of the health hazards of asbestos in the 1970s and the connection with lung cancer brought cancer and specifically lung cancer back on the agenda as an environmental and an occupational issue—one which was more specifically located than the vaguer environmental associations of the 1940s and 1950s.[15] The established connection between smoking and lung cancer drew tobacco into the discussion. Here was a precursor of the combination of environment and individual which passive smoking came to symbolize. It was significant, too, that this environmental concern surfaced as an occupational health issue, paralleling the earlier occupational emphasis of social medicine in the 1940s.

The issue of smoking and its impact on the environment had been on the policy agenda since the 1960s but it had no particular significance until the end of the 1970s. Let us first look at how the issue had been discussed in those years. The need to restrict smoking in public places was on the agenda of the RCP reports from the start and was always discussed in the various Cabinet and other governmental committees. But it usually fell foul of the 'social acceptability' argument, the lack of willingness to interfere with a public habit which might have electoral repercussions. In the early 1960s, for example, in the memoranda presented by officials to the Cabinet committee, the Home Office and the Scottish Office surveyed restrictions which might be possible in places of entertainment:

If it could be shown that smoking in an enclosed place is injurious to the health of other persons present a different situation might arise. But there is no evidence that this is so. The most that can be said is that smoking in cinemas may be a nuisance to other persons.

[14] C. Sellers, 'Worrying about the Water: Sprawl, Public Health and Environmentalism in Post World War Two Long Island', seminar paper at LSHTM, 7 April 2006.

[15] P. W. J. Bartrip, *The Way from Dusty Death. Turner and Newall and the Regulation of Occupational Health in the British Asbestos Industry, 1890–1970* (London: Continuum, 2001); G. Tweedale, *Magic Mineral to Killer Dust. Turner and Newall and the Asbestos Hazard* (Oxford: Oxford University Press, 2000).

Such restrictions would be ignored—as Young's comment on the DHSS shows they were even in the early 1980s. The civil servants suggested the encouragement of voluntary action—and their comments underline the 'cranky' image of non-smoking at this time. 'There could be non smoking restaurants as there are vegetarian restaurants, frequented only by persons who wish to partake of the fare provided.'[16] The perception of the issue as a moral one was in part because the major arguments against smoking in public places came from the National Society of Non Smokers (NSNS), who argued that such habits were selfish. 'Lines on the tobacco habit' published by the Society, typified this position:

> In how many houses all over the land
> Is tobacco the tyrant, for ever at hand
> Pervading each room and polluting the air?
> So long as they're at it, the smokers don't care
> How others may suffer who cannot avoid
> The horrible fumes with which they're annoyed.
> They do not, these smokers, consider at all
> What to *them* may be sweet, may be bitter as gall
> To those who prefer to breathe air clean and pure
> But who daily, and hourly, that smoke must endure.
> How *selfish* they are—what perversion of taste,
> Continuous bad manners, uncleanness and waste.[17]

Related initiatives, such as the Order of Fridayites whose members took a pledge to abstain from smoking on one day a week (usually either Thursday or Friday), gave the environmentalist case against smoking a fusty temperance tinge.[18]

Occasional initiatives were reported to restrict smoking in public space. But these were not always successful: the introduction of no smoking areas in the Classic cinema chain in the 1960s was widely ignored. In 1963, when Charles Fletcher suggested to Sir Basil Smallpiece, managing director of British Overseas Airways Corporation (BOAC), that the airline should introduce non-smoking sections on its

[16] National Archives, Cabinet Office papers, CAB 130/185 GEN 763/4, 2 April 1962, Home Office and Scottish Office memorandum, Restrictions on smoking in public places.
[17] National Archives, Ministry of Health, papers quoted in NSNS publicity material sent to MH, MH 55/2221.
[18] National Archives, Ministry of Health papers, MH 55/2221, also has details of the Fridayites.

aircraft, the matter was rejected as both commercially and practically impossible.

The problem is fundamentally one of priorities. To do as you firstly suggest—marking certain rows 'non-smoking' implies that we would allow passengers to choose their own seats when they embark. If we were to do this, not only should we get vigorous complaints from the smokers forced by lack of space into the non smoking rows, but we should be unable to provide for other reasonable seating requirements in the way that our present system permits ... Although a non-smoker myself, I believe that for long distance air travel the sort of seating preferences I have listed above have a higher priority than the non-smoker's dislike of being near to smokers. I am reinforced in this view by the very small number of complaints that we receive from non-smokers.[19]

The evidence on public attitudes to the environmental impact of smoking was somewhat contradictory. Although there seemed to be widespread toleration of public smoking, the sociologist Ann Cartwright's evaluation of the Edinburgh health education campaign at the end of the 1950s had shown greater public support for the nuisance effect of smoking than there was for the epidemiological case. The evaluation provided suggestive evidence of a greater degree of potential environmentalism in popular views than was reflected either in science or in policy. Cartwright's evaluation provided an illustration of public attitudes to smoking in the aftermath of the campaign conducted in Edinburgh on the basis of the Doll–Hill results in the 1950s. Most of those researched had heard of the theory about the relationship between smoking and lung cancer but few accepted it. The anti-smoking campaign had produced a rise in the proportion of the population who thought smoking was harmful to health but no change in behaviour—a classic failing of such health campaigns. The evaluation revealed popular attitudes which were distinct from the scientists' case. People thought smoking was harmful to health in ways which the campaign had not mentioned. They believed that smoking would harm the health of others. Twenty cigarettes a day was seen as the boundary between safety and danger and there was strong support for restrictions on smoking in public, although little enthusiasm for an advertising ban or an increase

[19] Wellcome Library for the History and Understanding of Medicine, ASH archive, Box 19 (old series), 24 January 1963, letter from Sir Basil Smallpiece to Charles Fletcher.

in duty.[20] These were results which suggested popular support for nuisance rather than for science. To some degree they were supported by the government social survey research on smoking. This focused to a greater extent on smokers and their attitudes rather than public attitudes and was informed by social psychology. However, the results there also underlined a high degree of support among non-smokers for the 'aesthetic' and 'nuisance' arguments on smoking. But many smokers who supported other negative statements about smoking did not agree. The survey report concluded that if these arguments were to be emphasized in publicity there was a danger of a boomerang effect in attitudes.[21] This was the research equivalent to the politicians' fears about electoral support. The key issue at this stage was the balance of emphasis to be struck and the dominant social culture which favoured smoking. In 1979, an industry spokesman, reviewing a speech by the director general of the World Health Organization (WHO) on tobacco and disease, summed this up: 'the social acceptability issue will be the central battleground on which our case in the long run will be won or lost.'[22]

The dominant culture of smoking was changing during the 1970s. Middle-class smokers began to give up while working-class ones continued to smoke. The RCP's 1977 report noted that the percentage of professional people and doctors smoking had dropped. The previous twenty years had seen the development of a social class gradient in smoking, although the proportion of women (and nurses) had continued to rise.[23] The Pizza Express chain, attractive to a middle-class clientele,

---

[20] A. Cartwright, F. M. Martin, and J. G. Thomson, 'Distribution and Development of Smoking Habits', *Lancet*, 274 (1959), 725–7; *eidem*, 'Efficacy of an Anti Smoking Campaign', *Lancet*, 275 (1960), 327–9; A. Cartwright, J. G. Thomson, and a group of Edinburgh DPH students, 'Young Smokers. An Attitude Study among Schoolchildren, Touching Also Parental Influence', *British Journal of Preventive and Social Medicine*, 14 (1960), 28–34; A. Cartwright, F. M. Martin and J. G. Thomson, 'Health Hazards of Cigarette Smoking, Current Popular Beliefs', *British Journal of Preventive and Social Medicine*, 14 (1960), 160–6.

[21] A. C. McKennell and R. K. Thomas, *Adults' and Adolescents' Smoking Habits and Attitudes*, Government social survey 353/B (London: HMSO, 1967).

[22] Quoted in Royal College of Physicians, *Smoking and the Young. A Report of a Working Party of the Royal College of Physicians* (London: RCP, 1992), 16.

[23] Royal College of Physicians, *Smoking or Health. A Report of the Royal College of Physicians. The Third Report from the RCP of London* (London: Pitman Medical, 1977); *idem, Health or Smoking? Follow-up Report of the Royal College of Physicians* (London: Pitman, 1983).

were the first restaurants successfully to introduce restrictions—in 1976. Restrictions on smoking in hospitals and the more general issue of restrictions on public places had always figured in the various RCP reports. But they had not been given any particular prominence. Charles Fletcher, in a letter to Daube in 1973, commented that 'we are interested in the health aspects of smoking, not the moral aspects of it ... we should be concerned about the inconvenience which smokers cause to non-smokers, but this is a very minor aspect of health.'[24] The scientific basis for such a moral or rights agenda appeared to be lacking as Fletcher's comment underlined. In the 1970s the activists found little science to support their position. In 1973 the ASH expert group had looked at the risks of pipe and cigar smoking and had considered 'so called "passive smoking"' using a recently published report from the US Public Health Service. It concluded

The present evidence indicates that there is virtually no risk to the healthy non-smoker apart from exceptional exposure to tobacco smoke in an unventilated room or a close car, but patients already suffering from chronic bronchitis or CHD may suffer adverse health effects.[25]

ASH placed greater emphasis on the nuisance argument at that stage. 'In public places, the right to be free from smoke should have a higher priority than the right to smoke. Non-smoking should be considered the normal practice, and special areas should be set aside for those who wish to smoke.'

As the public health case hardened during the 1970s, a new environmentalism started to creep into the language of the more militant activists and this constituency developed a more aggressive stance on the pollution of public space. Initially the argument remained a moral one, not based on science. The argument continued the moral argument of the earlier NSNS activists, but redefined it as a rights-based one. The rights of the non-smoker were at risk. This was an important development because it brought the anti-smoking activist position within the civil liberties arena which had standing in radical circles. In 1977, Mike Daube wrote in a letter to David Ennals, Labour Secretary of State at the DHSS, telling him about plans to hold a conference on 'The Rights of the Non-Smoker' at the King's Fund:

---

[24] Wellcome Library for the History and Understanding of Medicine, ASH archive, Box 19 (old series), 28 September 1973, Letter from Fletcher to Daube.
[25] HEA (later HDA and then NICE), leaflet archive. *Pipe and Cigar Smoking. Report of an Expert Group, 1973.*

part of the purpose of the conference is to ensure that attention paid to the rights of the non-smoker in future focuses on the serious social aspects of the campaign rather than the more eccentric elements which have received attention in the past.

The conference speakers included Stephen Lock, editor of the *British Medical Journal* (*BMJ*), on 'Whose Rights?', Professor John Colley on 'Involuntary Smoking', Eileen Crofton of Scottish ASH on 'The Hospital Patient', and Eva Alberman on 'The Unborn Child'. An ASH survey of twenty European countries had shown that Britain came seventeenth in provision for non-smokers. The purpose of the conference was to launch a new British campaign for the rights of non-smokers.[26] ASH and the public health coalition were launching an argument based on rights rather than science. They aimed to overturn the industry-promoted argument—that smokers harmed no one except themselves—by arguing that one person's freedom to smoke compromised another's right not to have to inhale. This was a broader argument than the nuisance–selfishness moral agenda of the NSNS. But it was not a scientific argument; the issue was defined as one of rights, not of 'scientific facts'. It symbolized the 'new activism' of anti-smoking in the 1970s but did not fit within the epidemiological discourse of risk. The new argument made some members of the radical wing of British public health uneasy. Sheila Adam, later a leading public health figure, commented in 1980

If the philosophy of 'victim blaming' is accepted then to blame the smoker may not only be unhelpful but unfair. The increasing interest in the issue of passive smoking ... is likely to lead to greater assertion on the part of non-smokers of their rights to a smoke-free environment ... it is important that the possible adverse effects of this change are anticipated.[27]

Then, in the early 1980s science appeared on the scene to provide the evidence needed. In 1981, papers by the Japanese epidemiologist Hirayama and others, published in the *BMJ*, showed that the non-smoking wives of heavy smokers had a much higher risk of lung

[26] Wellcome Library for the History and Understanding of Medicine, ASH archive, Box 36, 18 February 1977, Letter from Daube to David Ennals.

[27] HEA collection (later HDA, now NICE), S. Adam, 'Warning: Cigarettes Can Seriously Damage Your Health—Even If You Don't Smoke!', in Smoking and Smoking-Related Diseases, Proceedings of a seminar held 3–5 December 1980, NHS Training and Studies Centre, Harrogate. Unit for Continuing Education Department of Community Medicine, University of Manchester.

cancer.[28] A steady stream of publications and reviews of evidence occurred after that date. Epidemiological evidence from the American Cancer Society, the West of Scotland Prospective Study, Sweden, Japan, Greece, and elsewhere added weight to the case for passive smoking.[29] This gained acceptance in policy circles quite quickly. In the United States, the Surgeon General's report of 1986 accepted the health consequences of what it called 'involuntary smoking' and a National Academy report of the same year measured and assessed its health effects. In Britain, the government accepted an interim statement from the ISCSH on passive smoking in March 1987. In March 1988, the committee produced its fourth and last report.[30] In a section on exposure to environmental tobacco smoke (ETS), the committee accepted a small increase in the risk of lung cancer in non-smokers from exposure to ETS. The quantification of risk showed some imprecision:

> there might be 1 to 3 extra lung cancer cases per year per 100,000 non-smokers regularly exposed to ETS. Since there are no firm data on the numbers of people who fall into that category, no more than a rough estimate of the actual number of lung cancer deaths arising in this way could be made. It might however amount to several hundred out of the current annual total of about 40,000 lung cancer deaths in the United Kingdom, a small but not negligible proportion.

Passive smoking was slow to take off, but has proved to be a powerful policy fact in the twenty-first century. Its establishment and acceptance involved more than the simple broadening of the medical knowledge base, the revelation of science which had previously been unknown. It could be seen as a case study of the processes of scientific fact creation, and the sociologist Peter Jackson, using the theories of Ludwig Fleck, has outlined the process of the 'medicalisation of tobacco smoke'.[31] The distinction between the scientific effects of mainstream

---

[28] T. Hirayama, 'Non Smoking Wives of Heavy Smokers Have a Higher Risk of Lung Cancer: A Study from Japan', *British Medical Journal,* 282 (1981), 183–5.

[29] P. Lee, *Environmental Tobacco Smoke and Mortality. A Detailed Review of Epidemiological Evidence Relating Environmental Tobacco Smoke to the Risk of Cancer, Health Disease, and Other Causes of Death in Adults Who Have Never Smoked* (Basel: Karger, 1992).

[30] Independent Scientific Committee on Smoking and Health, *Fourth Report of the Independent Scientific Committee on Smoking and Health* (London: HMSO, 1988).

[31] P. W. Jackson, 'Passive Smoking and Ill Health: Practice and Process in the Production of Medical Knowledge', *Sociology of Health and Illness,* 16 (1994), 423–47; *idem,* 'The Case of Passive Smoking', in R. Bunton, S. Nettleton, and R. Burrows (eds.),

and sidestream smoke opened up a space for the emergence into the gaze of science of the previously invisible passive smoker. Jackson drew attention to the importance of the biochemical markers which demonstrated that once invisible social connections could be rendered visible through a reading of these markers in the body. His analysis took less account of the fact that this was also a highly charged 'policy fact' with considerable social, political, legal, and conceptual ramifications for the nature of public health. It marked a significant change in the way the knowledge base of public health was conceived.

Passive smoking emerged out of the earlier discussions in the 1970s round the unborn child and the 'first year of life' studies. It also drew on technological innovation which made it possible to measure the components of smoke inside the body. The broader context for such developments, also visible in the next chapter on the 'rise of addiction', was the changes in the status and compass of chronic disease epidemiology and the 'risk factor' as established originally through the Doll–Hill studies. By the 1980s, epidemiology by itself was no longer sufficient as a 'proof convincing' mode and alliances were being formed with other scientific disciplines which gave the epidemiological case added strength. These alliances prefigured a new style of science within public health which placed greater emphasis on biomedical research and led into the pharmaceutical emphasis of the 1990s. Some of the earlier work on passive smoking was undertaken in locations which had never been epidemiologically focused. Michael Russell, for example, whose work at the Addiction Research Unit had used a variety of styles including laboratory work, presented results in the *Lancet* in 1973 on the absorption by non-smokers of carbon monoxide from a room air-polluted by tobacco smoke.[32] In the early 1970s research studies had also concentrated on the risk to babies and to the unborn child. Studies in South Wales and the results of the National Child Development Study and the British Perinatal Mortality Survey were also published then, and expanded the concept of risk to encompass the unborn child. It was this research emphasis which had been reflected in the HEC's health education campaigns in the 1970s.

The Sociology of Health Promotion. Critical Analyses of Consumption, Lifestyle and Risk (London: Routledge, 1995).

[32] M. A. H. Russell, P. V. Cole, and E. Brown, 'Absorption by Non-smokers of Carbon Monoxide from Room Air Polluted by Tobacco Smoke', *Lancet*, 1 (1973), 576.

The developments were in part also made possible through new technology, ironically initially developed for research on the safer cigarette. Technological developments to measure the components of smoke had originally been set in train in the 1970s in order to research the 'safer cigarette' and to provide information on cigarette packets as part of the voluntary agreements. These technical developments also enabled risk to be recategorized. By the 1980s, the scientific investigations had developed the two categories of mainstream and sidestream smoke. Some substances were found to be present in greater quantities in undiluted sidestream than in mainstream smoke—nicotine, carbon monoxide, ammonia, and carcinogens. But the nature of the risk to the non-smoker—as we can see from the ISCSH report quoted above—was still imprecise. The 1983 RCP report recognized that such smoke would be diluted by the air in a room which would also contain both inhaled and exhaled smoke. The composition of this smoke would also depend on whether the smoker took it into his lungs. It concluded, 'Passive smoking is therefore difficult to assess quantitatively and there are no agreed standards for expressing the extent of pollution of indoor atmospheres by tobacco smoke or in constituents.'[33] A different type of technology served to clarify risk. Again the 'safer smoking' work of the 1970s provided the initial impetus. Martin Jarvis and Michael Russell, in their criticism of the ISCSH 1979 report for its failure to take account of 'compensatory smoking', had criticized the committee's obsession with machine-smoked yields. They stressed the importance of measuring smoke intake using other measures. The use of biochemical markers, initially carboxyhaemoglobin and then urinary cotinine, brought a definite connection between what was inhaled and levels of risk. Such markers had been little used before, with the exception of serum cholesterol, also important in the revived public health stance of the 1980s. Urinary cotinine in particular opened up the possibility of looking inside the body and drawing quantifiable connections between bodily ingestion of this marker for nicotine and the ingestion of ETS. As a leading smoking researcher commented, 'Until the arrival of cotinine passive smoking was pooh-poohed. The industry pooh-poohed it—but epidemiology and markers combined the evidence.'[34] Not all researchers in the field initially accepted the

[33] Royal College of Physicians, *Health or Smoking? Follow-up Report of the Royal College of Physicians* (London: Pitman, 1983).
[34] Interview with smoking researcher by Virginia Berridge, 4 July 1996.

validity of this style of evidence for public health. In correspondence on the subject in the *BMJ* in 1982, Michael Russell, whose research team had produced some of the early studies which combined epidemiological evidence with that from biological markers, commented, 'Epidemiologists have been slow to appreciate the value of intake measures, although their use could greatly strengthen the association with smoking habits of the disease processes they study.'[35] Epidemiology and laboratory science were to provide complementary explanations of risk—as we will see later for HIV/AIDS.

Not all epidemiologists greeted the new scientific fact with open arms—as Russell's comment made clear. Richard Peto, who worked on the doctors' study with Richard Doll, expressed this view in a public lecture at London School of Hygiene and Tropical Medicine (LSHTM) in 1995. 'It [passive smoking] doesn't kill many non smokers—that's a political nuisance to the smokers and the tobacco companies. So what—so do drivers. It's big numbers that count and that's smokers.'[36] But the main opposition came from the industry and researchers who were industry-funded. The main public opponent in Britain of the passive smoking case was the statistician Peter Lee, whose association with the tobacco industry went back to the days of the Harrogate laboratories. This enabled his critique to be dismissed as 'industry science' although he had had more informal links with orthodox scientists in the field. The concept of passive smoking brought further ruptures in the relationships between industry and orthodox science. 'They [the industry] wouldn't collaborate with me now. Passive smoking was the big watershed,' said one leading epidemiologist in the mid-1990s.[37] In an interview, David Poswillo, long-time member of the ISCSH and chair of its 1990s successor SCOTH (Scientific Committee on Tobacco and Health), traced the roots of the new environmentalism in public health and the outright hostility between industry and activists to the US asbestosis cases of the 1970s. These had hit the insurance market and caused major problems with Lloyd's 'names'. 'The tobacco companies could see the writing on the wall—insurers were helping them to get out of liability—there were agreements between insurers and tobacco companies.'[38] The industry

[35] M. Russell, reply to criticism by the epidemiologist Richard Peto, *British Medical Journal*, 285 (1982), 507.

[36] R. Peto, Public health lecture on smoking, LSHTM, 14 March 1995, author's notes.

[37] Interview with smoking researcher by Virginia Berridge, 4 July 1996.

[38] Interview with David Poswillo by Virginia Berridge, 24 April 1997.

had already attempted to counter the 'rights' argument through their establishment of pro-smoking groups (FOREST was set up in 1979). These promoted anti-nanny state arguments and also gained support from Labour MPs anxious about employment.[39] The industry also provided money, through the voluntary agreements in the early 1980s, for the setting up of two trusts to fund research. One, the Health Promotion Research Trust, was to fund health promotion research as long as it did not deal with smoking. The resultant furore led to the funding of one research project on smoking. The other trust, more significant in the long run, was the Tobacco Products Research Trust, the history of which we will return to in Chapter 9.

Passive smoking raised the importance of the law in public health and also revitalized occupational health. Occupational health, health in the workplace, began to resume the importance within public health which it had had within early social medicine. The asbestos issue of the 1970s had led the way and the scientific risk associated with passive smoking was also bound up in comparative discussions with this environmental hazard. But some of the landmark law court successes came from outside the UK. In 1988, an Australian bus driver, Sean Carroll, won compensation from Melbourne's State Transport Authority for lung cancer contracted via ETS. He was a non-smoker who had worked for the authority for twenty years. It was a case in Australia in 1991 too which marked a legal definition of the legitimacy of passive smoking. A judge there ruled that the tobacco industry had been guilty of misleading and deceptive advertising by claiming that there was no scientific proof that passive smoking was a health risk. The case was brought by the Australian Federation of Consumer Organisations against the Tobacco Institute of Australia, whose fateful advertisement had declared, 'There is little evidence and nothing which proves scientifically that cigarette smoke causes diseases in non-smokers.' The judgement in the case was critical of the Institute's witnesses, who had tended to criticize particular studies, while witnesses for the federation, it commented in a perceptive recognition of the scientific alliances which went to make the case,

tended to regard the separate items of scientific material—for example, epidemiological studies, the 'no threshold' for carcinogens theory, the presence of carcinogens in ETS, and cotinine levels in non-smokers—as constituent parts

---

[39] M. D. Read, 'The Politics of Tobacco', PhD thesis, University of Essex, 1989.

of a mosaic, each piece itself representing some evidence that environmental tobacco smoke causes cancer in non-smokers.[40]

In Britain, the occupational case became more prominent but the legal route was less productive. In 1988, the Health and Safety Executive's pamphlet, *Passive Smoking at Work,* read, according to the *BMJ*, 'as if it were written by the tobacco industry'. The 1974 Health and Safety at Work Act had placed a duty on the employer to provide a working environment for employees free of risks to health. However, the *BMJ* thought the booklet was trapped at the point of asking if a non-smoking policy should be adopted, rather than providing details of how it could be implemented.[41] But the anti-tobacco activist line hid a more complex reality. The Health and Safety Executive (HSE) wanted to encourage the adoption of voluntary policies at work, so their representative had argued. A civil servant who was involved commented,

Using FA powers for passive smoking risks was seen as anathema to inspectors as they knew it would alienate lots of employers and would mean that their efforts to deal with the traditional health and safety risks would be all the harder. So as always the response was a leaflet ... ASH were being very dogmatic that ventilation did not work and, if correctly applied, all the evidence from contaminant control in industry was that it could significantly reduce exposure and risk ... The subsequent adoption of company smoking policies was seen as a vindication of the HSE approach.[42]

Again the connection with asbestos came in—for Doll and Peto had argued that the risks of working in a building which had some asbestos were fifty to one hundred times lower than working in one where one was exposed to passive smoking.[43] The legal route proved more difficult in the UK and it was February 1993 before the first victory in an occupational case was recorded, when Stockport Borough Council paid £15,000 in an out-of-court settlement to Veronica Bland, who had developed chronic bronchitis after eleven years' exposure to smoking colleagues in the school meals section of the education division.[44] Swifter regulation of public rather than workplace space

[40] S. Chapman and S. Woodward, 'Australian Court Rules That Passive Smoking Causes Lung Cancer, Asthma Attacks and Respiratory Disease', *British Medical Journal,* 302 (1991), 943–5.
[41] '*Passive Smoking at Work*', *British Medical Journal,* 297 (1988), 1565.
[42] HSE civil servant e-mail, 5 September 2006.
[43] See Doll's comments, *British Medical Journal,* 293 (1986), 1376.
[44] 'UK Woman Wins First Settlement for Passive Smoking', *British Medical Journal,* 306 (1993), 351.

was achieved through safety concerns, in particular the Kings Cross fire of 1987, started by a smouldering cigarette stub, which brought about bans on smoking on the Underground. Safety rather than epidemiological risk brought the earliest restriction. In 1988, British Airways forbade smoking on domestic flights within the UK. Its new aircraft used more recirculated air so the only solution was to ban smoking.[45] It seemed a far cry from the 1970s when the British Airline Pilot Association (BALPA) had opposed proposals to ban pilots smoking in the cockpit.[46]

INNOCENT VICTIMS

The 'new environmentalism' of passive smoking provided a risk to the general population rather than just to the individual smoker. Smokers threatened others rather than just themselves. This widened the debate and provided a potentially powerful engine for driving policy—once the science was clarified. In the mid-1990s, a DH civil servant called the evidence 'iffy'—but a report published by the new SCOTH in 1998 gave the fact greater legitimacy. The concept also revived classic public health concerns about infectious disease, which were starting to emerge elsewhere on the public health agenda in the 1980s. Food safety and infection were emergent issues—and the Stanley Royd hospital infection case of 1984 and other cases were a powerful driver for a reorganized professional public health after the disastrous reorganization of the 1970s.[47]

Passive smoking, like HIV/AIDS later in the decade, also involved the 'innocent victim'. Here it was the victim of others' smoke. In the early research, women and children were those who were most at risk. The epidemiological population-based arguments mingled with others which stressed heredity; the inheritance of acquired characteristics argument was reborn in the late twentieth century, nearly a century after its significance within eugenics. The statistician Peter Lee's 1992 survey of passive smoking studies found twenty-nine studies, most of which dealt with the impact of male smoking in females.[48] But women

[45] *British Medical Journal*, 297 (1988), 1001.
[46] Wellcome Library for the History and Understanding of Medicine, ASH archive, Box 79, R.30, Rights of the non-smoker, 1975–7.
[47] See discussion of these episodes in Berridge, Christie, and Tansey (eds.), *Public Health in the 1980s and 90s.*
[48] Lee, *Environmental Tobacco Smoke and Mortality.*

did not long retain the status of innocent victim. The most high-profile victim of passive smoking in the UK was male, the comedian Roy Castle who died in 1994. Women later assumed a more active, and culpable, role in passive smoking as the locus of infection for the family. Smoking researchers, examining saliva cotinine concentrations in a representative population sample of non-smoking school children, found that 'Results show that school children with parents who smoke receive a significant dose. There is higher consumption in men, but mothers' smoking had a stronger influence on exposure than the father's.'[49] Enquiry into the connection between 'cot death' (SIDS) and smoking in the 1990s found an increased association of cot death with mothers who had smoked during pregnancy.[50] 'Passive smoking in utero' also appeared in the reports; 'women as mothers', and hence culpable, replaced the women as the innocent victim. The child, however, remained the victim throughout. The researcher Ann Charlton, in a pamphlet produced by the Association for Non Smokers' Rights in 1991, connected passive smoking with a huge range of birth defects and failures of development later in life.[51] In 1987, the *BMJ* published an article which purported to show the difference in appearance between babies borne to smokers and to non-smokers. The paper's authors concluded:

We believe that infants born to mothers who smoke can be distinguished from those born to non-smokers by their appearance. We and others could not, however, identify or quantify the differences being detected. Certainly it was not the most wrinkled or dimpled babies who were selected. Selection was by a subtle, subjective 'gut feeling'. Nevertheless, this finding remains useful.[52]

That such extraordinary findings, redolent of a combination of phrenology and heredity, could be published bears witness to the significance

[49] M. J. Jarvis, M. A. H. Russell, C. Feyerabend, J. R. Eiser, H. Morgan, P. Gammage, and E. M. Gray, 'Passive Exposure to Tobacco Smoke: Saliva Cotinine Concentrations in a Representative Population Sample of Non-Smoking Schoolchildren', *British Medical Journal*, 291 (1985), 927–9.

[50] P. J. Fleming, P. S. Blair, C. Bacon, et al., 'Environment of Infants during Sleep and Risk of Sudden Infant Death Syndrome: Results of a 1993–5 Case Control Study for Confidential Enquiry into Stillbirth and Death in Infancy', *British Medical Journal*, 313 (1996), 191–4; P. S. Blair, P. J. Fleming, D. Bensley, et al., 'Smoking and the Sudden Infant Death Syndrome: Results from 1993–5 Case Control Study for Confidential Enquiry into Stillbirth and Death in Infancy', *British Medical Journal*, 313 (1996), 195–8.

[51] A. Charlton, *Children and Passive Smoking* (Edinburgh: Association for Non Smokers' Rights, 1991).

[52] H. F. Stirling, J. E. Handley, and A. W. Hobbs, 'Passive Smoking in Utero: Its Effect on Neonatal Appearance', *British Medical Journal*, 295 (1987), 627–8.

of the passive smoking concept for childhood and for public health strategies.

ADVERTISING AND WOMEN

Women lost their initial status as innocent victims of passive smoking, but they retained that position in relation to advertising. This was another key issue for the new militant public health as a strategy both to use and to oppose when used by industrial interests. From the 1970s, in particular after the Norwegian advertising ban of 1973, a ban on tobacco advertising became an important aim for activist interests. In the 1980s the demand was linked to women and young girls with some policy success. This campaign was significant in that it presented a new view of women which aroused opposition. Its representation of media effect was also open to question.

It was feminist pressure which saw the women and advertising issue emerge within public health. WHO began tentatively to consider women and smoking from the late 1970s and the regular international conference on smoking also devoted a section to women from the early 1980s. The US Surgeon General's report on women and smoking in 1980 had a major impact on national interest. In Britain, feminist pressure carried the women issue forward through ASH, using psychology as the dominant scientific paradigm. In 1981, Bobbie Jacobson, a doctor and the deputy director of ASH, published *The Ladykillers: Why Smoking is a Feminist Issue.* Jacobson had noticed that about three-quarters of the requests the organization received each week from people wanting to stop smoking were from women. At the launch of the third RCP report in 1977, a woman journalist asked the male medical panel why smoking was rising among women. Only one replied—to say he had no idea.[53] Scottish initiatives were again important in driving this public health issue forward. Scottish ASH took up the women theme and began to produce women-centred materials. A Channel Four documentary in 1983 focused on women dying of lung cancer and in the same year, the first international conference on women's health in Edinburgh, organized by SHEG (Scottish Health Education Group) and WHO,

---

[53] B. Jacobson, *The Ladykillers: Why Smoking is a Feminist Issue* (London: Pluto Press, 1981). Illustration 11.

had cigarettes on the agenda.[54] Also in 1983, a women's group at ASH in London co-organized with the Health Education Council (HEC) the first national conference on women and smoking.[55] A group of about seven women, including Linda Seymour and Patti White of ASH, began to work together to produce 'non sexist, non patronising' anti-smoking material aimed at women.[56] In 1985, the HEC launched an initiative on smoking and women's health, followed by a joint drive to remove cigarette advertising from women's magazines. Jacobson and Amanda Amos' report *When Smoke Gets in Your Eyes*, published for the HEC and the British Medical Association (BMA), encouraged changes in the voluntary agreement covering cigarette advertising aimed at young girls and women.[57] The HEC also published *Women and Smoking—A Handbook for Action* in 1986, which placed emphasis on the social and political determinants of smoking. Such concerns were not integrated into the main campaign materials produced by the HEC.[58] According to Jacobson, Donald Reid, who was in charge of the smoking 'brief' at the HEC in the 1980s, was not enthusiastic about the women-centred initiatives, regarding men's smoking as still the major problem.[59]

The focus on women was inspired by feminist perspectives and had much in common with similar developments in the same years in the drug and alcohol fields, where feminist self-organization also brought the issues of women's drinking and drug taking onto policy agendas. These initiatives were, however, focused on treatment.[60] There were areas of overlap in particular through the concept of dependence, which was widely used in smoking circles. The feminist case laid stress on

[54] E. Crofton, *Some Notes on the Women's Committee of ASH. A Personal Account* (1999), ms copy in author's possession.

[55] A. Amos, 'In Her Own Best Interests? Women and Health Education: Review of the Last Fifty Years', *Health Education Journal*, 52 (1993), 141–50.

[56] For details of these activities see Wellcome Library for the History and Understanding of Medicine, ASH archive, SA/ASH, Box 62, P.27 project officer file, Women and smoking material, 1981–86. Also interview with former member of ASH women's group by Virginia Berridge, 12 February 1999.

[57] B. Jacobson and A. Amos, *When Smoke Gets in Your Eyes: Cigarette Advertising Policy and Coverage of Smoking and Health in Women's Magazines* (London: HEC and BMA Professional Division, 1985).

[58] Amos, 'In Her Own Best Interests?', makes this comment.

[59] B. Jacobson, *Beating the Ladykillers* (London: Gollancz, 1988), 138.

[60] There is discussion of the initiatives in relation to alcohol in B. Thom, *Dealing with Drink. Alcohol and Social Policy: From Treatment to Management* (London: Free Association Books, 1999), Chapter 8.

the passivity of women and their 'duping' by the mass media. The role of psychology was central. It was argued that media exploited women through mass advertising. They were persuaded to start smoking by low tar cigarette advertisements, and continued to smoke because they were less confident than men. Smoking, Jacobson argued, was a sign of anger at a subordinate role in society and it was such pressures which kept women smoking. The women and smoking arguments were an important component in the emergence of the fully fledged concept of addiction, which will be discussed in the following chapter. But the solution was abstention and will power. The second half of Jacobson's first and second editions were traditional self-help manuals with psychological strategies for behaviour modification and relapse prevention. The models of media effect used in this campaigning were common within public health—they stressed the 'brainwashing' of the population and in particular its female component, which fitted well with public health's 'anti-industry' line. The idea of an 'evil empire' plotting to brainwash individuals, with women as particularly susceptible, had an appealing public image. But media theorists did not agree and argued that such effects were not autonomous and were produced in a symbiotic relationship with those of the audience.[61]

The passive view of women also came under attack from researchers with a focus on health inequality. The origins of this critique, as we have discussed, lay in the HEC's smoking pregnant mother campaign and also in an offshoot of the feminist activity of the 1980s. The sociologist Hilary Graham published 'Women's Smoking and Family Health' in 1987 in *Social Science and Medicine*. Graham's attention had been drawn to the lone mothers smoking question when women she first interviewed in the 1970s were outraged at the HEC's smoking mother campaign. They resented the implication that they did not care and also resented the model's nakedness. From these interviews a different picture emerged. Smoking was not just a way of structuring caring but also a means of reimposing order when the structure broke down. 'It's the only thing I do for me', said one woman. Smoking was a way for poor mothers to cope. Graham drew attention to the paradoxical position of smoking for women. It contributed to a sense of well being while threatening physical health. It promoted family welfare, but increased

[61] Media 'effect' is discussed in J. Kitzinger, 'Resisting the Message: The Extent and Limits of Media Influence', in D. Miller, J. Kitzinger, K. Williams, and P. Beharrel (eds.), *The Circuit of Mass Communication* (London: Sage, 1998), 192–212.

risk of ill health. The research positioned smoking as mediating issues of gender and of class.[62] Unsurprisingly, it was not popular in public health circles in the late 1980s and early 1990s. Further attacks on the women as mothers arguments came from the sociologist Ann Oakley, who published an attack in the journal *Sociology of Health and Illness* on the assumptions behind the epidemiological constructions. If growth retardation was due to foetal hypoxia, asked Oakley, why did this occur in some classes and not in others? Smoking in pregnancy had been singled out as a problem rather than women's smoking as a whole. And this, too, had not been seen as a problem so long as smoking was a cross-class activity. In classic public health terms, it was only when the problem became confined to the working class that the rest of society began to fear infection.[63] Such views were important precursors of the revival of class and inequality issues in the late 1990s.

NEW NATIONAL AND INTERNATIONAL NETWORKS

Passive smoking, advertising, and the innocent victims arguments both symbolized and helped stimulate new networks in public health in the 1980s and 1990s. 'Advocacy coalitions' became important mechanisms for science-based activism and new players entered into alliance. For smoking the role of the BMA became prominent. The Association was reconstructing its rather fusty and doctor-focused image in the early 1980s with greater involvement in social campaigning and public health issues. It took up smoking in 1984. Dropping any idea of a risk reduction approach the BMA, in alliance with ASH and the HEC, took a media conscious high-profile approach. It developed virulent opposition to the risk reduction opportunities of the chewing tobacco Skoal Bandits in 1985, to tobacco advertising, and to charitable investment in tobacco companies. Jacobson and Amos' work on women's smoking was published jointly by the BMA and HEC. The BMA also launched *The Big Kill*, with great public relations flair at the same time. This was

[62] H. Graham, 'Smoking in Pregnancy: The Attitudes of Expectant Mothers', *Social Science and Medicine*, 10 (1976), 371–82; *eadem*, 'Women's Smoking and Family Health', *Social Science and Medicine*, 25 (1987), 47–56.

[63] A. Oakley, 'Smoking in Pregnancy: Smokescreen or Risk Factor?', *Sociology of Health and Illness*, 11 (1989), 311–35.

a statistical analysis of smoking-related deaths and disease published in fifteen regional volumes. The organization credited itself with having produced a much more hostile attitude to smoking as a result of the campaign; the anti-smoking campaign was re-energized. A key player in the activities was Pamela Taylor, who had arrived at the BMA almost by accident; she had revived its press office and set up a parliamentary unit. She recalled,

you had to create public opinion and that was the real excitement of working at the BMA at the time. It was if you like actually getting permission from society to fight the issues that we wanted to fight and a lot of the time we were better at doing that than the governments of the day.

Ethics became an important arena for the BMA under its secretary John Havard, but so too did tobacco control. This was Taylor's baby—

people really didn't want us—somebody said we were like the Americans—big and late—it was a very fair comment—anyway we did something pretty crass, on trying to quit smoking in the workplace ... so I remember going to talk to ASH and talking to them about the positioning the BMA could have, then I set up a thing called the Tobacco Alliance, and we had every player in the field, so people sat down because we were chairing who would not normally sit down together at all, and there were rivalries and so on, but ... we gave a platform to others ... which they could never have got on their own.[64]

The advent of National No Smoking Day in the early 1980s led to the cancer charities becoming involved. David Simpson, director of ASH in the 1980s, recalled that this was good publicity. 'They discovered that tobacco control was a mainstream public health activity ... cross party, not a left wing campaign. This was a huge education process—we spent time trying to widen the basis of the anti tobacco coalition.' The 1980s was in general a 'much less interesting time' after Young's departure but the coalition broadened and achieved both public relations successes and some policy ones too in particular over taxation, where the Conservative government continued price rises started by the Labour government. Again the advocacy coalition was important. 'We asked the Royal College presidents to write to the Chancellor—their letters would be heavy weight ones. They grew to love it—it was new for them.'[65] The activities of this coalition were described in a BMA report, *Smoking out the Barons*, published in 1986

[64] Interview with Pamela Taylor by Kelly Loughlin, 28 June 2000.
[65] Interview with David Simpson by Virginia Berridge, 8 July 2003.

by the BMA Public Affairs Division. This was typical of the focus of public health publication as it developed in the 1980s. The book was both a 'how to do it' manual—but also an 'instant history' of the campaign.[66] This historical regard became more important during the decade.

The coalition also developed significantly at the international and European levels during the 1980s, compared to the early 1970s when the civil servant Julia Dawkins and Charles Fletcher had been the only overseas representatives at the US InterAgency Council national conference.[67] The international dimension had first developed in the 1960s through the world conferences. Initially these had brought together public health people of all persuasions and industry interests. But the later conferences were more in line with the new public health emphasis on an absolutist approach. Godber gave a speech in Norway in February 1976 whose tone was typical: 'It's time to stop being gentle and persuasive with the merchants of death who make and sell these deadly things. Let's not ask for their cooperation—which we won't get—but tell them what their limits are.'[68] Tobacco activism became an international matter. The Australian influence was particularly strong; their tactics provided examples which were transferred cross-nationally. Nigel Gray, director of the Anti Cancer Council of Victoria, Australia, published *Lung Cancer Prevention: Guidelines for Smoking Control* in 1977 and the work of anti-smoking activists in Australia through organizations like MOP UP and BUGA UP were influential in the UK. The Australian activist Simon Chapman spent time in the UK on secondment to the HEC while finishing off a PhD thesis on cigarette advertising and smoking; his experience brought in knowledge of what was happening in other countries. The old international networks in health changed emphasis. Sir John Crofton remembered how the International Union against TB and Lung Disease (IUATLD) set up a tobacco and health committee. Crofton and other international associates tried to push the issue more strongly through WHO, since Halfdan Mahler, WHO director general in the 1980s, had previously

[66] British Medical Association Public Affairs Division, *Smoking Out the Barons* (Chichester: Wiley, 1986).

[67] Wellcome Library for the History and Understanding of Medicine, ASH archive, Box 29, Note from Julia Dawkins on the first national conference on smoking and health of the National InterAgency Council.

[68] Ibid., William Norman papers, R.18, Box 77, Godber file, Godber's speech to third world conference on smoking and health.

been concerned with TB and John Reid, the Scottish chief medical officer (CMO), was on the WHO Executive Board. Crofton, who was chair of the IUATLD committee, went with Le Maistre of the American Cancer Society to Geneva to meet Mahler with Simpson and Keith Ball in May 1986. It was agreed to convene a WHO Advisory Group, chaired by John Reid, to prepare a Global Action Plan on Tobacco and Health. The tobacco activist Judith McKay was the rapporteur. A resolution pressing WHO to produce the Action Plan was passed. Such initiatives went into decline under the director generalship of Nakajima in the late 1980s, but were to revive strongly and with a new focus on the international activities of the tobacco industry in the 1990s.[69]

Here was a process of internationalization which could be seen in other health policy areas—alcohol, drugs, all had strong and developing international health networks. Europe also developed as a coordinating mechanism during the 1980s. Symbolically, the first attempted community involvement in smoking dated back to the 1983 Asbestos Directive. Recognizing the connections between smoking and asbestos in the development of lung cancer, the EC sought to gain a ban on smoking in workplaces where there was also a risk of exposure to asbestos. The main stimulus to action came with the establishment in 1987 of the Europe against Cancer programme, initially a response to the Chernobyl explosion. This came into existence at the same time Europe was expanding its competence to take on public health and provided an important stimulus. Between 1989 and 1992, seven directives and one non-binding resolution on tobacco were adopted.[70] These processes of internationalization also represented more general flows of influence and knowledge within the overall ideology of public health. The concept of health promotion was disseminated at the international level during the 1980s as well. Seminal documents which launched this were the earlier Lalonde report of 1974, also *WHO's Global Strategy for Health for All by the Year 2000* of 1981 and its *Ottawa Charter for Health Promotion* in 1986. The concept of 'empowerment' of citizens gained importance and this newer form of public health emphasized advocacy, the social and economic context, much along the lines developed for

[69] Sir J. Crofton, unpublished memoirs, n.d.

[70] A. Gilmore and M. McKee, 'Tobacco Control Policy in the European Union', in E. Feldman and R. Bayer (eds.), *Unfiltered. Conflicts over Tobacco Policy and Public Health* (Cambridge, MA: Harvard University Press, 2004), 219–54; N. Bosanquet, 'Europe and Tobacco', *British Medical Journal*, 304 (1992), 370–2.

smoking.[71] It also developed a strong spatial dimension through the Healthy Cities initiative.

PROBLEMS FOR THE HEC

But the main supporter of the public health–health promotion case in Britain, the HEC, experienced major problems during the 1980s. It was at this interface between public health and government that the most acute tensions were felt in the first half of the decade and afterwards. David Player arrived as new director in 1984. As director of SHEG in Scotland he had led some high-profile and innovative campaigns on smoking, which had included taking on the sponsorship of the Scottish football team, which promptly became a no smoking team. Player made sure both the Scottish lion and the no smoking logo sailed across the grounds when Scotland played in Europe. He recalled, 'Jock Stein told the kids, "It's more important for you to stop smoking than for us to win the World Cup." We made a commercial and we played it every hour in the run up to the World Cup.'[72] On his arrival in London, Player wanted to recruit Daube, who had been working in Edinburgh as a senior lecturer, as head of Public Affairs. Daube was interviewed and voted the best candidate but was not appointed because of the opposition of civil servants. The incident became a cause célèbre with a Panorama programme on the subject, and a subsequent libel action brought by Ray Petch against Daube, who had accused him of blocking his appointment. Player felt all this was 'a setback ... I don't think I ever overcame it.' His buccaneering public health views were hardly to the liking either of civil servants or of ministers. Player called the funds provided for the Health Promotion Research Trust (HPRT) 'blood money'; he had conflicts with the food industry over diet. His involvement in the action group (set up with Mike Daube before Player left Scotland) Action on Alcohol Abuse was opposed by ministers and by civil servants. A representative of the Distillers Company called him the Ayatollah Komeini of Scotland, a description which Player clearly relished. The final straw came with Player's commissioning of

---

[71] Berridge, Christie, and Tansey (eds.), *Public Health in the 1980s and 90s.*

[72] RCP and Oxford Brookes video archive, Interview with David Player, February 1988.

the report *The Health Divide* as a follow-up to the Black report. The HEC Board refused to allow its premises to be used for the launch and Player turned the ban into a media event which gained the report as much publicity as its predecessor.[73] Clearly there had already been talk of what to do about the HEC—when Player attacked the HPRT a civil servant had commented in front of ministers and its Council, 'Can't you think of a better reason for us to wind up the HEC than attacking this poor man Sir John Butterfield?' (chair of the HPRT). In 1986 came the opportunity they had been looking for. The advent of HIV/AIDS provided the ideal opportunity for government to kill two birds with one stone—to appear to be doing something to counter the threat of AIDS and to get rid of Player and the HEC at the same time. In the Commons emergency debate of 1986, Norman Fowler announced that a new body would be set up to run AIDS public education. The new special health authority would 'enhance and strengthen the role of the HEC.' However, in private the view was different. A senior civil servant commented, 'the Health Education Council had fallen foul of Ministers ... that man had a mission to solve the problem of heart disease. Ministers had no time at all for the HEC, they didn't trust it with AIDS. The conclusion was to cut its throat and set up a new authority.'[74] Player did not find employment with the new Health Education Authority.

Its smoking programme continued. Although this suffered less political interference than the HIV/AIDS work was to experience, the smoking work was also shaped by political imperatives. One member of the smoking team remembered the teenage smoking programme of the late 1980s had been wrapped up in the Look After Your Heart programme because Ray Whitney, health minister at the time, had been in some political trouble and decided to have a heart disease campaign. Mrs Thatcher herself launched the campaign at the Queen Elizabeth II centre in Westminster in 1989, asking in an aside, 'Is this stuff about smoking and lung cancer really true?'[75] Smoking and young people, the team member pointed out, was politically popular as a campaigning strategy, although it produced few returns. Focusing on older people would have been more productive—more were inclined to give up in

---

[73] Player gives his version of these events in the witness seminar on the Black report in Berridge and Blume (eds.), *Poor Health*.

[74] Interview with senior civil servant by Virginia Berridge, from Berridge, *AIDS in the UK. The Making of Policy, 1981–1994* (Oxford: Oxford University Press, 1996).

[75] Interview with former HEA employee by Virginia Berridge, 31 October 1995.

their 30s and 40s when they started to cough—but this strategy had little political mileage.

INFECTION, HIV/AIDS, AND THE REVIVAL OF PUBLIC HEALTH

Passive smoking and its elaboration as a concept marked the beginning of the 1980s. The public health issue which defined its second half was HIV/AIDS. This drew on the revival of infection as a public health interest which had also marked the redefinition of smoking. The arrival of HIV as a policy issue in 1985–6 brought in its train a revived role for formal public health as an occupation. The CMO, Sir Donald Acheson, was chairing a committee on the future of public health at the same time as HIV/AIDS was a high political priority. The public health committee had its origins in part in the need to define public health in relation to the new role of general management in the NHS.[76] The image of public health in the report was subsequently criticized for its out-of-date style, for its reliance on medicine and on classic themes of infection which had characterized public health in the nineteenth century. But HIV/AIDS also fitted within a public health template which smoking had established during the 1980s—the threat of infection was there and the role of the 'innocent victim'. The syndrome was an epidemiological one but epidemiology increasingly allied itself with laboratory science. Advocacy groups were important and the issue was one of rights as well as of science. There was internationalism and the cross-national transfer of policy models. And, as with smoking, the solution lay in part with the mass media and mass media campaigns.[77] HIV/AIDS and smoking might appear on the surface to have little in common as public health issues. But together they epitomized the new and more militant public health ideology of the 1980s, its combination of environmentalism, infection, and heredity. By the end of the 1980s environmentalism and the individual were firmly back on an activist public health agenda, as a leaflet produced for the HEC symbolized.

You probably know that fresh clean air is needed to stay healthy. At one time fresh clean air could be taken for granted. Today, in many towns, this is no

[76] Berridge, Christie, and Tansey (eds.), *Public Health in the 1980s and 90s.*
[77] Berridge, *AIDS in the UK.*

longer the case. Factories and cars give out smoke and harmful chemicals. This is called pollution. A lit cigarette is like a chemical factory.[78]

In the 1990s the environmentalists within the smoking arena were to promote a harsher more punitive line as a strategy, the control of public space in line with the environmentalism of quarantine-based public health of earlier centuries.

[78] HEA leaflet archive, Smoking and Pollution, Pupils' booklet, Family Smoking Education project (London: HEC, 1986).

9

Medicating the Underclass?
Pharmaceutical Public Health
and the Discovery of Addiction

As the twentieth century drew to a close, smoking epitomized the conflicting tendencies within public health and the changes in its knowledge
base, the general tensions between environmentally conscious health
promotion ideas and the growing influence of pharmaceutical imperatives which stressed vaccination or drug interventions as preventive
measures. These tensions were also expressed in different policy agendas. An American clinical pharmacologist characterized the opposition:
'The environmentalists ... are hard line, want the end of smoking and
the undermining of industry ... the harm reduction people ... tend to
be clinical pharmacologists, centred on the role of nicotine.'[1]

Environmentalists and epidemiologists who supported the scientific
fact of passive smoking were joined by other scientists and activists from
the ranks of 'pharmaceutical public health'. The rise of the concept
of addiction to nicotine as a 'policy fact' signified the enhanced role
of pharmaceutical interests, the role of treatment and of medicalized
ideas; treatment became a public health strategy. The genetic concepts
which had fallen from favour in the 1950s and 1960s began to
make a reappearance. As smoking descended the social scale, the
options crystallized round the regulation of space and the medication
of individuals, contrasting environmental and medical strategies. These
changes were also part of complex moves in the substance use arena.
Illicit drugs and alcohol, psychiatric preserves which had used the
language of addiction since the late nineteenth century, moved more
closely within the ambit of public health. Tobacco, a mainstream public
health issue since the 1950s, in its turn moved closer to those substances

---

[1] Interview with US clinical pharmacologist by Virginia Berridge, 10 June 2005.

in concepts and approaches. Smoking and tobacco became an important 'cross-over point' for the incorporation of concepts of addiction into the public health mainstream. In the course of this accommodation, the definition of tobacco itself began to alter and boundaries round its status to shift. The rest of this chapter will examine the emergence of this new view of public health.

ENVIRONMENTALISM GOES TO WAR

First let us look briefly at how the environmental cause developed. Public health activists adhered throughout the 1990s to the environmentalist passive smoking case and to the absolutist agenda focused on taxation and the banning of advertising. There were attempts to use US-style litigation; these led to an increasing focus on historical archives as a new source of activist research. The use of industry documents also underlined tobacco's increasing internationalization as an activist cause.

In the early 1990s smoking formed part of the Conservative government's public health initiatives. An AIDS Action Group was a precursor of the Health of the Nation working party which did preparatory work for the *Health of the Nation* White Paper, which was published in 1992. This was criticized for its failure to consider issues of inequality and unemployment; instead, it stressed the role of individuals and their behavioural failures. A researcher who sat on the preparatory committees was critical of the document's disease focus, with smoking only a subfactor, but saw this as arising from the health politics of the time. 'The DH wanted to retain ownership. If they focussed on smoking, it would go to the DTI—so they used the disease focus.'[2] However, another researcher who sat on the working party was positive. 'Setting up the Health of the Nation working party was a radical move by the DH. It was the first time they'd looked at health rather than treatment and it came from the WHO Targets for Health.'[3] There was a paper on tobacco from the economist Joy Townsend which set out a programme for reducing tobacco use by 45%—it included an advertising ban, health education, and restrictions on smoking in public places. There was change between the first and final drafts of the White Paper with

---

[2] Interview with health services researcher by Virginia Berridge, 6 March 1997.
[3] Interview with health economist by Virginia Berridge, 7 March 2003.

much more explicit subtarget identification. Her demand for a 5% above inflation increase in tobacco tax went into the final White Paper as a target. But Kenneth Clarke stopped publication of the White Paper until after the election—'it was teaching your grandmother to suck eggs', in his view.[4]

Much energy also went into the question of an advertising ban, as Europe also began to take a role with its 1989 directive banning tobacco advertising on television.[5] The work of activists like Simon Chapman, Bobbie Jacobson, and Amanda Amos examining the impact of advertising and the role of advertising in women's magazines underlined the importance of the issue for the environmentalists.[6] The industry had long contended, in opposition to public health interests, that advertising had little effect on causing people to start smoking, it was simply a means to encourage brand switching. Public health research on the other hand tended to show that advertising did have an effect on the young and that sports sponsorship on television also had an impact. The publication of the 1992 Smee report by the chief government economist showed that banning advertising would be effective and was widely cited by the public health side. It showed that advertising affected total consumption and not just brand share.[7] However, from the political point of view banning advertising was a non-starter under the Conservative government. Adjournment debates were regularly held on tobacco advertising throughout the early 1990s, with little effect.[8] In 1994, the Labour MP Kevin Barron's Tobacco Advertising Bill reached its second reading, but got no further and a new voluntary agreement was signed. [9]

The failure of the ban strategy was not for want of trying by public health researchers. The researcher Richard Peto was placed beside Virginia Bottomley, then minister of Health, at a lunch in Oxford specifically so that he could raise the advertising ban with her 'but she just kept veering away from it. Then she said she had

[4] Ibid.

[5] A. Gilmore and M. McKee, 'Tobacco Control Policy in the European Union', in E. Feldman and R. Bayer (eds.), *Unfiltered. Conflicts over Tobacco Policy and Public Health* (Cambridge, MA: Harvard University Press, 2004), 234.

[6] British Medical Association Public Affairs Division, *Smoking out the Barons* (Chichester: Wiley, 1986).

[7] C. Smee, *Effect of Tobacco Advertising on Tobacco Consumption: A Discussion Document Reviewing the Evidence* (Economic and Operational Research Division, Department of Health, 1992).

[8] In 1991 and 1993.   [9] Hansard, vol. 243, cols 445–514.

to speak to her neighbour at lunch—but he wanted to talk about it too!'[10] The Conservative politician Michael Heseltine wrote to John Major pressing for the ban—and the letter was leaked to public health researchers—but little could happen while Kenneth Clarke, with tobacco industry interests, remained Secretary of State. Virginia Bottomley, who replaced William Waldegrave in 1992, was reported as saying that 'I can either have an advertising ban or Health of the Nation—so I'll go for the latter.'[11] Activists increasingly looked to Europe or to a change of government for action on the ban. The advertising ban had become a part of the public health agenda which was beyond scientific argument. As one researcher commented (in 1997), 'The evidence isn't strong enough to secure a ban—it's not an argument, it's a moral issue.'[12]

The science of passive smoking was formalized during the 1990s. A new expert committee was the vehicle. The Scientific Committee on Tobacco on Health (SCOTH) was set up in 1994. The committee revitalized the defunct Independent Scientific Committee on Smoking and Health (ISCSH) and brought on board some of the behavioural scientists who had been separately corralled into another committee, the Committee for Research into the Behavioural Aspects of Smoking and Health (CRIBASH), which had looked at the impact of sports spon-sorship and advertising. Not all public health interests were enamoured of the new arrangements. 'SCOTH was set up as a front when the ban on tobacco advertising was being talked out in the early 90s. The government could say they were doing something.'[13] The chair of the new committee was David Poswillo, an oral surgeon who had also been a member of the ISCSH. The committee brought in psychologists such as Martin Jarvis from the smoking section of the Addiction Research Unit at the Institute of Psychiatry. There were tensions—members spoke of a row over a draft report which was too positive about the benefits of smoking. During an interview with one committee member I noticed a quotation on his filing cabinet from Poswillo dated 5 July 1994. 'We had a pleasant and agreeable meeting with the Tobacco Manufacturers' Association and I would not want to press for data

[10] Interview with Richard Peto by Virginia Berridge, 22 April 1997.
[11] Interview with two public health researchers by Virginia Berridge, 12 February 1999.
[12] Interview with GP researcher by Virginia Berridge, 19 March 1997.
[13] Interview with public health epidemiologist by Virginia Berridge, 22 April 1997.

that might change this relationship.'[14] Some committee members had wanted sales figures. Poswillo saw it differently during an interview. 'The new committee is more broadly based—with a GP, epidemiology, psychology, behavioural groups, the addiction side of things. It's a proper scientific committee looking at tobacco and health. It's almost as ideal as you'd wish to have. It's difficult in constraining them from marketing and promotion—unless there's scientific evidence on this.'[15]

Environmental tobacco smoke (ETS) was high on the committee's list. The main purpose of its report on smoking, finally published in 1998 after the Labour government had come to power and after four years' work, was to give policy closure to the scientific controversy. Despite industry 'spoiling' tactics in the media round a World Health Organization (WHO) report on the same subject published just before the British one, the report's judicious acceptance of passive smoking as a 'scientific fact' gave legitimacy to the policy proposals for restrictions on smoking in public places.[16] It was noticeable, however, that the Department of Health press release quoted Peto on the threat of active, rather than passive, smoking. 'Active smoking is the really big risk—half of all active smokers are killed by the habit unless they are able to quit, but so many UK smokers have now managed to stop that tobacco deaths before age 70 have halved, from 80,000 in 1965 to 40,000 in 1995.'[17] A civil servant working on tobacco called the scientific evidence on passive smoking 'iffy'.[18] Martin Jarvis spoke in a lecture at LSHTM in 1999 of the 'symbolic value' of ETS but commented, 'You're quite hard pressed to say there's one individual who got lung cancer because of passive smoke.'[19] The government's White Paper *Smoking Kills*, published the same year as the SCOTH report, concentrated on voluntary agreements and a Public Places Charter was proposed.

Litigation, despite the success of some workplace cases, was in general unsuccessful in the UK as an environmentalist public health strategy. In

---

[14] Ibid.
[15] Interview with David Poswillo by Virginia Berridge, 24 April 1997.
[16] Department of Health press release 98/086, 11 March 1998, re SCOTH report on passive smoking. There had earlier been differences between the UK and US industries over Project Whitecoat set up by Philip Morris to keep the passive smoking controversy alive through industry-funded scientists. In 1988, the UK industry had qualms about whether this was the appropriate way to proceed. See M. Jarvis, 'Passive Smoking' paper given at London School of Hygiene and Tropical Medicine (LSHTM), 28 January 1999.
[17] Department of Health press release 98/086, 11 March 1998, re SCOTH report on passive smoking.
[18] In a comment to the author, 1995.   [19] Jarvis, 'Passive Smoking' paper.

1992 for the first time, in the wake of the US Supreme Court decision in the *Cipollone* v. *Liggett Group* product liability case, there was marked interest in filing such suits in the UK. Two firms of solicitors reported that they were inundated with enquiries after they advertised for test cases to bring a similar law suit against the UK tobacco industry. Suit was eventually filed on behalf of fifty-five lung cancer victims on the grounds that the companies had known since the 1950s that it was the tar in the cigarettes that was causing the cancers, and that they could have taken steps to reduce tar intake. Legal aid was granted and then withdrawn because the case was not considered to have a good chance of success. Legal proceedings were continued on a conditional fee basis and the case came to court—against Imperial and Gallaher in February 1999. But the majority of claimants had exceeded the three-year time limit for personal injury claims and the case did not proceed. Further attempts were equally unsuccessful.

Legal action brought a new style of research into the picture—the use of historical documents. Proving the industry had ignored risks needed evidence—and that evidence could only come from the past. This was primarily a US development, where whistleblowers within the industry and industry documents released as part of the various court settlements brought huge amounts of archival material into the public domain. A website at the University of California publicized the material.[20] In the UK British American Tobacco Company documents in a repository in Guildford became the object of public health research interest and the Commons Health Committee report on the industry in 2000 was unusual in making access to archives a major plank of its policy recommendations.[21] Public health researchers did activist history in the UK—a different situation from the United States where professional historians lined up for or against the tobacco companies in the law courts. This use of history, which is discussed more fully elsewhere, was also indicative of the narrowing gap between research and advocacy. In the 1950s and afterwards Bradford Hill had clearly demarcated research results and policy advocacy, advising the young Richard Doll against policy involvement. By the 1980s the gap had narrowed for government and for the public health arena. Governments wanted relevant research

---

[20] S. A. Glantz, L. A. Bero, P. Hanauer, and D. E. Barnes, *The Cigarette Papers* (Berkeley and Los Angeles: University of California Press, 1996). See also http://www.library.ucsf.edu/tobacco.

[21] House of Commons, Health Committee, *The Tobacco Industry and the Health Risks of Smoking, vol. i: Report and Proceedings of the Committee* (London: HMSO, 2000).

and so too did public health. Two leading public health researchers at the Health Education Authority interviewed in the late 1990s spoke of the past tensions between the scientific community whose focus was treatment and 'the advocates' for whom research was a means to action. 'The advocates are saying it's a public discussion, changing hearts and minds. He [a leading scientist] was saying none of it is proven and I can show you something that works ... But now, there's a coming together of the scientific approaches and the mass approaches ... I wanted to put science into practice.'[22]

Scientific research and advocacy were closely entwined. Meanwhile, one of the activist groups which had first brought science into the public and policy domain was in trouble in the 1990s. Action on Smoking and Health (ASH) was less of a force that it had been. 'ASH never really recovered from Geoffrey Finsberg', said one participant.[23] Its workplace consultancy struggled. And there were also internal problems and personality difficulties with a series of directors after Simpson left in 1990. One observer remarked, 'The members were "the great and the good", the doctors and they were becoming elderly. The information function had come to dominate, not campaigning ... There were "old suits" on the ASH Board.' An attempt to mimic the 'parent's movement', important in the United States with an organization called Parents Against Tobacco, disintegrated with disagreements between the director of ASH, David Pollock, and the veteran social campaigner Des Wilson. Cultural clashes when styles did not suit, staff resignations, financial problems, all meant that ASH was in 'complete breakdown' at one stage in the mid-1990s and did not begin to recover until the end of the decade.[24]

Breakdowns in relationships within charities were common enough, but one issue in the 1990s was that the action seemed to be moving elsewhere. Smoking and tobacco were becoming global rather than national issues for the environmentalist wing of public health. Public health saw its role in this area, as in others, on the global stage. David Simpson, for example, director of ASH in the 1980s, set up an international information and activist agency in the 1990s. Passive

[22] Interview with two public health researchers by Virginia Berridge, 12 February 1999.
[23] Ibid. Finsberg was George Young's replacement in the early 1980s as a health minister.
[24] These comments are composited from a number of interviews with researchers in the field and with former staff members of ASH.

smoking and tobacco control were sometimes twinned with climate change as a global environmental issue. International agencies like WHO had a long track record with tobacco, but the arrival in 1998 of a new Norwegian director general, Gro Harlem Bruntland, put tobacco firmly back on the agenda. A WHO official commented in 1995, 'The policy group at WHO see tobacco and AIDS as the big issues.'[25] Other non-health-related agencies began to give it attention in the 1990s too. The World Bank published a report on tobacco and developing countries in 1993 which researchers in the UK saw an important influence. Smuggling came on to the agenda as an international issue and formed part of the moves towards an International Framework Convention on Tobacco, which dominated the end of the decade. The researcher Richard Peto symbolized the changes from national to global. He had worked jointly with Doll on the follow-up studies of British doctors smoking, the forty-year series still being published in the 1990s, but he increasingly turned his attention to China and to the damage wrought, and to come, through smoking. Such changes of focus on the part of agencies and researchers were themselves a response to the changed stance of the international tobacco companies, which sought markets in developing countries and in Eastern Europe where state tobacco monopolies were abandoned and private enterprise moved in after the collapse of communism.[26]

THE MEDICALIZATION OF SMOKING: ADDICTION AND TREATMENT

Environmentalism was not the only public health tactic in the 1990s. 'The lifestyle approach is being supplemented by pharmacological measures,' commented one participant. The scientific knowledge base of public health was changing quite markedly and drawing on different disciplines; new models involved treatment as well as prevention; the characterization of the smoker underwent fundamental shifts; and the particular meaning and nature of tobacco itself was also changing. These were complex interactions that heightened an awareness of

---

[25] Interview with WHO official by Virginia Berridge, 5 December 1995.
[26] A. Gilmore, C. Radu-Loghin, I. Zatushevski, and M. McKee, 'Pushing up Smoking Incidence: Plans for a Privatised Tobacco Industry in Moldova', *Lancet*, 365 (2005), 1354–9.

perceptions of smoking which had been around, in the background, for some years, but which attained policy significance at the end of the 1990s. Epidemiology as a 'stand alone' public health discipline came under increasing criticism and began to draw on alliances with other, previously separate, scientific areas. A new medical view that stressed the addictive nature of smoking and nicotine emerged; and the policy implications saw a revival, often unwittingly, of some of the debates and strategies of the 1970s. Such views were rooted in the rise of different scientific networks since the 1950s and in particular the development of psychopharmacology, which from the 1980s began to form alliances with epidemiology to make new public health arguments. The rest of this chapter will examine the catalysts of this change: the rise and transformation of treatment; changes in the concepts of dependence and addiction; the new view of the smoker; and the particular role of nicotine.

THE RISE AND TRANSFORMATION
OF TREATMENT

Smoking, as discussed in earlier chapters, had emerged as a public health issue in the 1950s via the route of chronic disease epidemiology. There was no real model of treatment for disease. Let us go back and see how this developed. Commenting on Doll's appointment in the 1960s as Regius Professor of Medicine at Oxford, a statistician remarked, 'They wanted an eminent doctor who didn't want beds—being an epidemiologist he didn't need beds.'[27] Smoking had little 'pre-history' in terms of a medical model. Before the epidemiological associations, there had been some discussion of the connection between smoking and disease. But there was no organized treatment sector as had been the case with alcohol and drugs since the late nineteenth century. In those cases, the concept of inebriety had been significant and there had been political pressure for a state-funded treatment system through the Inebriates Acts.[28] Revived ideas of disease and treatment in the post-second World War years for these substances, alcohol in particular, had not drawn smoking in. Early discussions of smoking and treatment illustrate the

---

[27] Interview with public health statistician by Virginia Berridge, 10 January 1995.
[28] V. Berridge, 'Punishment or Treatment? Inebriety, Drink and Drugs, 1860–1914', *Lancet*, 364 (2004), 4–5.

blurred boundaries between medical, psychiatric, and public health concepts. While doctors in the alcohol field were discussing the need for treatment facilities, Medical Officers of Health were considering and running the early health education campaigns. Treatment as a concept and practice did filter into the smoking arena, focusing initially on the hospital clinic. The model was self-control, however, rather than active medical treatment. One of the pioneers was the National Society of Non Smokers (NSNS), which had opened stop smoking clinics in Liverpool, London, Manchester, and Leicester, but most closed down in the 1950s. Dr Wood had been initially responsible for the only National Health Service (NHS) clinic, located at the Central Middlesex.[29] Keith Ball then ran the clinic, building on the early anti-smoking interest and social medicine sentiment in the hospital. The clinic was evaluated as part of the new research-based emphasis of public health. In 1965, Ball reported on the first year's results from the anti-smoking clinic, which he had been running since 1962. The clinic ran once a week in the evening for seven weeks. It used group activities; patients were not normally seen individually. The programme consisted of films and graphic diagrams, together with group discussion and self-monitoring of a gradual cutting down to smoking cessation, which usually came halfway through the course. The model was that of the self-help group, familiar through other organizations like Alcoholics Anonymous or Weight Watchers. It dealt with populations of smokers rather than individuals. There was no real treatment on offer. Ball reported, 'Some need a prop in the shape of a pill, though none so far tried has been conspicuously helpful. Others find dummy cigarettes of use. All are encouraged to find a simple alternative to smoking when the desire is strong—deep breathing, going for a walk, polishing the floor, sucking mints, and sniffing smelling salts have all been found helpful.'[30] When officials reported to the Cabinet committee on smoking in 1964, they found thirty anti-smoking clinics in operation, all using different methods.[31] Success rates were hardly encouraging at around 20% of those who went through the Central Middlesex programmes.

[29] National Archives, Ministry of Health papers, MH 55/2236.1962, Anti-smoking clinics.
[30] K. Ball, B. J. Kirby, and C. Bogen, 'First Year's Experience in Anti Smoking Clinic', *British Medical Journal*, 1 (1965), 1651–3.
[31] National Archives, Cabinet Office papers, CAB 130/185/763, 15 June 1964, Smoking and Health, Examination by officials, Report to Ministers.

But the hospital model remained influential in the 1960s and early 1970s. Keith Ball wrote in the *British Journal of Hospital Medicine* in 1970 that the hospital doctor was in a strong position to help his patient stop smoking. 'The chest and heart physician is the best informed individual on the effects of cigarette smoking and to him falls a wider challenge—the control of smoking in the community. ... We hospital physicians have a real responsibility in this matter.'[32] Ball's connection between the hospital-based doctor and the community mirrored the concurrent developments within the occupation of public health which was moving from the community into hospital-based medicine. The hospital emphasis paralleled similar developments in the alcohol field. The Ministry of Health memorandum on the hospital treatment of alcoholism was published in 1962 and the Standing Mental Health Advisory Committee thought that smoking might follow a similar route. However, there were differences. Psychiatric involvement would not be needed and the clinics could be attached to hospital chest medicine departments. Dr Burn of Salford who ran an anti-smoking clinic in Huddersfield wrote to the *Lancet* in 1962 urging the new hospital alcoholism clinics to take on smoking and drugs—but also stressing the role of the public health team. In 1962, Aubrey Lewis, Dean of the Institute of Psychiatry, planned to set up an experimental anti-smoking clinic at the Maudsley Hospital in conjunction with the Medical Research Council (MRC) Social Psychiatry Unit which would evaluate the results.[33] Overall, anti-smoking clinics expanded in the 1970s: by the end of the decade there were fifty, accompanied by an expansion of commercial anti-smoking aids.[34] Health professionals were seen as the 'storm troops' of cultural change, building on the epidemiological doctors study and the hospital was also important as the location for public health initiatives involving them. At the 1971 world conference it was suggested that clinics might be run specially for teachers, also seen as key opinion formers. A survey in the mid-1970s of the smoking habits of health professionals and of school teachers found that all groups, with the exception of nurses, had lower smoking

[32] Wellcome Library for the History and Understanding of Medicine, ASH archive, Box 19 (old series), K. Ball, 'Cigarette Smoking and the Responsibility of the Physician', *British Journal of Hospital Medicine* (December 1970), 865–6.
[33] National Archives, Ministry of Health papers. These initiatives are all in the MH 55/2236 file.
[34] Royal College of Physicians, *Smoking or Health* (London: Pitman Medical, 1977), 27.

prevalence than in the general population.[35] A 1977 Department of Health and Social Security (DHSS) circular instituted non-smoking in health premises.[36]

But smoking treatment remained problematic throughout the 1970s. The dominant mode was the anti-smoking group rather than the clinic, and self-help manuals and programmes proliferated. The Health Education Council (HEC) was the source of many. Typical was *The Smoker's Guide to Non Smoking: Why You Should Stop, How to Go about It, A Plan of Action, Your Questions*, published in 1979 as part of a campaign called Look after Yourself.

Is there some miracle cure nobody's told you about?
Sadly no.
There's no foolproof formula for giving up. No easy way.
You might as well face the fact: stopping smoking is often a bit of a battle.
But in a battle you can win if you apply a little psychology …
This booklet will help you in two ways:
Firstly it will help you *make up your mind* to actually *do something* about giving up … and also it will help by providing you with a carefully prepared *plan of action*. But remember, no one else can win this battle for you. It's you who must take command.[37]

The text, like many others of similar import, implied a model of self-help and moral purpose, free of professional intervention. But there was a professional input, that of psychology—and psychologists were key members of staff in some of the clinics. They contributed to the elaboration of the concept of dependence, which, as we will see below, was so important for smoking in the 1970s. The other component of the 'modern' public health ideology of the period was also there—the mass media. The media were not just a vehicle for advertising: television programmes were also important in inculcating the motivation to quit. The organization of these programmes operated through the networks of the new public health ideology. In 1977, the DHSS gave ASH a grant to manage the responses to a Granada TV programme on stopping smoking—half a million people wrote in for

[35] DHSS, *Smoking and Professional People* (London: DHSS, 1979).
[36] Department of Health circular, DHSS HC(77)3, March 1977, Health Services management, Non Smoking in health premises.
[37] Health Education Council leaflet archive, Health Education Council, *The Smoker's Guide to Non Smoking: Why You Should Stop, How to Go about It, a Plan of Action, Your Questions* (London: HEC, 1979), 81.

help.[38] As Hilton has commented, the sociability of tobacco smoking was beginning to be replaced by an alternative sociability. Increasing numbers of the population were beginning to buy into the 'public health' culture of trying to give up or to avoid a health risk.[39] But this was not a solitary matter, rather a group exercise consolidated and legitimated by techniques of psychology and mass media management. Trying to stop smoking through such means was, it is difficult to recollect, 'modern' and 'trendy' in the 1970s, part of the culture of a middle-class generation which looked to health consumerism and to self-help guides.[40]

A NEW ROLE FOR THE GENERAL PRACTITIONER

The specialist hospital model never quite took off for smoking. But a new treatment development at the end of the 1970s impacted both on alcohol and on smoking. This was the emphasis on the role of the general practitioner in giving advice on levels of alcohol consumption, and on smoking cessation. Such an emphasis on a primary care-led response was also located in other issues; general practice was redefining itself and in search of a new role; governments were seeking lower cost health care in the wake of the oil crisis of 1973. The inculcation of self-control was medicalized through these developments and general practice took on part of the public health mantle, a tension in roles which had been apparent since the interwar years. Two key papers, both emanating from the same research unit, defined the new approach. Michael Russell's paper in the *British Medical Journal* in 1979 demonstrated that GP advice against smoking would be more effective than increasing the fifty special anti-smoking clinics.[41] This paralleled similar arguments in the alcohol field, where Griffith Edwards' 'A Plain Treatment for Alcoholism', published in 1977, was also making the research case for brief interventions.[42] The authors of both papers were members

[38] Wellcome Library for the History and Understanding of Medicine, ASH archive, Box 36.

[39] M. Hilton, 'Smoking and Sociability', in S. Gilman and Z. Xun (eds.), *Smoke. A Global History of Smoking* (London: Reaktion Books, 2004), 126–33.

[40] For example *Our Bodies, Ourselves*, the Boston Women's Health Collective text republished in the UK in 1978. It was first published in the United States in 1971.

[41] M. A. H. Russell, C. Wilson, C. Taylor, and C. D. Baker, 'Effect of General Practitioners' Advice against Smoking', *British Medical Journal*, 2 (1979), 231–5.

[42] G. Edwards and J. Orford, 'A Plain Treatment for Alcoholism', *Proceedings of the Royal Society of Medicine*, 70 (1977), 344–8.

of the Medical Research Council-funded Addiction Research Unit at the Institute of Psychiatry, a location which, as we will see, was significant from the 1970s at many levels for the perceptions of tobacco and responses to it. Russell's research was taken forward by the GP researcher Godfrey Fowler in Oxford. When the 1990 GP contract was renegotiated for example, GPs were given extra payments as part of their new contracts for their anti-smoking activities and for running anti-smoking groups and clinics.[43] But there was still no real treatment to offer and so medicalization was uncertain and indeterminate. All this was to change in the 1980s and 1990s.

TAX AND CLASS: THE STATUS OF THE SMOKER

The contest for legitimacy between smokers and non-smokers took a decisive turn in the 1980s and 1990s in favour of non-smokers. The culture of smoking as normal, its rituals, its cross-class ubiquity, all began to change. Two key factors were the impact of the taxation-oriented high-duty policies first initiated under Denis Healey as Chancellor in the late 1970s and the arguments of health economists on tax and class. These had rather a different impact than the economists had supposed. Economists, it will be remembered, had argued that smoking was a waste of working-class life and that high taxation, long resisted by politicians on electoral grounds, would be a means of improving the living standards as well as health of those working-class people who gave up. Taxation helped encourage giving up, there was no doubt. But its impact, it was realized in the 1980s and 90s, also helped to establish a class gradient in smoking and potentially amplified rather than reduced inequality. A different style of research pointed to these unintended consequences of policy. The joint committee on research into smoking set up by the MRC and the Social Science Research Council (SSRC) had recommended in its 1978 report that a new study of smoking attitudes, behaviour, and motivation be undertaken. The joint committee had a panel on attitudes to smoking heavily influenced by the work of the psychologist Fishbein and his theory of reasoned action. The survey was carried out by the Office of Population Censuses and Surveys (OPCS) Social

---

[43] D. Florin, 'How Does Science Influence Policy? Health Promotion for Coronary Heart Disease by General Practitioners', MD thesis, University of London, 1997.

Survey Division for the DHSS by the social psychologists Alan Marsh and Joan Matheson, and was published in 1983. It noted the contest for legitimacy which was taking place. Two status groups were in conflict. 'If the norms of non-smokers are officially endorsed, the smoker will clearly drop in status ranking.'[44] Their work showed how popular attitudes to smoking had changed since the 1950s and 1960s. However, rather than a complete reversal of belief, there was an accommodation to the emerging 'scientific facts'. People still believed in the long-standing relationships with cough, breathlessness, and bronchitis. There had been a big increase in belief in the association of smoking with heart disease. But, as in Cartwright's survey of the 1950s, belief in the connection with lung cancer had seen only a modest rise—and people thought the risk was smoking over twenty a day, exactly the figure which had come from the Edinburgh research thirty years previously.

Marsh continued some smoking work and then moved to a career in family poverty research at the Policy Studies Institute, an independent research agency. His work there revealed that poor people had continued to smoke—but this was a difficult finding even to talk about, let alone publicize. Marsh was invited to the HEC/ASH group on women's smoking of which Hilary Graham was also a member. The group's work had just led to a book, *Her Share of Misfortune,* and more data were needed: Marsh's research result seeped out. A private conference was called to discuss the finding—'high powered people came': here was a challenge to smoking policy and its taxation basis. The finding was controversial for other aspects of government poverty policy: 16% of income support was returning to government through tobacco taxes. Marsh's instinct had been to hush the matter up in case benefits were axed. The argument was finally published in 1994 in a book by Marsh and Stephen McKay, *Poor Smokers.*[45] Media management helped. The authors took advice from journalists on how to avoid the 'undeserving poor' line which the media could have used. 'Nick Timmins said—stress how difficult the circumstances are ... there was a brilliant article in *The Independent* "they can't afford to give up and they can't bear not to" ... There's not a single more difficult task in social policy than

---

[44] Quoted in A. Marsh and J. Matheson, OPCS Social Survey Division, *Smoking Attitudes and Behaviour. An Enquiry Carried out on Behalf of the DHSS* (London: HMSO, 1983).
[45] A. Marsh and S. McKay, *Poor Smokers* (London: Policy Studies Institute, 1994).

persuading the poor not to smoke.'[46] Marsh put a positive spin on the result as well. 'I'm not against taxation policy—they are hauling millions a year from the poorest smokers—surely they should return it in serious interventions?' The research also fitted with the growing research interest in inequalities which dated from the time of the Black report and was gathering pace in the early 1990s. It amplified Hilary Graham's women-focused arguments about smoking and its impact on the poor. It also identified a clear group of smokers who were no longer the cultural norm. As Marsh commented, 'Thirty per cent of smokers are boxed up in the bottom ten per cent of income distribution.' This was a growing cause for policy concern: the cost of smoking was increasing rather then reducing inequality. But it also demonstrated that a cultural gulf had opened up. Smoking was now 'the defiant badge of the underclass'.[47] Poor smokers were 'the last refuge of normative smoking. People here are still expected to smoke.'[48] Those who knew the history of public health sensed that a change was in the air; threats from the working class to the middle class had been the engine of public health change in the nineteenth century. Once a habit was associated with the poor, it was much easier to adopt a more punitive approach.

THE RISE OF ADDICTION

Marsh's original work on smoking in the 1980s had been informed by social psychology and he saw it as undermining 'the medical model'. Paradoxically, however, in the 1990s the existence of 'poor smokers' and their resistance to traditional public health intervention helped affirm a new medical argument—that smokers had continued to smoke because they were addicted and could not give up. What they needed was treatment—and by the 1990s a treatment was indeed potentially available.[49] Anti-smoking researchers, using tobacco industry documents, argued that the 'fact' of smoking or nicotine as addictive had been known since the 1960s to the industry, which had hidden it—and it was only thirty years later that the full truth was revealed. However, the story of the rise of addiction as both a scientific fact and a policy truth was a good deal more complex than such a 'heroes and villains'

---

[46] Interview with Alan Marsh by Virginia Berridge, 3 November 1997.
[47] Ibid.   [48] Marsh and McKay, *Poor Smokers*, 82.
[49] See following section on nicotine.

framework can accommodate. This was not just a question of hidden secret research but rather a process which throws light on both the changing nature of public health and of perceptions of tobacco use.The following section of this chapter analyses the changes in definitions of dependence and addiction post-Second World War and the scientific networks which sustained those ideas, along with their differing institutional and national locations; the changes in the meaning and nature of tobacco, in particular the rise of nicotine and its boundary change into both 'drug' and 'medicine' and the contest for legitimacy between those two definitions; and the meaning of such changes both for smoking policy and for the knowledge basis of public health in general.

If smoking had little pre-history of treatment, the same was true of addiction, which had never been a central concept in tobacco discourse. This discussion is of course not positing a universal transhistorical approach to the concept but sees it rather as the product of particular historical contexts which create and categorize such definitions. Such historical processes of definition have been widely discussed among historians in relation to illicit drugs and alcohol, where the concepts were related to the parallel development of ideas of insanity in the nineteenth century. Here, historians have tried to escape from, and to critique, earlier 'Whig' notions of inevitable progress to a present-day understanding of addiction, seeing the significance of the concept as rooted in changing policy and social contexts and scientific networks.[50] This style of work has remained so far separate from the study of the rise of the concept of addiction for smoking. Here anti-smoking activism has portrayed a 'lifting of the veil', the revelation of something which was universal and ahistorical—a representation which has affinities with the old Whig 'march of progress' of scientific understanding—with a new conspiratorial turn.

Smoking had a different 'addiction history'. It was not a mental hygiene issue in the nineteenth century and it barely fitted into the concept of inebriety with its hereditarian framework. Dr Norman Kerr, president of the Society for the Study of Inebriety (the ancestor of the

---

[50] For examples of the literature on the social construction of addiction, see R. Porter, 'The Drinking Man's Disease: The "Pre-history" of Alcoholism in Georgian Britain', *British Journal of Addiction,* 80 (1985), 383–96; H. Levine, 'The Discovery of Addiction. Changing Conceptions of Habitual Drunkenness in America', *Journal of Studies on Alcohol,* 39 (1978), 143–74; M. Valverde, *Diseases of the Will. Alcohol and the Dilemmas of Freedom* (Cambridge: Cambridge University Press, 1998).

current Society for the Study of Addiction) writing about tobacco in 1888, did not see it in this way.

A crave I have noted, but it is a self-originated crave, the physical effect of the narcotic action on the nervous system ... Though no defender of tobacco, which it cannot be denied is a mere luxury, injurious to the health of many, even when used in moderation, I am driven to the conclusion that in the philosophical and practical meaning of the term, there is no true tobacco inebriety or mania.[51]

Anti-smoking, like the movements associated with alcohol and drugs, had moved easily between medical and moral concepts at the turn of the century. Like those substances, tobacco had also been associated with the debates on national deterioration, in particular because of use by young boys. But tobacco was never fully integrated into the inebriety–emergent addiction model. Even W. E. Dixon's major article on the tobacco habit in the late 1920s, at a time when medical theories of addiction were in full spate—and were of policy significance in the drugs area—shied away from fully embracing it. 'The true addict is held in bondage by the fear of withdrawal, and the craving which follows it. With tobacco this does not exist; the loss of one's smoke is an annoyance, but hardly a tragedy.'[52] Unlike alcohol and drugs, tobacco was not poised for the post-Second World War 'rediscovery of addiction' when concepts of disease and treatment seemed to offer new and exiting ways forward. For those substances, scientific studies emphasized the compulsive use of the substances as a disease (alcoholism or drug addiction) requiring medical intervention, leading to the establishment of psychiatric hegemony. For smoking, the scientific routes post-war had been different as we have seen, coming through epidemiology and the rise of chronic disease. Of course, the idea of the cigarette as enslaving was commonplace, and it was also common for middle-class jesting talk to speak of addiction and bondage in connection with the cigarette. But such talk had no institutional, or professional hegemony, as it did for drugs and alcohol.

What did assert a form of professional hegemony in the 1970s was the concept of dependence, whose emergence needs some contextualizing.

---

[51] N. Kerr, *Inebriety* (London: H. K. Lewis, 1888). M. Raw and G. Edwards, 'The Tobacco Habit as Drug Dependence', *British Journal of Addiction*, 86 (5) (1991), 483–4, use this quotation and Kerr's admission that he had been a heavy smoker to argue for a personal motivation behind the lack of an inebriety model for smoking in the nineteenth century. It would more likely seem to be representative of the culture of middle-class male smoking.

[52] W. E. Dixon, 'The Tobacco Habit', *British Journal of Inebriety*, 25 (1927–8), 99–121.

The role of the international sphere was important. In the interwar years the old League of Nations had been an important agent of biological standardization and also of the dissemination of pan-European statistical indices for research and community diagnosis.[53] In the post-war years, the WHO had taken on such a role and had grown in importance as an organization which standardized and disseminated concepts of disease, both tangible and intangible, such as 'habit' and 'addiction'. A WHO expert committee, originally on 'habit-forming drugs', later changed to 'Committee on drugs liable to produce addiction', wrestled in the 1950s with the differences between addiction and habit so far as alcohol and drugs were concerned. The definitions adopted by WHO emphasized the basic biochemical level of addiction; a redefinition in 1957, for example, saw addiction as generally a physical craving accompanied by psychological factors. This biochemical emphasis was congruent with the main tendencies in science at the time. In 1964, WHO adopted the term 'drug dependence', which brought habit and addiction into the same model. Dependence was defined as 'a state arising from repeated administration of a drug on a periodic or continuous basis' with characteristics which varied according to the type of drug involved. It could be 'psychic and sometimes physical'; the biochemistry was the real driving force. Alcohol, for political reasons, was seen as occupying an intermediate position between habit-forming and addiction-producing drugs, while illicit drugs, where economic interests were less strong, gained definitional boundaries which significantly extended the boundaries of disease.[54] In 1977 new concepts were elaborated for alcohol — the 'alcohol dependence syndrome' and 'alcohol-related disabilities', the former combining physical and psychological dependence and the latter developed in order to support US drives for reimbursable treatment under insurance cover for alcohol.[55] The former definition rapidly made its way

[53] L. Murard, 'Atlantic Crossings in the Measurement of Health; from US Appraisal Forms to the League of Nations Health Indices', in V. Berridge and K. Loughlin (eds.), *Medicine, the Market and the Mass Media. Producing Health in the Twentieth Century* (Abingdon: Routledge, 2005), 19–54. P. Weindling (ed.), *International Health Organisations and Movements, 1918–39* (Cambridge: Cambridge University Press, 1995).

[54] V. Berridge, 'Dependence: Historical Constructs and Concepts', in G. Edwards and M. Lader (eds.), *The Nature of Drug Dependence* (Oxford: Oxford University Press, 1990), 1–18 ; R. Room, 'The World Health Organisation and Alcohol Control', *British Journal of Addiction,* 79 (1984), 85–92; V. Berridge, *The Society for the Study of Addiction: Alcohol and Drug Treatment and Control 1884–1988* (London: Society for the Study of Addiction, 1990), Published as special issue of *Addiction,* 85 (8) (1990), 983–1097.

[55] Room, 'The World Health Organisation and Alcohol Control'.

into the ICD (International Classification of Disease) and became part of the WHO Mental Health Division's general concern for the classification of psychiatric disorders, while the latter, renamed alcohol-related problems, became the conceptual arena for public health–prevention-related strategies within WHO and represented the growing involvement of a range of other professional groupings within the alcohol field.[56] Smoking shared in some of these international developments and a category of dependence for smoking was added to the ICD in 1974.

In the UK in the 1970s there were important developments with new scientific networks round smoking and other substances. The Addiction Research Unit (ARU) at the Institute of Psychiatry was established in 1967 with MRC funding out of an earlier alcohol project, under the directorship of the psychiatrist Griffith Edwards. Edwards pioneered working with psychologists. He was joined in the late 1960s by the general physician and psychiatrist Michael Russell, who led work on smoking which was also MRC funded. This incipient alliance across the substances was significant and so was Russell's work more generally. His work at the ARU during the 1970s and 1980s pioneered many of the scientific and policy initiatives to dominate the smoking debate of the late 1990s—the economics of smoking and taxation policy; general practitioner intervention; the critique of the low tar–low nicotine policy; and work on nicotine and addiction and its commercial and policy application. Although his views had not been popular within public health circles in the 1970s—he opposed the emphasis on health education, mass media, and abstention; critiqued the low tar–low nicotine policy; but supported harm reduction for smoking more generally—they were rediscovered through the heightened importance assumed by nicotine and the concept of addiction at the end of the century. While the location of his team within an 'addiction'-focused psychiatric institution meant that the science–policy prescriptions had little impact on public health, many of Russell's ideas assumed new importance through their reintroduction from different scientific locations

    [56] See also B. Thom, *Dealing with Drink. Alcohol and Social Policy: From Treatment to Management* (London: Free Association Books, 1999), 16–17. G. Edwards and M. M. Gross, 'Alcohol Dependence: Provisional Description of a Clinical Syndrome', *British Medical Journal,* 1 (1976) 1058; G. Edwards, M. M. Gross, M. Keller, J. Moser, and R. Room, *Alcohol Related Disabilities* (Geneva: WHO, 1977); G. Edwards, 'Problems and Dependence: The History of Two Dimensions', in M. Lader, G. Edwards, and D. C. Drummond (eds.), *The Nature of Alcohol and Drug Related Problems* (Oxford: Oxford University Press, 1992).

and networks and from the United States at a time when biomedical inputs were becoming more acceptable in general across the whole public health field.

Edwards and Russell initially aimed to combine the substances in a common approach and to cement an alliance with psychology, which at this time was in the process of emancipating itself from psychiatry and securing its position as a high status profession within the health service in general as well as in the alcohol field.[57] Here was an early attempt to bring together the substances—drugs, alcohol, and smoking tobacco—under the same conceptual banner and with a strong alliance between psychology and psychiatry. In 1976 the two men co-edited a book, *Alcohol Dependence and Smoking Behaviour*, which demonstrated the desire for research and thinking which crossed and tore down the 'substance barriers'. WHO was also encouraging what was called the 'combined approach' to substance use and abuse in the 1970s, but 'there is at every level a continued reluctance to admit smoking to full membership of the drug club.' Edwards and Russell recognized that smoking came with a different conceptual history. They were dealing with 'smoking as presenting a set of problems uncontaminated by our preconceptions relating to illegal drug use, or by the latent moral judgements which cluster around alcoholism.'[58]

Psychologists were important storm troops of new ideas. But there were problems for a combined approach across the substances. A former staff member commented, 'The psychologists in the field were brought in by Mike and Griff... it's a natural field for psychologists... Drugs and alcohol had the connection with psychiatry... these [with smoking] were brought together by Griffith and Mike—it was adopt a child who never fitted with the rest of the family... Smoking is not a psychiatric field.'[59] There was a conflict of objectives between the substances. The psychologists brought in to work on alcohol mostly aimed for harm reduction—the ideas around controlled drinking were important and controversial in the 1970s. For smoking, their aim was different—to work towards abstention. One psychologist who worked at the ARU commented:

[57] See also ibid. 142.
[58] G. Edwards, M. A. H. Russell, D. Hawks, and M. Macafferty, *Alcohol Dependence and Smoking Behaviour* (Farnborough: Saxon House and Lexington Books, 1976), xii, 205–6.
[59] Interview with smoking psychologist by Virginia Berridge, 7 November 1995.

Smoking was seen as learned behaviour ... we used rapid smoking techniques—make them ill—rather naïve behavioural approaches. There was a study on electric aversion therapy—that was the fashion in the 1970s ... Raw [another psychologist] was looking at cue exposure—resisting temptation to smoking in the presence of cue like having a drink of a coffee, this was grounded in the principles of learning theory. Smoking was an over learnt behaviour. Abstinence was seen as the appropriate treatment goal—controlled smoking never took off.[60]

Russell's work brought the physical and psychological aspects together for smoking as his colleagues were doing for alcohol and drugs. He gave the strongest elaboration of the theory of cigarette dependence in a 1971 paper: 'Cigarette Smoking is probably the most addictive and dependence producing form of object specific self-administered gratification known to man.'[61]

In the 1980s developments within psychology moved away from the dependence model towards theories of behaviour change which had more affinity with the public health educational model. The social psychologist Alan Marsh argued that the rapid fall in smoking was not explained by the overarching theory of nicotine dependence but was a more complex psychological model which he called the 'attitude model'. The development of 'affect control' was of crucial importance, something which young smokers grew to attribute to smoking. But this was a habit which could be unlearnt—smoking habits could be destabilized for smoking was a 'learned dependence'.[62] Such a stance gave a more positive role to the public health tactic of health education, but this was health education which did not stress damage (which simply made smokers fatalistic) but rather the health advantages of giving up. Marsh's work, which was elaborated through the work he did for the OPCS Social Survey Division, was recognizably in the earlier tradition of McKennell and Thomas' work on the personality types of smokers and took this social psychology line forward in new directions. He was the research director of the Economic and Social Research Council (ESRC) in the late 1980s and this social psychology model informed much of the ESRC's AIDS funding. Smoking for psychologists became a case study of the wider issue of behaviour change with models also applied to

[60] Interview with smoking psychologist by Virginia Berridge, 26 June 1996.
[61] M. A. H. Russell, 'Cigarette Dependence: I. Nature and Classification', *British Medical Journal*, 2 (1) (1971), 330–1.
[62] A. Marsh, 'Smoking: Habit or Choice?', *Population Trends* (autumn 1984), 14–20.

drugs and alcohol. The work of American psychologists Prochaska and Di Clemente was of great significance. A psychologist commented, 'The stages of change model was first applied to smoking in the late 1970s. Psychologists became less linked to treatment. There's less emphasis on clinical approaches and more on community and public health.'[63] Dependence came under attack through this line of work which had greater affinity with the public health model.

The concept was also under more general criticism in the alcohol and drugs field in the 1980s: the habit–disability component of the earlier theoretical discussions emerged as a more amorphous entity called 'problem alcohol' or 'problem drug' use. The public debate on illicit drugs still used the concept of addiction, seen as inevitable and timeless, but researchers in those areas started to move towards 'problem' definitions which supported the involvement of a wider range of non-medical players in the scientific and policy field and undermined medical and psychiatric hegemony.[64] Meanwhile in the smoking field the concept of addiction became more firmly established for the first time in the 1980s and 1990s. In the early twenty-first century, however, as we will see, a revision of concepts led to increasing overlap across the substances, the goal which Edwards and Russell had aimed at thirty years earlier.

The key to these developments was the rising importance of the relatively new field of psychopharmacology and its discovery within the field of public health epidemiology. Here I will set out the development of the field and the following section on nicotine will explore the substance-specific dimensions of the 'discovery'. The early development of psychopharmacology had been in relation to psychiatry in the years between the 1940s and 1960s with the rise of the amphetamines, the use of LSD in the treatment of mental illness, and the rise of the ben-zodiazepines.[65] Such developments were far from the epidemiological interests of the public health field of the period which was consciously moving away from the 'medical model'. However, there had been a 'push' from the pharmaceutical industry in the rise of public health interest in the 1950s. The reorientation of drug research away from the malarials had led to the discovery of substances like beta-blockers which

[63] Interview with smoking psychologist by Virginia Berridge, 26 June 1996.
[64] G. Stimson, 'Research on British Drug Policy', in V. Berridge (ed.), *Drugs Research and Policy in Britain. A Review of the 1980s* (Aldershot: Avebury, 1990), 260–81.
[65] D. Healy, *The Psychopharmacologists* (London: Altman, 1996).

became important as public health strategies later on.[66] For tobacco and its incipient alliance with illicit drugs the crucial development was work at Aberdeen by Hughes and Kosterlitz, the discovery of the opiate receptors in the mid-1970s, and the pharmacological impact this had on concepts of addiction. Hughes wrote in the late 1980s,

The pharmacological approach to addiction in its broadest sense involves the use of drugs as tools to probe all aspects of tolerance and dependence, and inevitably overlaps with the behavioural approach. Over recent years cooperation between pharmacologists, biochemists and psychologists with new theories has led to major advances towards defining the neural substrates for various dependent related processes. These advances in psychopharmacology build on the premise that it is the rewarding or reinforcing consequences of drug action which are responsible for the initiation and maintenance of drug abuse.[67]

In the UK work on pharmacology was funded by the MRC's committee on the pharmacology of drugs of dependence, chaired by the Oxford pharmacologist William Paton. From the mid-1970s onwards it began to develop an interest in the psychopharmacology of smoking with a grant to Michael Russell to work on nicotine in 1977 and further work funded on nicotine by Stolerman and Kumar at the Institute of Psychiatry in the early 1980s.[68] The Newcastle psychopharmacologists Heather Ashton and Rob Stepney in *Smoking Psychology and Pharmacology* published in 1980 described how smokers could actually manipulate their nicotine intake through smoking in order to affect mood—either to combat mental lethargy or to soothe stress. Smokers relied on smoking as a psychological tool to maintain their emotional balance almost from hour to hour. It was difficult to give up something which was so useful. 'Some smokers seem consciously to exchange a greater risk of physical illness for a lower risk of mental illness.'[69] This work was outside the public health mainstream at the time, but it was to move to a more central role in the 1990s. One leading researcher then saw it as an import from the United States which was being modified in policy

[66] V. Quirke, 'From Evidence to Market: Alfred Spinks's 1953 Survey of New Fields for Pharmacological Research, and the Origins of ICI's Cardio-vascular Programme', in Berridge and Loughlin (eds.), *Medicine, the Market and the Mass Media*, 146–71.
[67] J. Hughes, 'The Nature of Addiction: The Pharmacological Approach', in Berridge (ed.), *Drugs Research and Policy in Britain*, 237–59.
[68] See Medical Research Council, *Annual Reports*, e.g. 1972–3 (London: HMSO, 1973), 30–1; 1976–7 (London: HMSO, 1977), 17.
[69] Marsh, 'Smoking: Habit or Choice?'.

terms in the British context. In 1995 he said, 'In the 90's, the addiction model is making the running in policy—we are importing it and may affect it dramatically.'[70] American researchers such as Avram Goldstein and Charles O'Brien were the cutting edge of addiction research: their interests across the the substances served to consolidate the addiction model.[71]

What was important in this process was a reordering of scientific networks and relationships in which the transnational transfer of concepts was important. Addiction was 'in the air' in a number of different scientific networks in the 1980s. Some, such as health economics, had links with the field of smoking and of public health; others like psychology had established links both with the addiction field and with public health. In the early 1980s psychopharmacology was not the only scientific arena which was speaking the language of addiction. The SSRC had a committee on addiction whose report in 1982 brought together the networks for alcohol and tobacco.[72] Interest arose in addiction over a wide front: the neuro-sciences and their dopamine systems, economic theories, and nicotine research. There were different models of disease—the chronic disease model with occasional relapse, or the brain disease model.[73] Of particular importance as a symbolic link between disease and public health models was the popularity of theories of addiction in the health economics field. Gary Becker's theory of 'rational addiction' elaborated in a 1988 paper argued that addiction was an economically rational act.[74] An economist explained that it had led to a rash of theories and debate. 'Whether you were addicted or not depended on how you viewed your time, and this was related to social class, whether you looked to the future or not ... It could be used as a right wing individualist theory but it's used for the idea of "citizen" now—that you take responsibility for other people.'[75] A school within psychology was also looking at the 'attribution of addiction' and found

[70] Interview with smoking psychologist by Virginia Berridge, 31 January 1995.

[71] L. Knowlton, 'Investigating Addiction Responses and Relapses', *Psychiatric Times*, 18 (2), (2001), <http://www.psychiatrictimes.com> accessed 2 August 2006.

[72] Social Science Research Council, *Research Priorities in Addiction: A Report from a Subcommittee of the SSRC* (London: SSRC, 1982).

[73] Talk by Richard J. Bonnie at 'Altered States' conference, New School for Social Research, New York, February 2001, author's notes.

[74] G. S. Becker and K. M. Murphy, 'A Theory of Rational Addiction', *Journal of Political Economy*, 96 (1988), 675–700.

[75] Interview with health economist by Virginia Berridge, 15 January 1998.

that the language of addiction was in widespread use among the public at large. A psychologist explained,

Dick Eiser [a psychologist who had worked at the ARU] was interested in attribution theory—how people explain their own behaviour ... many non-smokers would label smokers as addicts—they were stupid and irrational ... Smokers labelled themselves as addicts—Dick's idea was that it served a function. Labelling was seen as a cop out—they didn't have to do anything.[76]

The rise of the concept of addiction must be seen within the context of this reordering of public health-related sciences and the role of distinct national forms of research and research funding. The MRC's support for psychopharmacology, for example, arose from its long-standing support for 'basic' research rather than for public health. Different scientific and policy 'lessons' were also drawn in the UK. These focused on the role of nicotine and it is to the complex discussions of this drug, which dominated much of the dependence and addiction changes outlined above, that we now turn.

NICOTINE: DRUG OR MEDICINE?

The role of nicotine and the rise of the concept of addiction has often been characterized as a case study of the duplicity of the tobacco industry. The industry knew, back in the 1960s, from their internal research that this substance was addictive—but in the United States maintained it was not, until revelations from industry documents demonstrated their prior knowledge.[77] This storyline is a compelling activist tale, with both heroes and villains: but it misrepresents the complexity of scientific interests which led to the rise of addiction, as we have seen earlier. Using industry documents alone leads to misunderstanding of the wider range of interests at stake in research on nicotine and the policy and practice implications which were drawn. The rise of addiction as a public health concept and the discussion of the role of nicotine also had much to do with the repositioning of public health science in the 1980s.

Public health had a problem. There were dramatic falls in the prevalence of smoking in the early part of the1980s, but such steep declines

---

[76] Interview with smoking psychologist by Virginia Berridge, 26 June 1996.
[77] P. Pringle, *Dirty Business. Big Tobacco at the Bar of Justice* (London: Aurum Press, 1998).

did not continue and in some age and gender groupings—young women from twenty to twenty-four—smoking actually began to rise again in the 1990s.[78] Public health people needed reasons to explain this stalling. One compelling argument was that smokers were addicted and could not give up. Such an argument also carried powerful potential weight in anti-industry battles, since it effectively disposed of industry arguments about 'free will' and individual rights. The arguments based on human rights were also under attack from another direction through the scientific fact of passive smoking. Addiction provided another building block for public health to box in the industry: increasingly there was no scientific hiding place. And the revelations about 'secret knowledge' were potentially powerful in the law courts. But this was an American story and in the UK the scientific and policy history was different in significant respects, not least the policy implications of the science.

The nicotine story also illustrated how the nature and meaning of tobacco was changing in the 1980s and 1990s, in ways which brought the substance closer to illicit drugs and the addiction model. Tobacco, the 'borderline substance' as it was termed in government drug regulation circles, was being pulled in two directions through the increased focus on nicotine. Like morphine in the nineteenth and early twentieth century, it was both 'medicine' and 'dangerous drug'. The story of the opiates then demonstrated clear parallels with that of tobacco later on.[79] The development of methadone as a synthetic alternative to the opiate alkaloids had offered a further opportunity for the rise of 'treatment' models under professional control. There were similar developments round tobacco/nicotine and nicotine replacement therapy in the late twentieth century. However, the different 'professional history' of tobacco/nicotine meant that its prescribing status and professional ownership was different and non-medical interests such as pharmacy were also involved.

The role of nicotine in addiction had been discussed since the nineteenth century both among the public and in medical circles. J. M. Barrie's *My Lady Nicotine* was among the best-known examples, while Lennox Johnston's paper in *The Lancet* in 1952 in which he had

---

[78] See ASH fact sheet no. 1: *Smoking Statistics: Who Smokes and How Much*, <http://www.ash.org.uk>, accessed 31 July 2006.

[79] V. Berridge, 'Changing Places: Illicit Drugs, Tobacco and Nicotine in the Nineteenth and Twentieth Centuries', in E. M. Tansey and M. Gijswijt-Hofstra (eds.), *Biographies of Remedies: Drugs, Medicines and Contraceptives in Dutch and Anglo-American Healing Cultures* (Amsterdam: Rodopi, 2002), 11–34.

described how he had substituted cocaine hydrochloride for nicotine addiction was often quoted.[80] In the 1960s, as we have seen, research on nicotine had been seen as a positive aspect of tobacco smoking and had led to the programme of work at the Harrogate laboratories under Alan Armitage, the results of which had been published in *Nature*. As we saw in Chapter 3 the Harrogate scientists asked the Royal College of Physicians (RCP) for advice on their nicotine research and the work was presented to the public health scientists. Document 46 of papers presented to the committee at its meeting on 15 May 1969 was Alan Armitage's 'The Role of Nicotine in the Tobacco Smoking Habit'.[81] A leading pharmacologist remembered the work:

There weren't many other centres—the labs of the Tobacco Research Council in Harrogate had produced a study in the late 1960s, they did good work on nicotine pharmacology, through animal studies, the role of nicotine in the smoking habit. They published a paper in *Nature*—they were arguing that people smoked to obtain the effects of nicotine—it would have useful effects on the brain and behaviour—they were saying that smoking is drug use.[82]

After this work came to an end, Michael Russell began work on nicotine and dependence at the Institute of Psychiatry with MRC funding. Here throughout the 1970s he mapped out the argument about the role of nicotine in addiction. A colleague remembered, 'There was a lot of research—addiction was nicotine self administration ... His first papers were in 1970 and 1971—he was the pioneer for nicotine in the UK, the most significant voice in the whole world.'[83]

Technological developments were a crucial part of the research. A blood nicotine assay was developed in cooperation with Colin Feyerabend of the National Poisons Unit at New Cross hospital, which enabled the amount of nicotine and other substances to be quantified.

The assay was the crucial development—technology influences the way the field developed. It influenced a whole lot of research possibilities. Evidence pointed to nicotine as crucial ... Studies on smokers' blood nicotine levels and the yield of the cigarette showed that yield was immaterial. People were smoking more to get nicotine.[84]

[80] L. Johnston, 'Cure of Tobacco Smoking', *Lancet* 2 (1952), 480–2.
[81] Royal College of Physicians archive, Minutes of committee.
[82] Interview with Institute of Psychiatry psychopharmacologist by Virginia Berridge, 14 October 1997.
[83] Interview with smoking psychologist by Virginia Berridge, 31 January 1995.
[84] Ibid.

The same was true of snuff takers—their blood nicotine levels were similar to those of smokers. Papers were published on blood levels with nicotine in the *BMJ* in 1980 and papers on blood levels with snuff in the *Lancet* at the end of the 1970s and in 1982. These technical developments which made it possible to visualize inside the body paralleled those in public health which were bringing the effects of smoking on the unborn foetus into view.

For the first time they went hand in hand with the possibility of an effective 'treatment' for smoking. Russell was interested in nicotine as a possible therapeutic agent. Nicotine gum was one possibility and the research unit did work on its absorption, which was published in 1975–6.[85] There was also a clinical trial of nicotine gum whose publication in 1982 created widespread interest and which was used as the pivotal study for the Federal Drug Agency's (FDA) registration of nicotine gum as a therapeutic substance. The trial clearly confirmed the usefulness of the gum in smoking treatment and withdrawal: abstinence was 47% in the nicotine gum group compared with 21% in the placebo group.[86]

This was a significant stage in the medicalization of smoking and of the active principle nicotine. Until this point, the treatment model was not at all central, in part because there was little to offer. In June 1957, Henry Blythe, 'stage and consultant hypnotist' in Torquay, had written to the Ministry of Health offering two new ten-inch LPs, 'Stop Smoking' and 'Slim While You Sleep'.[87] Lobeline had been tried by other clinics and it was possible that aversion therapy or electric shock treatment might be considered. Not all were as cynical as the Deputy CMO, Goodman, who in a 1961 minute, asked, 'Is there, and is there likely to be, any drug which has a significant effect in helping people to stop cigarette smoking? (short, of course, of a big dose of potassium cyanide).'[88] When the consumer magazine *Which* published a report on

[85] M. A. H. Russell, C. Wilson, U. A. Patel, C. Feyerabend, and P. V. Cole, 'Plasma Nicotine Levels after Smoking Cigarettes with High, Medium and Low Nicotine Levels', *British Medical Journal*, 2 (1975), 414–16.

[86] M. J. Jarvis, M. Raw, M. A. Russell, and C. Feyerabend, 'Randomized Controlled Trial of Nicotine Chewing Gum', *British Medical Journal*, 285 (1982), 537–40; also M. Raw, M. J. Jarvis, C. Feyerabend, and M. A. H. Russell, 'Comparison of Nicotine Chewing Gum and Psychological Treatment for Dependent Smokers', *British Medical Journal*, 16 (August 1980), 481–2.

[87] National Archives, Ministry of Health papers, MH 55/2222.

[88] National Archives, Ministry of Health papers, MH 55/2227, 6 July 1961, Minute from Goodman to Goulding.

smoking in 1971, it noted that the Standing Joint Committee on the Classification of Proprietary Preparations (the Macgregor committee) had considered Lobidan (an ethical lobeline preparation) in 1970 and given it the lowest possible rating—as not of proven efficacy—smokers were better advised to try without.[89]

Also in 1971, at the second world conference on smoking in London, two Swedish researchers from the department of clinical physiology at the University of Lund, presented their results on 'nicotine containing chewing gum as a substitute for smoking'. The chewing gum had been developed initially because of a request from the Swedish navy. The strict no smoking policy on submarines caused problems for officers and crew during long periods at sea. Nicotine withdrawal among the sailors prompted mood swings, lowered efficiency, and had a detrimental effect on overall morale. Dr Claes Lundgren, an expert in military respiratory medicine, approached a Swedish pharmacologist named Ove Ferno in December 1967 to ask for his help in developing a tobacco substitute. Lundgren had noticed that submariners could chew tobacco on the boats without too much of a problem and the action of chewing tobacco reduced their craving for cigarettes. He believed that nicotine was the primary reason behind the need to smoke and suggested an oral tobacco substitute which would prevent the user from being exposed to the harmful constituents of cigarettes. Initially nicotine was delivered through an aerosol delivery system, but this was so unwieldy and foul tasting that it was quickly abandoned. It was important to develop a mode of delivery which would prevent over-rapid absorption and toxic effects. As the director of research at Leo pharmaceutical company in Helsingborg, Ferno was able to push ahead with the nicotine replacement therapy (NRT) project. Technical problems had been more or less ironed out by the time the gum was presented at the third world conference in 1975. That conference began a collaboration between Ferno and Michael Russell which gave the product (now named Nicorette) a much higher international profile. Other products like nicotine nasal spray were also developed by collaboration between the two.[90]

Nicotine thereby began a process of change to a potential medicine, but this process of boundary change took nearly twenty years. The gum

[89] Reference to *Which* report in National Archives, Cabinet Office papers, CAB 152/16/10 part 3.
[90] 'Conversation with Ove Ferno', *Addiction*, 89 (10) (1994), 1215–26.

was registered first in Switzerland in 1979, in Canada in 1979, the UK in 1980, Sweden in 1981, and the United States in 1984. But the regulation of the 'treatment' entailed complex debates and negotiations over the status and nature of the substance. In Sweden, for example, the regulatory authority decided in 1974 that an agent acting against the desire to smoke could not be termed a medical drug. Chewing gum containing nicotine was classified as a foodstuff, as chewing tobacco and snuff had been for a long time. However, if such agents could be proved to cure a disease *caused* by smoking then they could be classified as drugs. Leading figures in the anti-smoking field in Sweden emphasized that nicotine gum had to be controlled as a prescription-only drug. Then in 1977 the Swedish food authorities ruled that the gum could not be classified as a food. It was left as neither one thing or another. After intense lobbying, the gum was classified as a drug and registered in 1981. A similar sequence of events occurred in the UK with the gum available only on private prescription until the late 1980s. It was the only prescription-only medicine which was not available on the NHS. The Borderline Substances committee of the Department of Health had said that it could not be given on an NHS prescription because it had not been proven effective in general practice. A GP in Manchester prescribed some on the NHS in the mid-1980s and was brought before a disciplinary tribunal. Michael Russell spoke in his defence, arguing that smoking was an addiction and needed treatment.

These convoluted struggles over nicotine and its treatment applications were far from the public health mainstream in the early 1980s. Russell was a forthright opponent of health education strategies and a strong supporter of nicotine as a means of harm reduction. This was at that time anathema to the public health camp. He recalled, 'I gave a talk fifteen years ago at a respectable conference in Edinburgh—if you could get people to switch to snuff you could prevent lung cancer and bronchitis—all for a small risk. People don't like it if you raise these issues.'[91] Russell, with wider experience of the debates in the addiction field, could see the issues involved in nicotine maintenance. In a 1991 editorial in the *Lancet* entitled 'Nicotine Use after the Year 2000', he argued the case for nicotine maintenance.

What distinguishes nicotine from other widely abused drugs is that its effects are subtle and do not cause socially disruptive intoxication, provoke violence, or

91 Interview with Michael Russell by Virginia Berridge, 16 February 1995.

impair performance. Yet deaths due to tobacco far outnumber those caused by all other drugs. The central paradox is that, while people smoke for nicotine they die mainly from the tar and other unwanted components in the smoke. Why have governments persisted in allowing the manufacture, extensive advertising, and promotion of such a lethally contaminated drug delivery system as the cigarette, while putting so little pressure on the tobacco industry to develop more purified forms of nicotine delivery?[92]

Such arguments carried little weight with a public health lobby which still regarded safer smoking (in whatever form) as a discredited strategy and abstention as the only aim. Russell's location in psychiatry, his differing professional background, and his pharmaceutical industry links were seen with disfavour. The gum also suffered, from the other point of view, because it did not seem like a 'medicine'. One of Russell's colleagues commented:

By establishing the efficacy of nicotine replacement we're moving towards the public health model of brief interventions in primary care. That's a more acceptable message that has filtered through ... Nicotine is less acceptable. People found it difficult to accept it as a form of drug addiction. They felt it was counter productive to label it as an addiction, because it absolved people from responsibility. The GP intervention was influential ... Mike Russell's programme was coherent and relevant, ... but he was seen as too much of a loose cannon ... the association with the Maudsley was a problem—it wasn't a mental health issue.[93]

The scientific message might have been right, but it was coming from the wrong messengers at the wrong time.

By the 1990s this had changed. More research had expanded the boundaries of knowledge on nicotine. But it was more than simply knowing more. This time the research was differently located within different scientific networks and the policy agenda was also in a state of flux. The concept of addiction was reimported from the United States where there had been an expansion of work in psychopharmacology since the 1970s. Murray Jarvik's group at Albert Einstein College in New York, which had worked on the effects of drugs on animals and on memory, turned its attention to work on nicotine in the early 1970s. The project was supported by the American Cancer Society which had

    [92] [M. A. H. Russell], 'Nicotine Use after the Year 2000', *Lancet,* 337 (1991), 1191–2.
    [93] Interview with smoking psychologist by Virginia Berridge, 31 January 1995.

not funded basic pharmacology previously. There was little nicotine research in the United States—it was not a popular area. A researcher remembered,

It was seen as not being a proper drug—interest in opiate dependence was rising... people interested in nicotine pharmacology—there were those who felt nicotine was an old drug and the basic pharmacology had been investigated. Others saw that nothing was known about the role of nicotine in smoking. There were parallels with cannabis but studies there were impeded by the lack of an active principle—it was difficult to do good laboratory work.[94]

Work by Goldstein and others at Stanford brought work on morphine, heroin, and methadone together with that on nicotine and caffeine.[95] In the United States, addiction was both a public health problem and an infectious disease, and nicotine shared in these developments. A British researcher commented, 'The Americans weren't into nicotine addiction at all—talking to them was hard work. ... But there's an increase of interest in nicotine as a drug now. Now they dominate, there are so many people and lots of groups. They were slow to catch up and now they are reinventing the wheel.'[96]

Most of the British work which developed along these lines focused on dependence rather than on nicotine per se, but it was a scientific growth area from the 1990s. A psychopharmacologist remembered that in the mid-1960s the area had been 'a backwater' and even at the end of the 1980s there were only two or three groups—but a period of rapid expansion in work on dependence in the UK began in the 1990s.[97]

In Britain, work on nicotine did begin in the late 1980s, but in a rather different context. The vehicle was the Independent Scientific Committee on Smoking and Health. By the 1980s, the committee had a new chairman, Dr, later Sir, Peter Froggatt, and a desire to see whether its policy programme was actually beneficial to the health of smokers. In the voluntary agreement of November 1980 there was provision for the tobacco industry (through the Tobacco Advisory Council, TAC) to provide the ISCSH with £1 million a year for three years for

---

[94] Interview with Institute of Psychiatry psychopharmacologist, 14 October 1997. See also interview with Neil Benowitz, 10 June 2005.

[95] A. Goldstein, *Addiction. From Biology to Drug Policy*, 2nd edn (Oxford: Oxford University Press, 2001); 1st edn (1993) has a section 'The Drugs and the Addicts', which brings all these substances together.

[96] Interview with smoking psychologist by Virginia Berridge, 31 January 1995.

[97] Interview with Institute of Psychiatry psychopharmacologist, 14 October 1997.

independent monitoring research as proposed by ISCSH on the effects on health of product modification. The Tobacco Products Research Trust (TPRT) was set up in 1982 as a charity, as the best means of administering an arm's length arrangement. This model of arm's length industry funding was subsequently used by the government and the TAC in the setting up shortly after this of another Trust, the Health Promotion Research Trust. That proved to be a much more controversial body, funded by the industry with £11 million for three and a half years to sponsor health promotion in fields other than smoking. Those working for the TPRT were aghast. 'We were astonished that they had all this money we could have done with—their logo looked very similar and there was a lot of confusion for about a year. But they were the Trust that really got the stick—their research was more woolly, it was all lifestyle factors.'[98]

A balancing act developed between the industry, research administrators, and researchers. One of the first researchers to have money from the Trust was Walter Holland, a leading health service researcher from St Thomas', a member of the ISCSH with a long track record in smoking research. Holland had planned a randomized controlled trial of low tar cigarettes during the lifetime of the previous Hunter committee, but the trial had not taken place. In the 1980s this work was funded by the TPRT. The research had to wait until the manufacturers had the technology to manipulate the tar and nicotine content of cigarettes into different combinations. Its pilot caused a furore, Holland recalled, when health visitors were used to hand out cigarettes. The result showed that 'people adjusted to get their normal fix. The low tar policy was a waste of time.'[99]

Although the industry refused to allow the expansion of the original terms of reference and at one point threatened legal action, the work of the Trust did broaden to include animal studies and the mechanisms of disease, and also some consideration of ETS.[100] Researchers had initially been distrustful, but this distrust was overcome, and studies were funded more rapidly from 1986 onwards, with the ISCSH acting as the referee body. Six priority areas were identified; they ranged from compensatory smoking through the effect of smoking on the foetus and

---

[98] Interview with Cheryl Swann, administrator of Tobacco Products Research Trust, by Virginia Berridge, 6 June 1997.
[99] Interview with Walter Holland by Virginia Berridge, 9 March 1997.
[100] Interview with Cheryl Swann by Virginia Berridge, 6 June 1997.

child to the role of tar and nicotine. By July 1996, thirty-seven projects had been completed with over a hundred publications and others were pending. The Trust was also associated, either directly or in association with the Department of Health, with a number of scientific symposia, on compensatory smoking, for example.[101]

Its work on the role of nicotine was of major importance, not just in scientific terms, but in opening a new era in the science–policy relationship in smoking policy. Its work on product modification led to an interest in nicotine as well as in tar. The third report of the ISCSH in 1984 had drawn attention to the possible toxicity of nicotine and its role in initiating and maintaining smoking as a habit. A major symposium in 1986 organized by the CIBA Foundation and the MRC and sponsored by the TPRT drew together the results of research. Sir Peter Froggatt and the researcher Nicholas Wald summarized the key results. The evidence showed that nicotine levels should be brought down, but that the toxicity of cigarettes might be reduced more if nicotine yields were reduced less than tar ones. Dependence, or addiction to nicotine, they recognized as a double-edged issue. It was a reason to maintain nicotine levels in cigarettes (which were otherwise less harmful) or to lower them in order to wean people off the habit.[102] This work marked a significant new stage in the framing of policy, with the arrival of addiction, which had been discussed for some while, as a much more important science–policy concept. In the British context, although not in the United States to such a great extent, there was a revival of harm reduction alongside abstention strategies in the late 1980s. The recognition of a group of smokers who would not, or could not, give up helped to underpin policy interest in the concept of addiction and the strategies which could be used to combat it.

The work of the TPRT came to an end through a variety of factors. The EU directive of 1992 which established upper levels of tar in cigarettes called the work of the ISCSH in that direction into question; it was no longer needed. Its demise left the TPRT operating on its own until 1995, and it finally wound up in 1996. (Its funds were transferred to the Foundation for the Study of Infant Deaths.) At its height in 1987, 60% of all research funding on smoking in the UK (£1.42 million) was

---

[101] C. Swann and Sir P. Froggatt, *The Tobacco Products Research Trust, 1982–1996* (London: RSM Press, 1996).

[102] Sir P. Froggatt and N. J. Wald, 'The Role of Nicotine in the Tar Reduction Programme', in N. Wald and P. Froggatt (eds), *Nicotine, Smoking and the Low Tar Programme* (Oxford: Oxford University Press, 1989), 229–35.

provided by the Trust.[103] But by the late 1980s policy relationships were changing again. The industry provided no new funds after 1987; those involved spoke of a more 'them and us' relationship than the one they had been used to in the earlier days of the ISCSH and the Trust. But the TPRT, with its work on nicotine and low tar in particular, had made a major contribution to scientific understanding of the operation and possible strategies for modification of these substances within tobacco. One researcher who had spanned the various committees commented, 'Froggatt made real efforts to take account of nicotine. The position on this gradually shifted in the 1980s ... He got Nick Wald on board. He's an epidemiologist and knows about smoking behaviour ... He'd not been in this area—he was into prenatal diagnosis, screening for Down's.'[104] The involvement on the same committee of public health researchers like Walter Holland also ensured that the message this time was coming through different scientific channels. The ARU unit also changed its location in the 1990s, moving to a new health behaviour unit within a public health department at UCL, which again underlined the shift in scientific networks.

Addiction and the role of nicotine was thus beginning to be established as a scientific and as a 'public health fact' by the mid-1990s. But it also emerged as a 'policy truth' by the end of the decade in the UK. The US Surgeon General's report of 1988 on nicotine addiction was important symbolically in giving the US policy stamp of approval. In the United States, however, nicotine researchers initially argued for an abstentionist model, for the reduction of nicotine, and for low tar–low nicotine cigarettes. In the UK, on the other hand, everything focused on tar and no specific targets were set for nicotine. During the 1970s and 1980s tar to nicotine levels improved, but this stopped in the 1990s. But in the UK, addiction and the use of nicotine as treatment benefited from political change and a heightened policy awareness of inequalities. By the mid-1990s both Nicorette nasal spray and Nicotinell chewing gum were prescribable on the NHS but GPs had to justify the circumstances under which the prescriptions were written. Direct advertising of the gum came in 1998 and gum of both strengths along with transdermal patches were on sale direct to the public. In the government's White Paper *Smoking Kills,* published in 1998, NRT was given a central role in

[103] Swann and Froggatt, *Tobacco Products Research Trust.*
[104] Interview with smoking psychologist by Virginia Berridge, 31 January 1995.

the battle against smoking and inequality, which were linked together. NRT was to be free for a limited period to those on low incomes and there was the possibility of NRT in pregnancy for the heaviest smokers; joint research with the pharmaceutical industry was to be developed. The Royal College of Physicians issued a report on nicotine addiction in 2000, which showed a woman on the front cover desperately pulling on a cigarette.[105]

The public health lobby also began seriously to consider harm reduction as a strategy. The Health Education Authority, usually the bastion of abstentionist public health sentiment, published a report on regulating nicotine delivery systems. Recent innovations from the tobacco industry (the smokeless cigarette and nicotine delivery devices) led to public health calls for a nicotine regulatory authority which would consider all these varied modes under one regulatory umbrella.[106] Such calls also paralleled events in the United States where the FDA's attempts to regulate fell foul of court action disputing federal competence in the area. A public health researcher commented, 'Advocates are now willing to debate these approaches. ... It has brought reduction of risk back on the agenda ... Russell's ideas of the '70's are back on the agenda.'[107] A talk given by Martin Jarvis on 'smoking and deprivation' at LSHTM in 1996 symbolized the marriage of concepts of addiction, public health, and policy priorities:

Deprived smokers are the most dependent smokers ... What are the implications for treatment? There has been much thrust towards a health education message. Get the poor to take smoking seriously. That kind of idea is not supported by the data—we need to find interventions which target dependence more effectively. Make the prescription for nicotine reimbursable.[108]

Addiction, treatment, perhaps maintenance, industrial alliances of a different sort were more central to government agendas by the end of the 1990s. Sir Donald Acheson, former chief medical officer, chaired a government enquiry into inequality in health and commented that NRT was one of the top three most effective modes for dealing with inequality.

[105] Royal College of Physicians, *Nicotine Addiction in Britain* (London: Royal College of Physicians, 2000). Illustration 12.
[106] M. Raw, *Regulating Nicotine Delivery Systems: Harm Reduction and the Prevention of Smoking Related Disease* (London: Health Education Authority, 1997).
[107] Interview with HEA researcher by Virginia Berridge, 10 November 1997.
[108] M. Jarvis, 'Smoking and Deprivation', paper given at LSHTM, 23 May 1996.

The close relationship between pharmaceutical industry products and public health policy interventions was a more general development of the 1990s. Statins for the prevention of heart disease, and methadone as a preventive for HIV and for injecting drug use were paralleled as pharmaceutical-based initiatives by the rising focus on vaccines and drug interventions for diseases of the developing world. 'Medicating the underclass' was what one participant in the National Drug Treatment conference called it in 2006.[109] Pharmaceutical public health was indeed on the agenda.

[109] Taken from my notes of the conference.

Conclusion

In April 2006, Prime Minister Tony Blair appeared dressed in a track suit to publicize the need for healthy exercise and eating. For Harold Macmillan or Burke Trend, prime minister and Cabinet secretary fifty years earlier, to have taken part in such an event would have been unthinkable. But the staged event emphasized the change in the ideology of public health and in the policy response, which is the subject of this book. By 2006, exercise and eating were important public issues, poised perhaps to displace smoking, which was seen as an issue on the way to resolution. The change in public health over a fifty-year period to the state promotion of healthy individual lifestyles could not have been better illustrated. Blair in a speech on the role of the state in public health later that summer drew attention to the dilemmas of intervention in public health matters for politicians. Many of those debates had also taken place fifty years earlier: Blair was clearly unaware that the politicians of the 1950s had also agonized over the same issues.[1]

The main purpose of this book has been to analyse the changing outlook, the discourse and ideology of public health, not to give a political history of smoking. But it is worth drawing attention to the undoubted change for the smoking issue brought about by the advent of a Labour government in 1997. The excitement among public health activists at an early conference on smoking in that year was palpable as Frank Dobson, the minister of Health, and Tessa Jowell, the first ever minister for Public Health, announced the proposed implementation of the long-desired advertising ban.[2] A White Paper on smoking appeared

---

[1] Tony Blair, Speech on Healthy Living (26 July 2006), <http://www.number10.gov.uk/output/Page 9921.asp>, accessed 6 October 2006.

[2] My notes of conference, 'Dying for a Fag', London, 14 July 1997. Speakers included Richard Branson, Frank Dobson, Tessa Jowell, and the Irish EU commissioner responsible for employment and social affairs.

the following year. [3] The ban was nevertheless long in coming, with some political difficulties with Formula One racing along the way, and the first phase of the Act was implemented in 2003. In general, however, public health has had a higher profile under the Labour government, and the publication of the Wanless report on the subject in 2004 was notable for making the economic argument for public health and its origin as a Treasury document.[4] This was in marked contrast to the Treasury's disinclination to consider such issues in the 1970s. The stance of ministers was in general different. When the 2001 EU Tobacco Directive was under discussion, industry representatives did not find Labour ministers receptive to attempts at lobbying, even those with whom they had had earlier contacts over the issue of cigarette smuggling.[5] The increasing European dimension of many smoking and tobacco-related issues was undoubtedly important. So, too, was 'policy transfer', the transfer and influence of policies across national boundaries. A particular example of this process was the agreement for a smoking ban in pubs and clubs, agreed in 2005 and influenced by the imposition of such a ban in Irish drinking outlets and the proposal to do the same in Scotland.[6] These events were all high profile in the media. Less visible but equally important, nicotine replacement therapy (NRT) continued its career as an over-the-counter (OTC) and prescription-based drug for the treatment of nicotine addiction. At the time of writing, it is prescribable by nurses and by pharmacists.[7] NRT underlined the enhanced role of primary care in treatment.

These events underlined the continuing tensions in public health between different approaches and concepts. The 'coercive permissiveness' of the 1960s continued in the emphasis on healthy lifestyles, but had taken an environmental turn with a concern for the regulation of public space. Here the early twenty-first century was in sharp contrast to the 1950s, with public attention focused on public space rather than

---

[3] *Smoking Kills. A White Paper on Tobacco*, Cm4177 (London: Department of Health, 1998).

[4] Wanless Report, *Securing Good Health for the Whole Population: Final Report* (London: HM Treasury, 2004), <http://www.hm-treasury.gov.uk/consultations_and_legislation/wanless/consult_wanless04_final.cfm>.

[5] S. Mandall, *Tobacco Industry Efforts to Influence the 2001 Tobacco Products Directive*, MSc student project, LSHTM, 2006.

[6] This brief treatment does not cover the parliamentary circumstances, which were a good deal more complex.

[7] S. Anderson, 'Community Pharmacists and Tobacco in Great Britain: From Selling Cigarettes to Supporting Smoking Cessation', draft paper, 2006.

the private and family realm, the regulation of domestic space and the home being the traditional concern of public health. Regulation of the underclass was a strong theme which united public health initiatives round public space in relation to drugs, alcohol, and smoking. Public health retained the emphasis on the role of the individual lifestyle, but increasingly this contained a strengthened criminal justice and punitive approach with a particular emphasis on the regulation of public behaviour by young people.

'Systematic gradualism' had been the other tactic in public health, particularly apparent in the 1950s–70s with the harm reduction initiatives in relation to the modification of tobacco or its replacement by New Smoking Material. Such initiatives had drawn on industrial alliances, most notable with the tobacco industry. Contrary to the received view, this industry seems to have been notable for its disunity for much of that period, at least until the changes of ownership of the late 1970s and 1980s. By the end of the century, systematic gradualism came to prominence again, in changed circumstances. The 'rise of addiction' as a concept owed much to the realization that a significant section of the lower-class population was continuing to smoke. Alongside the regulation of behaviour through criminal justice initiatives came a new 'medical model' which saw the future of public health in medication and in the provision of drugs as part treatment, part preventive strategies. NRT for smoking had its parallels in methadone for drug addiction and statins for the prevention of heart disease. ASH, in a change of stance, endorsed this medical harm reduction strategy.

Health was marketed to individuals in different ways in the early twenty-first century. In the 1960s the great change had been in the willingness of doctors and subsequently politicians to speak to the public, and subsequently their use of the tools of mass persuasion to do so. By the end of the century, there was a different type of marketing. This was the availability of treatments and commercial preventive substitutes, a strategy which had been tried and failed in the 1970s. By the end of the century, this had a new life through alliances with the pharmaceutical industry.

By the end of the century, many of the public health tactics and concepts which were novel and unusual in the 1950s and 1960s were so commonplace as to be unremarkable. People expected doctors to give advice on lifestyle conditions and politicians to give advice on how the population should eat and drink. Government itself had become a public health activist. The reorientation of epidemiology post-war to concepts of risk in relation to chronic disease were part of everyday currency, although they had been novel and lacking in legitimacy in the 1950s. The science of public health had not remained static, however, and by the end of the century, epidemiology was in question as a 'stand alone' public health science and drawing on new alliances with laboratory science which it had eschewed in the 1950s.

Marketing public health in the post-war years involved the incorporation of these scientific changes in a complex repositioning between expertise and the state. Doctors positioned themselves in relation to the public, but also to the state. The raft of new expert committees which came into being in the 1970s and after provided a means of cementing 'communities of interest' between government and public health–medical expertise. The new health pressure groups, moving away from a mass membership model to a media and government-based (and funded) one, also symbolized the changing relationships between voluntarism, expertise, and the state. A cadre of public health activists who had little relationship to the formal, medical public health profession in health services was emergent. In fact it is noticeable how little this formal profession appears in the analysis given here. Even within central government, the formal role of public health, personified in the person of the chief medical officer (CMO), came less into the story than in the days of Godber's tenure for much of the period covered by this book, with the recent exception of a more visible role under the Labour government.[8]

The role of evidence was central to this repositioning and reordering of public health discourse. Historians of evidence-based medicine have drawn attention to the post-war rise of the randomized controlled trial. The story outlined here also points to the increasing importance of social science and its techniques within public health. The social sciences became technical tools for the public health field as evidence and evaluation also moved centre stage in policy discourse. This is a different history of the 'evidence base'.

Commentators on the post-war public health profession have drawn attention to a tension between its activist role and its redefinition as technician manager. The story outlined here has elements of both those characterizations. But it also tells a different story with different tensions.

---

[8] In the history of the CMO written by Sheard and Donaldson, the subject of smoking makes no appearance after the initial consideration of the 1950s and 1960s. Yellowlees took fewer initiatives and Acheson was occupied with HIV/AIDS.

It moves from public health's obsession with itself as an occupation to a wider brief. If we examine the concepts of post-war public health, then it is the relationships between marketing and the public, between medical and lifestyle, addiction or behavioural approaches and the scientific alliances which underpin them, which are also central to changes in that history of the post-war half-century. Of course, that outlook and discourse is not static and change is currently under way. Historians are not generally in the business of predicting the future. In the early twenty-first century, however, there have been signs of a further emergent stage in public health ideology. Advertising and mass media have become less important as dominant public health tactics than they had been in the 1960s and 1970s when they had been seen as new and modern.[9] Some scientists and policy makers have looked to a health future in which the boundaries between 'licit' and 'illicit' substances will be blurred and where the medication of populations will be the norm.[10] Certainly the story of tobacco outlined here shows the fluidity of the boundary changes between what has been seen as a medicine and what has been termed a drug—with the 'dangerous' connotations of that word. Tobacco has always been a 'borderline substance' in policy terms. At the same time as that substance has been losing cultural legitimacy, cannabis seems to have been gaining both medical and cultural status.[11] This process of the rise and fall of substances has been apparent outside the UK as well. In China the decline of opium smoking at the turn of

[9] A conclusion made in V. Berridge and K. Loughlin, *Records Relating to the Health Education Council, Health Education Authority, and Health Development Agency. Thematic Mapping Exercise, July/August 2006.* Report prepared for NICE. The removal of the public education function from the Health Education Authority when it became the Health Development Agency was one indication of this. The Health Development Agency was then amalgamated into NICE.

[10] This tendency within scientific and public policy emerged strongly in the 2005 Office of Science and Technology Foresight initiative on the future of psychoactive substances in which I was involved. See http://www.foresight.gov.uk. It can also be seen in other current policy initiatives such as the reclassification of drugs under the Misuse of Drugs Act, in the public and media discussion of 'happiness', and in relation to other drugs like the role of statins in the prevention of heart disease. See L. A. Reynolds and E. M. Tansey, *Cholesterol, Atheroselerosis and Coronary Disease in the UK, 1950–2000,* Wellcome Witnesses to Twentieth Century Medicine, vol. xxvii (London: Wellcome Trust Centre for the History of Medicine at UCL, 2006).

[11] V. Berridge, 'Changing Places: Illicit Drugs, Tobacco and Nicotine in the Nineteenth and Twentieth Centuries', in E. M. Tansey and M. Gijswijt-Hofstra (eds.), *Biographies of Remedies: Drugs, Medicines and Contraceptives in Dutch and Anglo-American Healing Cultures* (Amsterdam: Rodopi, 2002), 11–34. See also S. Taylor, 'Remedicalising Cannabis; Science, Politics and Policy', upgrading document (LSHTM, 2006).

the nineteenth century had been accompanied by the rise of cigarette smoking.[12] Alongside this pharmaceutical future, the environmental legacy of public health has been represented by a growing emphasis on the regulation of public space, although not yet of the family, through the criminal justice system. The future of public health ideology and the resolution of such complex tensions remain to be seen.[13]

[12] H. Cox, *The Global Cigarette. Origins and Evolution of British American Tobacco, 1880–1945* (Oxford: Oxford University Press, 2000); F. Dikotter, L. Laamann, and Z. Xun, *Narcotic Culture. A History of Drugs in China* (London: Hurst and Company, 2004).

[13] This book has not examined the argument that public health now has a new role through the fight against terrorism. This point of view seems to have had greater salience in the United States rather than in the UK. See D. Rosner and G. Markowitz, *Are We Ready? Public Health since 9/11* (Berkeley: University of California Press, 2006).

APPENDIX

Who Has Smoked and How Much

The following has been adapted from ASH fact sheet, no 1, March 2006.

NUMBER OF ADULT SMOKERS

The highest recorded level of smoking among men was 82% in 1948, when surveys started. Among women, smoking prevalence remained fairly constant between 1948 and 1970 and peaked at 45% in 1966. Overall prevalence among adults (aged 16 and over) fell steadily between the mid-1970s and early 1980s, faster among men than women, until there was effectively no difference between the sexes. After 1982, the rate of decline slowed, with prevalence falling by only about one percentage point every two years until 1990, since when it has levelled out. However, an analysis of data taken from the government's monthly Omnibus survey demonstrated that between 1999 and 2002 there was a decline in adult smoking of around 0.4% per annum. This rate of decline has continued. There are about 12 million adult cigarette smokers in Great Britain and another 2.3 million men who smoke pipes and/or cigars. There are about 11 million ex-smokers.

Table A.1. Prevalence of Cigarette Smoking by Gender

	1974	1978	1982	1986	1990	1994	1998	2002	2004
Men	51	45	38	35	31	28	28	27	26
Women	41	37	33	31	29	26	26	25	23
All	45	40	35	33	30	27	27	26	25

Values given in percentages.

MEASURING SMOKING RATES

Periodically the government sets targets to reduce smoking prevalence in the population. The latest targets are to reduce adult smoking rates to 21% or less by 2010, with a reduction in prevalence among routine and manual groups to

26% or less. However, a review of the future of the National Health Service concludes that in order to achieve optimum health outcomes, smoking rates would need to be reduced to 17% of adults by 2011.

CIGARETTE SMOKING AND AGE

Smoking prevalence is highest in the 20–4 age group for both men and women (36 and 29%, respectively) but thereafter in older age groups there are progressively fewer smokers. Smoking continues to be lowest among people aged 60 and over. Although they are more likely than younger people to have ever been smokers, they are much more likely to have stopped smoking.

Table A.2. Prevalence of Cigarette Smoking by Age

	Age 16–19	Age 20–4	Age 25–34	Age 35–49	Age 50–9	Age 60+
1978	34	44	45	45	45	30
1988	28	37	36	36	33	23
1998	31	40	35	30	27	16
2000	29	35	35	29	27	16
2004	24	32	31	29	24	14

Values given in percentages.

CIGARETTE SMOKING AND SOCIO-ECONOMIC GROUP

There is a strong link between cigarette smoking and socio-economic group. In 2004, 33% of men and 30% of women in routine and manual occupations smoked compared to 20% of men and 17% of women in managerial and professional occupations. There has been a slower decline in smoking among manual groups, so that smoking has become increasingly concentrated in this population. As in previous General Household Surveys (GHS), the 2004 data revealed an association between socio-economic group and the age at which people started to smoke. Of those in the managerial and professional households, 29% had started smoking before they were 16, compared with 44% of those in routine and manual households.

TOBACCO CONSUMPTION

Consumption of manufactured cigarettes among adult male smokers rose from 14 per day in 1949 to 19 per day in 1955, and remained at about this level until

Table A.3. Prevalence of Cigarette Smoking by Socio-economic Classification Based on Current or Last Job of the Household Reference Person, Persons Aged 16 and over

	Large employ- ers and higher managerial	Higher profes- sional	Lower manager- ial and profes- sional	Inter- mediate	Small employ- ers/own account	Lower supervis- ory and technical	Semi- routine	Routine
Men	19	16	22	26	25	30	34	33
Women	13	11	20	22	20	26	30	33

Values given in percentages.

1970 when there was an increase to 22 per day by 1973. Among female smokers, consumption rose steadily from 7 cigarettes per day in 1949 to a maximum of 17 per day in 1976. Since the mid-1970's cigarette consumption has fallen among both men and women. Although the prevalence of cigarette smoking changed little during the 1990s, the GHS has shown a continuing fall in the reported number of cigarettes smoked. The fall in consumption has occurred mainly among younger smokers, whilst the number of cigarettes smoked among those aged 50 and over has changed very little since the mid-1970s.

Table A.4. Daily Consumption of Manufactured Cigarettes per Smoker, 1949–2004

Year	Men	Women
1949	14.1	6.8
1959	18.4	11.0
1969	18.9	13.7
1979	21.6	16.6
1990	16.8	13.9
2000	15	13
2002	15	13
2004	15	13

BIBLIOGRAPHY
UNPUBLISHED OFFICIAL SOURCES

BBC written archives

J. Morris, 'Twentieth Century Epidemic: Coronary Thrombosis', Transcript of BBC third programme talk, 1 December 1955.

Bristol Record Office

Wills archive

Health Education Authority later Health Development Authority and currently part of NICE

Leaflet archive
Post campaign evaluation reports

The National Archives

Cabinet Office
Customs and Excise
Ministry of Health/Department of Health and Social Security
Ministry of Pensions and National Insurance
Treasury

Personal unpublished accounts

E. Crofton, *Some Notes on the Women's Committee of ASH. A Personal Account by Eileen Crofton* (1999).
Sir John Crofton autobiography, ms copy

Royal College of Physicians

Committee to report on smoking and atmospheric pollution

Web sources

Legacy tobacco documents collection, University College San Francisco, Little to Hartnett 25 April 1956, Council for Tobacco Research Collection, http://legacy.library.ucsf.edu/cgi/getdoc?tid=dqf1aa00&fmt=pdf& ref=results
Legacy Tobacco documents library, Note on meeting with Sir Alexander Todd FRS at Cambridge 1 February 1960. 19600204.
H. R. Bentley, Note on the Recommendations for Labelling Cigarette Packets Legacy documents, American Tobacco collection, 1962, http://legacy. library.ucsf.edu/tid/ujd01a00

United States District Court for the District of Columbia. United States of America versus Philip Morris USA INC. United States written direct examination of Allan M. Brandt, PhD, http://www.usdoj.gov/civil/cases/ tobacco2/20040920%20Allan%20M%20Brandt%20Ph.D520Written% 20Direct.pdf, accessed 23 November 2004.

Wellcome Library for the History and Understanding of Medicine
ASH archive

REPORTS

Department of Health and Social Security (DHSS), *Report of the Standing Scientific Liaison Committee (on the Scientific Aspects of Smoking and Health) to the Secretary of State for Social Services on the Publication of Tar and Nicotine Yields of Packeted Cigarettes* (London: DHSS, 1972).
_____ *Smoking and Professional People* (London: DHSS, 1979).
Expenditure Committee, *First Report from the Expenditure Committee 1976–77 Session, Preventive Medicine, vol i: Report* (London: HMSO, 1977).
_____ *First Report from the Expenditure Committee 1976–77 Session, Preventive Medicine, vol. ii: Minutes of Evidence* (London: HMSO, 1977).
Independent Scientific Committee on Smoking and Health, *First Report: Tobacco Substitutes and Additives in Tobacco Products: Their Testing and Marketing in the United Kingdom* (London: HMSO, 1975).
_____ *Second Report of the Independent Scientific Committee of [sic] Smoking and Health. Developments in Tobacco Products and the Possibility of 'Lower Risk' Cigarettes* (London: HMSO, 1979).
_____ *Fourth Report of the Independent Scientific Committee on Smoking and Health* (London: HMSO, 1988).
Health Committee, *Second Report. The Tobacco Industry and the Health Risks of Smoking, Volume II, Minutes of Evidence and Appendices* (London: The Stationery Office Limited, 2000).
Health Education Council, *Annual Reports.*
Ministry of Health, Central Health Services Council, Scottish Health Services Council, *Health Education. Report of a Joint Committee of the Central and Scottish Health Services Councils* (London: HMSO, 1964).
Prevention and Health. Everybody's Business: a Reassessment of Public and Personal Health (London: HMSO, 1976).
Public Health in England: the Report of the Committee of Inquiry into the Future of the Public Health Function (Acheson Report) (London: HMSO, 1988).
Royal College of Physicians, *Smoking and Health* (London: Pitman, 1962).
_____ *Air Pollution and Health* (London: Pitman, 1970).
_____ *Smoking and Health Now* (London: Pitman, 1971).
_____ *Smoking or Health* (London: Pitman Medical, 1977).

Royal College of Physicians, *Health or Smoking? Follow up Report of the Royal College of Physicians* (London: Pitman, 1983).
—— *Smoking and the Young. A Report of a Working Party of the Royal College of Physicians* (London: RCP, 1992).
—— *Nicotine Addiction in Britain* (London: RCP, 2000).
Smoking Kills. A White Paper on Tobacco. Cm4177 (London: Department of Health, 1998).
Social Science Research Council, *Research Priorities in Addiction: a Report from a Subcommittee of the SSRC* (London: SSRC, 1982).
Tobacco Manufacturers Standing Committee, *First Annual Report for the Year Ended 31 May 1957 and Subsequent Reports.*
Tobacco Research Council, *Review of Activities.*
Wanless Report, *Securing Good Health for the Whole Population: Final Report* (London: HM Treasury, 2004), http://www.hm- treasury. gov.uk/consultations_and_legislation/wanless/consult_wanless04_final.cfm.

HANSARD. PARLIAMENTARY DEBATES

PERIODICALS

British Medical Journal
Lancet

INTERVIEWS

London, Royal College of Physicians, Royal College of Physicians /Oxford Brookes video interview collection.
Personal interviews by Virginia Berridge with fifty 'key informants'.

PUBLISHED SOURCES

Abraham, J., *Science, Politics and the Pharmaceutical Industry: Controversy and Bias in Drug Regulation* (London: UCL Press, 1995).
Adam, S., 'Warning: Cigarettes Can Seriously Damage Your Health—Even if You Don't Smoke!', in *Smoking and Smoking Related Diseases. Proceedings of a Seminar Held 3–5 December 1980, NHS Training and Studies Centre, Harrogate* (Manchester: Unit for Continuing Education Department of Community Medicine, University of Manchester).
Alford, B. W. E., *W.D. and H.O. Wills and the Development of the U.K. Tobacco Industry 1786–1965* (London: Methuen, 1973).
Amos, A., 'In Her Own Best Interests? Women and Health Education: Review of the Last Fifty Years', *Health Education Journal*, 52 (1993), 141–50.
Anderson, S., 'Drug Regulation and the Welfare State. Government, the Pharmaceutical Industry and the Health Professions in Great Britain, 1940–80',

in V. Berridge and K. Loughlin (eds.), *Medicine, the Market and the Mass Media: Producing Health in the Twentieth Century* (Abingdon: Routledge, 2005), 192–217.

_____ 'Community Pharmacists and Tobacco in Great Britain: From Selling Cigarettes to Supporting Smoking Cessation', draft paper, 2006.

Anon., *The Imperial Story, 1901–2001* (Bristol: Imperial Group, n.d. ?2001).

Armitage, A. K., and Hall, G. H., 'Further Evidence Relating to the Mode of Action of Nicotine in the Central Nervous System', *Nature*, 214 (1967), 977.

_____, _____, and Morrison, C. F., 'Pharmacological Basis for the Tobacco Smoking Habit', *Nature*, 217 (1968), 331.

Armstrong, D., *Political Anatomy of the Body. Medical Knowledge in Britain in the Twentieth Century* (Cambridge: Cambridge University Press, 1983).

_____ *A New History of Identity: A Sociology of Medical Knowledge* (Basingstoke: Palgrave, 2002).

Armstrong, E. A., 'Diagnosing Moral Disorder: The Discovery and Evolution of Fetal Alcohol Syndrome', *Social Science and Medicine*, 47(12) (1998), 2025–42.

ASH fact sheet number 1: *Smoking statistics: Who Smokes and How Much* <http://www.ash.org.uk>, accessed 31 July 2006.

Ashton, M., 'The Power of Persuasion', special supplement on the role of the ACMD, *Druglink* 9(5), no pagination.

Atkinson, A. B., and Townsend, J., 'Economic Aspects of Reduced Smoking', *Lancet* (3 September 1977), 492–4.

Austoker, J., *A History of the Imperial Cancer Research Fund, 1902–1986* (Oxford: Oxford University Press, 1988).

Baggott, R., *Alcohol, Politics and Social Policy* (Aldershot: Avebury, 1990).

_____ *Public Health. Policy and Politics* (Basingstoke: Palgrave, 2000).

Baggott, R., Allsop, J., and Jones, K., *Speaking for Patients and Carers: Health Consumer Groups and the Policy Process* (Basingstoke: Palgrave, 2005).

Bartley, M., *Authorities and Partisans* (Edinburgh: Edinburgh University Press, 1992).

Bartrip, P. W. J., *The Way from Dusty Death. Turner and Newall and the Regulation of Occupational Health in the British Asbestos Industry, 1890–1970* (London: Continuum, 2001).

'Beating Biases in Therapeutic Research: Historical Perspectives' conference at Osler-McGovern Centre, Green College, Oxford, 5–6 September 2002. Some papers and an edited transcript of the discussion at this meeting have been published in *International Journal of Epidemiology*, 32(6) (2003), 922–48.

Bentley, H. R., and Berry, E. G. N., *The Constituents of Tobacco Smoke; An Annotated Bibliography. Tobacco Manufacturers Standing Committee Research Paper number 3* (London: TMSC, 1959).

Berlivet, L., ' "Association or Causation?" The Debate on the Scientific Status of Risk Factor Epidemiology, 1947–c. 1965', in V. Berridge (ed.), *Making Health Policy. Networks in Research and Policy after 1945* (Amsterdam: Rodopi, 2005), 39–74.

——— 'Uneasy Prevention. The Problematic Modernisation of Health Education in France after 1975', in V. Berridge and K. Loughlin (eds.), *Medicine, the Market and the Mass Media. Producing Health in the Twentieth Century* (Abingdon: Routledge, 2005), 95–122.

Berridge, V., 'Dependence: Historical Constructs and Concepts', in G. Edwards and M. Lader (eds.), *The Nature of Drug Dependence* (Oxford: Oxford University Press, 1990), 1–18.

——— 'The Society for the Study of Addiction, 1884–1988', *British Journal of Addiction*, special issue, 85(8) (1990), 983–1087.

——— 'Researching Contemporary History: AIDS', *History Workshop Journal*, 38 (1994), 227–34.

——— *AIDS in the UK. The Making of Policy, 1981–1994* (Oxford: Oxford University Press, 1996).

——— 'Doctors and the State: The Changing Role of Medical Expertise in Policy-Making', *Contemporary British History*, 11(4) (1997), 66–85.

——— 'Science and Policy: The Case of Post War British Smoking Policy', in S. Lock, L. Reynolds, and E. M. Tansey (eds.), *Ashes to Ashes: The History of Smoking and Health* (Amsterdam: Rodopi, 1998), 143–63.

——— 'Passive Smoking and its Pre-history in Britain: Policy Speaks to Science?' *Social Science and Medicine*, special historical issue, Science Speaks to Policy, 49(9) (1999), 1183–95.

——— *Health and Society in Britain since 1939* (Cambridge: Cambridge University Press, 1999).

——— 'History in Public Health: Who Needs It?', *Lancet*, 356 (2000), 1923–5.

——— 'Constructing Women and Smoking as a Public Health Problem in Britain 1950–1990's', *Gender and History*, 13(2) (2001), 328–48.

——— 'Jerry Morris', *International Journal of Epidemiology*, 30 (2001), 1141–5.

——— 'Smoking and Public Health', in G. Davenport, I. McDonald, and C. Moss-Gibbons (eds.), *The Royal College of Physicians and its Collections. An Illustrated History* (London: Royal College of Physicians, 2001), 57–9.

——— 'Changing Places: Illicit Drugs, Tobacco and Nicotine in the Nineteenth and Twentieth Centuries', in E. M. Tansey and M. Gijswijt-Hofstra (eds.), *Biographies of Remedies: Drugs, Medicines and Contraceptives in Dutch and Anglo-American Healing Cultures* (Amsterdam: Rodopi, 2002), 11–34.

——— 'The Origin of the Black Report: A Conversation with Richard Wilkinson', in V. Berridge and S. Blume (eds.), *Poor Health. Social Inequality before and after the Black Report* (London: Frank Cass, 2003), 120–2.

——— 'Post-war Smoking Policy in the UK and the Redefinition of Public Health', *Twentieth Century British History*, 14(1) (2003), 61–82.

—— (ed.), *Drugs Research and Policy in Britain. A Review of the 1980s* (Aldershot: Avebury, 1990).

—— 'Historical and Policy Approaches', in M. Thorogood and Y. Coombes (eds.), *Evaluating Health Promotion. Practice and Methods*, 2nd edn (Oxford: Oxford University Press, 2004), 11–24.

—— (ed.), *Making Health Policy. Networks in Research and Policy after 1945* (Amsterdam: Rodopi, 2005).

—— 'Making Health Policy: Networks in Research and Policy after 1945', in V. Berridge (ed.), *Making Health Policy. Networks in Research and Policy after 1945* (Amsterdam: Rodopi, 2005), 5–36.

—— and Blume, S. (eds.), *Poor Health. Social Inequality before and after the Black Report* (London: Frank Cass, 2003).

—— and Hickman, T., 'History and the Future of Psychoactive Substances', position paper for the Foresight Brain Science, Addiction and Drugs Project, 2005, <http://www.foresight.gov.uk/Previous_Projects/Brain_Science_Addiction_and_Drugs/Reports_and_Publications/Science Reviews/Index.htm>.

—— and Loughlin, K. (eds.), *Medicine, the Market and the Mass Media. Producing Health in the Twentieth Century* (Abingdon: Routledge, 2005).

—— and —— Introduction to *Medicine, the Market and the Mass Media: Producing Health in the Twentieth Century* (Abingdon: Routledge, 2005).

—— and —— 'Smoking and the New Health Education in Britain, 1950s to 1970s', *American Journal of Public Health*, 95(6) (2005), 956–64.

—— and —— *Records Relating to the Health Education Council, Health Education Authority, and Health Development Agency. Thematic Mapping Exercise, July/August 2006*. Report prepared for NICE.

—— and Starns, P., 'The "Invisible Industrialist" and Public Health: The Rise and Fall of "Safer Smoking" in the 1970s', in V. Berridge and K. Loughlin (eds.), *Medicine, the Market and the Mass Media: Producing Health in the Twentieth Century* (Abingdon: Routledge, 2005), 172–91.

—— and Taylor, S., *Epidemiology, Social Medicine and Public Health* (London: Centre for History in Public Health, 2005).

—— Christie, D., and Tansey, E. M. (eds.), *Public Health in the 1980s and 90s: Decline and Rise?* (London: Wellcome Centre, 2006).

Betteridge, J., 'Post War Broadcasting and Changes in Political Public Life', seminar paper given at the media history seminar Institute of Historical Research, 10 October 1995.

Blair, P. S., Fleming, P. J., Bensley, D., et al., 'Smoking and the Sudden Infant Death Syndrome: Results from 1993–5 Case Control Study for Confidential Enquiry into Stillbirth and Death in Infancy', *British Medical Journal*, 313(1996), 195–8.

Blythe, G. M., '*A History of the Central Council for Health Education, 1927–1968*', MLitt thesis, Oxford University, 1987.

Booth, C. C., 'Smoking and the Gold Headed Cane', in C. C. Booth (ed.), *Balancing Act: Essays to Honour Stephen Lock* (London: Keynes Press, 1991), 49–55.

Booth, M., Hartley, K., and Powell, M., 'Industry: Structure, Performance and Policy', in A. Maynard and P. Tether (eds.), *Preventing Alcohol and Tobacco Problems, vol. i, The Addictions Market* (Aldershot: Avebury, 1990), 151–78.

Bosanquet, N., 'Europe and Tobacco', *British Medical Journal*, 304 (1992), 370–2.

Brandt, A., 'The Cigarette, Risk and American Culture', *Daedalus*, 119 (1990), 155–76.

Briggs, A., *A History of the Royal College of Physicians, vol. iv* (Oxford: Oxford University Press, for the Royal College of Physicians, 2005), 1370–99.

British Medical Association Public Affairs Division, *Smoking Out the Barons* (Chichester: Wiley, 1986).

Bruun, K., Lumio, M., Makela, K., Pan, L., Popham, R., Room, R., Schmidt, W., Skog, O., Sulkunnen, P., and Osterberg, E., *Alcohol Control Policies in Public Health Perspective* (Helsinki: Finnish Foundation for Alcohol Studies, WHO Regional office for Europe, Addiction Research Foundation of Ontario, 1975).

—— (ed.), *Alcohol Policies in United Kingdom* (Stockholm: Studies in Swedish Alcohol Policies, 1982).

Bryder, L., *Below the Magic Mountain. A Social History of Tuberculosis in Twentieth Century Britain* (Oxford: Oxford University Press, 1988).

Bufton, M. W., 'British Expert Advice on Diet and Heart Disease c1945–2000', in V. Berridge (ed.), *Making Health Policy. Networks in Research and Policy after 1945* (Amsterdam: Rodopi, 2005), 125–48.

Bulmer, M., 'Social Science Research and Policy-Making in Britain', in M. Bulmer (ed.), *Social Policy Research* (Basingstoke: Macmillan, 1978).

—— 'The Policy Process and the Place in It of Social Research', in M. Bulmer (ed.) *Social Policy Research* (Basingstoke: Macmillan, 1978), 3–30.

—— 'Social Science Expertise and Executive—Bureaucratic Politics in Britain', *Governance,* 1 (1988), 26–49.

—— Bales, K., and Sklar, K. K. (eds), *The Social Survey in Historical Perspective, 1880–1940* (Cambridge: Cambridge University Press: 1991).

Burnham, J., 'American Physicians and Tobacco Use: Two Surgeons General, 1929 and 1964', *Bulletin of the History of Medicine,* 63 (1989), 1–31.

Bynner, J. M., *Medical Students' Attitudes towards Smoking. A Report on a Survey Carried out for the Ministry of Health* (London: HMSO, 1967).

—— *The Young Smoker. A Study of Smoking among School Boys Carried out for the Ministry of Health,* Government Social Survey, 383 (London: HMSO, 1969).

Cartwright, A., Martin F. M., and Thomson, J. G., 'Distribution and Development of Smoking Habits', *Lancet,* 2 (1959), 725–7.

———, ——— and ——— 'Efficacy of an Anti-smoking Campaign', *Lancet,* 1 (1960), 327–9.

———, ——— and ——— 'Health Hazards of Cigarette Smoking. Current Popular Beliefs', *British Journal of Preventive and Social Medicine,* 14 (1960), 160–6.

——— Thomson, J. G., and a group of Edinburgh DPH students, 'Young Smokers. An Attitude Study among Schoolchildren, Touching Also Parental Influence', *British Journal of Preventive and Social Medicine,* 14 (1960), 28–34.

Castle, B., *The Castle Diaries, 1964–1976* (London: Weidenfeld and Nicolson, 1980).

Chadarevian, S. de, 'Using Interviews to Write the History of Science', in T. Soderquist (ed.), *The Historiography of Contemporary Science and Technology* (Amsterdam: Harwood Academic Publishers, 1997), 51–70.

Chalmers, I., 'Fisher and Bradford Hill: Theory and Pragmatism?', *International Journal of Epidemiology,* 32 (2003), 922–48.

Chapman, S., and Woodward, S., 'Australian Court Rules That Passive Smoking Causes Lung Cancer, Asthma Attacks and Respiratory Disease', *British Medical Journal,* 302 (1991), 943–5.

Charlton, A., *Children and Passive Smoking* (Edinburgh: Association for Nonsmokers' Rights, 1991).

Clark, Sir Fife, *The Central Office of Information* (London: Allen and Unwin, 1970).

Cochrane, A., *Effectiveness and Efficiency: Random Reflections on Health Services* (London: RSM Press, 1972; repr. 1991).

Communication Research Ltd, *Anti-smoking in Pregnancy Campaign: Pre and Post Campaign Study* (Communication Research Ltd., May 1974); ditto (June 1975).

Courtwright, D. T., 'Drug Wars: Policy Hots and Historical Cools', *Bulletin of the History of Medicine,* 74 (2004), 440–50.

Coventry, P. A., and Pickstone, J. V., 'From What and Why Did Genetics Emerge as a Medical Specialism in the 1970s in the UK? A Case History of Research, Policy and Services in the Manchester Region of the NHS', *Social Science and Medicine,* 49 (1999), 1227–38.

Cox, G., *Pioneering Television News* (London: John Libbey, 1995).

Cox, H., *The Global Cigarette. Origins and Evolution of British American Tobacco, 1880–1945* (Oxford: Oxford University Press, 2000).

Crossley, N., 'Transforming the Mental Health Field: The Early History of the National Association for Mental Health', *Sociology of Health and Illness,* 20(4) (1998), 458–88.

Crossman, R., *The Diaries of a Cabinet Minister, vol. iii, Secretary of State for Social Services 1968–1970* (London: Hamish Hamilton and Jonathan Cape, 1977).

Crown, J., 'The Practice of Public Health Medicine: Past, Present and Future', in S. Griffiths and D. Hunter (eds.), *Perspectives in Public Health* (Abingdon: Radcliffe Medical Press, 1999), 214–22.

Croxson, B., 'From Private Club to Professional Network: An Economic History of the Health Economists' Study Group, 1971–1997', *Health Economics*, 7 (Suppl. 1) (1 August 1998), S9–S45.

Cueto, M., *Missionaries of Science: The Rockefeller Foundation and Latin America* (Bloomington: Indiana University Press, 1994).

Daemmrich, A., *Pharmacopolitics: Drug Regulation in the United States and Germany* (Chapel Hill and London: University of North Carolina Press, 2004).

Daly, J., *Evidence Based Medicine and the Search for a Science of Clinical Care* (Berkeley: University of California Press, 2005).

Daube, M., 'The Politics of Smoking: Thoughts on the Labour Record', *Community Medicine* (1979), 306–14.

Daunton, M. J., *Just Taxes. The Politics of Taxation in Britain, 1914–1979* (Cambridge: Cambridge University Press, 2002).

Davis Smith, J., Rochester, C., and Hedley, R. (eds.), *An Introduction to the Voluntary Sector* (London: Routledge, 1995).

Deakin, N., 'The Perils of Partnership, the Voluntary Sector and the State, 1945–1992', in J. Davis Smith, C. Rochester, and R. Hedley (eds.), *An Introduction to the Voluntary Sector* (London: Routledge, 1995).

Denham, A., and Garnett, M., *Keith Joseph* (Chesham: Acumen, 2001).

Diack, L., and Smith, D., 'The Media and the Management of a Food Crisis. Aberdeen's Typhoid Outbreak in 1964', in V. Berridge and K. Loughlin (eds.), *Medicine, the Market and the Mass Media. Producing Health in the Twentieth Century* (Abingdon: Routledge, 2005), 79–94.

Dikotter, F., Laamann, L., and Xun, Z., *Narcotic Culture. A History of Drugs in China* (London: Hurst, 2004).

Dixon, W. E., 'The Tobacco Habit', *British Journal of Inebriety*, 25 (1927–8), 99–121.

Doll, Sir R., 'Conversation with Sir Richard Doll', *British Journal of Addiction*, 86(4) (1991), 365–77.

—— 'The First Reports on Smoking and Lung Cancer', in S. Lock, L. Reynolds, and E. M. Tansey (eds.), *Ashes to Ashes: The History of Smoking and Health* (Amsterdam: Rodopi, 1998), 130–40.

—— 'Tobacco: A Medical History', Appendix 1, Memorandum by Health Education Authority, Minutes of Evidence taken before the Health Committee, 18 November 1999, p. 26, House of Commons, session 1999–2000, Health Committee, *Second Report, The Tobacco Industry and the Health Risks of Smoking*, Volume II, Minutes of Evidence and Appendices (London: The Stationery Office, 2000), 27–II.

Doll, R., and Hill, A. B., 'Smoking and Carcinoma of the Lung. Preliminary Report', *British Medical Journal*, 2 (1950), 739–48.

——— and ——— 'The Mortality of Doctors in Relation to Their Smoking Habits. A Preliminary Report', *British Medical Journal*, 1 (1954), 1451–5.

——— and ——— 'Lung Cancer and Other Causes of Death in Relation to Smoking. A Second Report on the Mortality of British Doctors', *British Medical Journal*, 2 (1956), 1071–81.

——— Peto, R., Boreham, J., and Sutherland, I., 'Mortality in Relation to Smoking: 50 Years' Observation on Male British Doctors', *British Medical Journal*; 328 (2004), 1519–33.

Donaldson, R. J., *Off the Cuff. Reminiscences of My Half Century Career in Public Health* (Richmond: Murray Print, 2000).

Duke, K., 'Getting beyond the "Official Line": Reflections on Dilemmas of Access, Knowledge and Power in Researching Policy Networks', *Journal of Social Policy*, 31(1) (2002), 39–59.

Dwork, D., *War is Good for Babies and Other Young Children. A History of the Infant and Child Welfare Movement in England, 1898–1918* (London: Tavistock, 1987).

Edwards, G., Russell, M. A. H., Hawks, D., and Macafferty, M., *Alcohol Dependence and Smoking Behaviour* (Farnborough: Saxon House and Lexington Books, 1976).

——— and Orford, J., 'A Plain Treatment for Alcoholism', *Proceedings of the Royal Society of Medicine*, 70 (1977), 344–8.

——— and Anderson, P., Babor, T. F., et al., *Alcohol Policy and the Public Good* (Oxford: Oxford University Press, 1994).

Elliot, R., ' "Destructive but Sweet": Cigarette Smoking among Women, 1890–1990', PhD thesis, University of Glasgow, 2001.

——— *Women and Smoking in Britain 1890–2000* (Abingdon: Routledge, forthcoming).

Emery, F. E., Hilgendorf, E. L., and. Irving, B. L., *The Psychological Dynamics of Smoking. Tobacco Research Council Research Paper Number 10* (London: TRC, 1968).

ESRC, *SSRC/ESRC—The First Forty Years* (London: ESRC, 2005).

Eyler, J., *Sir Arthur Newsholme and State Medicine, 1885–1935* (Cambridge: Cambridge University Press, 1997).

Eysenck, H. J., *Smoking, Health and Personality* (London: Weidenfeld and Nicolson, [1965]).

Fanu, J. Le, *The Rise and Fall of Modern Medicine* (London: Little, Brown, 1999).

Fee, E., and Morman, E. T., 'Doing History, Making Revolution: The Aspirations of Henry E. Sigerist and George Rosen', in R. Porter and D. Porter (eds.), *Doctors, Politics and Society: Historical Essays* (Amsterdam: Clio Medica, 1993), 275–311.

Fendley, A., *Commercial Break. The Inside Story of Saatchi and Saatchi* (London: Hamish Hamilton, 1995).

Ferno, Ove, 'Conversation with Ove Ferno', *Addiction*, 89(10) (1994), 1215–26.

Fisher, J. B., *R. A. Fisher: The Life of a Scientist* (New York: Wiley, 1978).

Fisher, R. A., 'Dangers of Cigarette Smoking', *British Medical Journal*, 2 (1957), 43.
_____ 'Alleged Dangers of Cigarette Smoking', *British Medical Journal*, 2(1957), 297–98.
_____ 'Lung Cancer and Cigarettes', *Nature*, 182 (1958), 108.
_____ 'Cancer and Smoking', *Nature*, 182 (1958), 596.
_____ *Smoking, the Cancer Controversy: Some Attempts to Assess the Evidence* (Edinburgh, 1959).
Fitzpatrick, M., *The Tyranny of Health: Doctors and the Regulation of Lifestyle* (London: Routledge, 2001).
_____ 'Take Two Aspirins and Thank Your Caring PM', *Times Higher*, 19–26 December 2003, 28–9.
Fleming, P. J., Blair, P. S., Bacon, C., et al, 'Environment of Infants during Sleep and Risk of Sudden Infant Death Syndrome: Results of a 1993–5 Case Control Study for Confidential Enquiry into Stillbirth and Death in Infancy', *British Medical Journal*, 313 (1996), 191–4.
Fletcher, C., *Common Sense about Smoking* (London: Penguin, 1963).
_____ 'Conversation with Charles Fletcher', *British Journal of Addiction*, 87(4) (1992), 527–38.
_____ 'The Story of the Reports on Smoking and Health of the Royal College of Physicians', in S. Lock, L. Reynolds, and E. M. Tansey (eds.), *Ashes to Ashes: The History of Smoking and Health* (Amsterdam: Rodopi, 1998), 203.
Florin, D. A., 'How Does Science Influence Policy? Health Promotion for Coronary Heart Disease by General Practitioners', MD thesis, University of London, 1997.
Freeman, J., and Johnson, V., *Waves of Protest: Social Movements Since the Sixties* (Lanham, MD: Rowman and Littlefield, 1999).
Froggatt, P., 'Determinants of Policy on Smoking and Health', *International Journal of Epidemiology*, 18(1) (1989), 1–9.
_____ and Wald, N. J., 'The Role of Nicotine in the Tar Reduction Programme', in N. Wald and P. Froggatt (eds.), *Nicotine, Smoking and the Low Tar Programme* (Oxford: Oxford University Press, 1989), 229–35.
Gilmore, A., and McKee, M., 'Tobacco Control Policy in the European Union', in E. Feldman and R. Bayer (eds.), *Unfiltered. Conflicts over Tobacco Policy and Public Health* (Cambridge, MA: Harvard University Press, 2004), 219–54.
Gilmore, A., Radu-Loghin, C., Zatushevski, I., and McKee, M., 'Pushing up Smoking Incidence: Plans for a Privatised Tobacco Industry in Moldova', *Lancet*, 365 (2005), 1354–9.
Glantz, S. A., Slade, J., Bero, L. A., Hanauer, P., and Barnes, D. E., *The Cigarette Papers* (Berkeley: University of California Press, 1996).
Glennerster, H., *British Social Policy since 1945* (Oxford: Blackwell, 1995).
Goldstein, A., *Addiction. From Biology to Drug Policy*, 2nd edn (Oxford: Oxford University Press, 2001).

Goodman, J., *Tobacco in History. The Cultures of Dependence* (London: Routledge, 1993).

Graham, H., 'Smoking in Pregnancy: The Attitudes of Expectant Mothers', *Social Science and Medicine*, 10 (1976), 371–82.

——— 'Women's Smoking and Family Health', *Social Science and Medicine*, 25 (1987), 47–56.

Grant, M., *Propaganda and the Role of the State in Inter-war Britain* (Oxford: Oxford University Press, 1995).

Gray, A., 'The Decline of Infectious Diseases: The Case of England', in A. Gray (ed.), *World Health and Disease*, Health and Disease series, Book 3 (Milton Keynes: Open University Press, 1993).

Gummett, P., *Scientists in Whitehall* (Manchester: Manchester University Press, 1980).

Hamlin, C., *Public Health and Social Justice in the Age of Chadwick. Britain, 1800–1854* (Cambridge: Cambridge University Press, 1998).

Harrison, B., *Drink and the Victorians. The Temperance Question in England, 1815–1872* (London: Faber and Faber, 1971).

HEA (later HDA, now NICE), *Smoking and Smoking Related Diseases. Proceedings of a Seminar held 3–5 December 1980, NHS Training and Studies Centre, Harrogate* (Manchester: Unit for Continuing Education Department of Community Medicine, University of Manchester).

——— *Pipe and Cigar Smoking. Report of an Expert Group, 1973.*

Healy, D., *The Psychopharmacologists* (London: Altman, 1996).

Heggie, V., 'Reimagining the Healthy Social Body; Medicine, Welfare and Health Reform in Manchester, 1880–1910', PhD thesis, University of Manchester, 2005.

Higgs, E., 'Medical Statistics, Patronage and the State: The Development of the MRC Statistical Unit, 1911–1948', *Medical History*, 44 (2000), 323–40.

Hilgartner, S., *Science on Stage. Expert Advice as Public Drama* (Stanford: Stanford University Press, 2000).

Hilton, M., ' "Tabs", "Fags", and the "Boy Labour Problem" in Late Victorian and Edwardian Britain', *Journal of Social History*, 28 (1995), 587–607.

——— 'Constructing Tobacco: Perspectives on Consumer Culture in Britain, 1850–1950', PhD thesis, University of Lancaster, 1996.

——— *Smoking in Popular British Culture, 1800–2000* (Manchester: Manchester University Press, 2000).

——— *Consumerism in Twentieth Century Britain. The Search for a Historical Movement* (Cambridge: Cambridge University Press, 2003).

——— 'Smoking and Sociability', in S. Gilman and Z. Xun (eds.), *Smoke. A Global History of Smoking* (London: Reaktion Books, 2004), 126–33.

——— and Nightingale, S., ' "A Microbe of the Devil's Own Make": Religion and Science in the British Anti-Tobacco Movement, 1853–1908', in S. Lock, L. Reynolds, and E. M. Tansey (eds.), *Ashes to Ashes: The History of Smoking and Health* (Amsterdam: Rodopi, 1998), 41–77.

Hirayama, T., 'Non Smoking Wives of Heavy Smokers Have a Higher Risk of Lung Cancer: A Study from Japan', *British Medical Journal,* 282 (1981), 183–5.

Holland, W. W., 'A Dubious Future for Public Health?', *Journal of the Royal Society of Medicine,* 95 (2002), 182–8.

_____ and Stewart, S., *Public Health, the Vision and the Challenge* (London: Nuffield Provincial Hospitals Trust, 1998).

_____ and Wood, R., 'Policies on Prevention: The Hazards of Politics', *Proceedings of the Royal College of Physicians of Edinburgh,* 25 (1995), 189–203.

Hughes, J., 'The Nature of Addiction: The Pharmacological Approach', in V. Berridge (ed.), *Drugs Research and Policy in Britain. A Review of the 1980s* (Aldershot: Avebury, 1990), 237–59.

Hunter, D. J., *Public Health Policy* (Cambridge: Polity Press, 2003).

_____ 'Public Health Policy', in J. Orme, J. Powell, P. Taylor, T. Harrison, and G. Buckingham (eds.), *Public Health for the Twenty-First Century* (Maidenhead: Open University Press, 2003).

Hunter, R. B., *Smoking and Health. The Philosophy of the Committee. Paper Presented to the Royal College of Physicians, Edinburgh, 21 April 1976* and reprinted as a pamphlet.

Jackson, M., 'Cleansing the Air and Promoting Health. The Politics of Pollution in Post War Britain', in V. Berridge and K. Loughlin (eds.), *Medicine, the Market and the Mass Media. Producing Health in the Twentieth Century* (Abingdon: Routledge, 2005), 221–43

Jackson, P. W., 'Passive Smoking and Ill Health: Practice and Process in the Production of Medical Knowledge', *Sociology of Health and Illness,* 16 (1994), 423–7.

_____ 'The Case of Passive Smoking', in R. Bunton, S. Nettleton, and R. Burrows (eds.), *The Sociology of Health Promotion. Critical Analyses of Consumption, Lifestyle and Risk* (London: Routledge, 1995).

Jacobson, B., *The Ladykillers: Why Smoking is a Feminist Issue* (London: Pluto Press, 1981).

_____ and Amos, A., *When Smoke Gets in your Eyes: Cigarette Advertising Policy and Coverage of Smoking and Health in Women's Magazines* (London: HEC and BMA Professional Division, 1985).

Jarvis, M. J., and Russell, M. A. H., 'Comment on the Hunter Committee's Second Report', *British Medical Journal,* 280 (1980), 994–5.

_____ _____ Feyerabend, C., Eiser, J. R., Morgan, H., Gammage, P, and Gray, E. M., 'Passive Exposure to Tobacco Smoke: Saliva Cotinine Concentrations in a Representative Population Sample of Non Smoking Schoolchildren', *British Medical Journal,* 291 (1985), 927–9.

_____ Raw, M., Russell, M. A., and Feyerabend, C., 'Randomized Controlled Trial of Nicotine Chewing Gum', *British Medical Journal,* 285 (1982), 537–40.

Jefferys, M., 'Social Medicine and Medical Sociology, 1950–1970: The Testimony of a Partisan Participant', in D. Porter (ed.), *Social Medicine and Medical Sociology in the Twentieth Century* (Amsterdam: Rodopi, 1997), 120–36.

——— and Westaway, W. R., ' "Catch Them Before They Start!" ' A Report on an Attempt to Influence Children's Smoking Habits', *Health Education Journal*, 19 (1961), 3–17.

Johnston, L., 'Cure of Tobacco Smoking', *Lancet*, 2 (1952), 480–2.

Jones, G., *Social Hygiene in Twentieth Century Britain* (London: Croom Helm, 1986).

Kandiah, M. D., 'Television Enters British Politics: The Conservative Party's Central Office and Political Broadcasting, 1945–55', *Historical Journal of Film, Television and Radio*, 15 (1995), 265–84.

Kerr, N., *Inebriety* (London: H. K. Lewis, 1888).

Kitzinger, J., 'Resisting the Message: The Extent and Limits of Media Influence', in D. Miller, J. Kitzinger, K. Williams, and P. Beharrel (eds.), *The Circuit of Mass Communication* (London: Sage, 1998), 192–212.

Knowlton, L., 'Investigating Addiction Responses and Relapses', *Psychiatric Times*, 18(2) (2001), <http://www.psychiatrictimes.com>, accessed 2 August 2006.

Kogan, M., and Henkel, M., *Government and Research. The Rothschild Experiment in a Government Department* (London: Heinemann Educational Books, 1983).

Lee, P., *Environmental Tobacco Smoke and Mortality. A Detailed Review of Epidemiological Evidence Relating Environmental Tobacco Smoke to the Risk of Cancer, Health Disease, and Other Causes of Death in Adults Who Have Never Smoked* (Basel: Karger, 1992).

Leedham, W., and Godfrey, C., 'Tax Policy and Budget Decisions', in A. Maynard and P. Tether (eds.), *Preventing Alcohol and Tobacco Problems, vol. i, The Addictions Market* (Aldershot: Avebury, 1990), 96–132.

Levene, A., Powell, M., and Stewart, J., 'Patterns of Municipal Health Expenditure in Interwar England and Wales', *Bulletin of the History of Medicine*, 78, 3 (2004), 635–69.

Levine, H., 'The Discovery of Addiction. Changing Conceptions of Habitual Drunkenness in America', *Journal of Studies on Alcohol*, 39 (1978), 143–74 .

Lewis, J., *The Politics of Motherhood. Child and Maternal Welfare in England, 1900–1939* (London: Croom Helm, 1980).

——— *What Price Community Medicine? The Philosophy, Practice and Politics of Public Health since 1919* (Brighton: Harvester/Wheatsheaf, 1986).

——— 'The Origins and Development of Public Health in the U.K.', in W. W. Holland et al. (eds.), *The Oxford Textbook of Public Health*, 2nd edn (Oxford: Oxford University Press, 1991), 23–33.

Loughlin, K., ' "Your Life in Their Hands": The Context of a Medical–Media Controversy', *Media History*, 6 (2000), 177–88.

Loughlin, K., 'Networks of Mass Communication: Reporting Science, Health and Medicine in the 1950s and 1960s', in V. Berridge (ed.), *Making Health Policy. Networks in Research and Policy after 1945* (Amsterdam: Rodopi, 2005), 295–322.

—— 'Publicity as Policy: The Changing Role of Press and Public Relations at the BMA, 1940s–1980s', in V. Berridge (ed.), *Making Health Policy. Networks in Research and Policy after 1945* (Amsterdam: Rodopi, 2005), 275–94.

—— 'Spectacle and Secrecy: Press Coverage of Conjoined Twins in 1950s Britain', *Medical History,* 49 (2005), 197–212.

McKennell, A. C., *A Comparison of Two Smoking Typologies. Tobacco Research Council Research Paper Number 12* (London: TRC, 1973).

—— and Thomas, R. K., *Adults' and Adolescents' Smoking Habits and Attitudes,* Government social survey 353/B (London: HMSO, 1967).

McKeown, T., *The Role of Medicine: Dream, Mirage or Nemesis?* (London: Nuffield Provincial Hospitals Trust, 1976).

—— and Record, R. G., 'Reasons for the Decline of Mortality in England and Wales during the Nineteenth Century', *Population Studies,* 16 (1962), 94–122.

McLaurin, S., and Smith, D. F., 'Professional Strategies of Medical Officers of Health in the Post-war Period—2: "Progressive Realism": The Case of Dr R. J. Donaldson, MoH for Teesside, 1968–1974', *Journal of Public Health Medicine,* 24(2) (2002), 130–5.

Macmillan, H., *The Macmillan Diaries. The Cabinet Years, 1950–1957*, ed. P. Catterall (London: Macmillan, 2003).

McPherson, K., and Coleman, D., 'Health', in A. H. Halsey (ed.), *British Social Trends since 1900. A Guide to the Changing Social Structure of Britain,* 2nd edn (Basingstoke: Macmillan, 1988), 398–461.

Magnello, E., and Hardy, A. (eds.), *The Road to Medical Statistics* (Amsterdam: Rodopi, 2002).

Mandall, S., *Tobacco Industry Efforts to Influence the 2001 Tobacco Products Directive*, LSHTM MSc student project, 2006.

Marks, H. M., *The Progress of Experiment. Science and Therapeutic Reform in the United States, 1900–1990* (Cambridge: Cambridge University Press, 1997).

Marsh, A., *The Dying of the Light. Smoke Free Europe: 7* (WHO Euro and BMA, n.d. but *c*.late 1980s).

—— 'Smoking: Habit or Choice?', *Population Trends* (autumn 1984), 14–20.

—— and McKay, S., *Poor Smokers* (London: Policy Studies Institute, 1994).

Marsh, D., and Rhodes, R. A. W. (eds.), *Policy Networks in British Government* (Oxford: Clarendon Press, 1992).

Matthews, J. Rosser, *Quantification and the Quest for Medical Certainty* (Princeton: Princeton University Press, 1995).

Merriman, R.J., *Attitudes towards Smoking: Indications for Further Research: Report of the Panel on Attitudes towards Smoking (Subcommittee of the Joint MRC/SSRC Committee on Research into Smoking)* (London: SSRC, 1981).

Miller, P., and Rose, N., 'The Tavistock Programme: The Government of Subjectivity and Social Life', *Sociology*, 22 (1988), 171–92.

Morris, J. N., 'Coronary Thrombosis: A Modern Epidemic', *The Listener*, 8 December 1955, 995–6.

——— *Uses of Epidemiology* (Edinburgh: Livingstone, 1957).

——— and Titmuss, R. M., 'Epidemiology of Juvenile Rheumatism', *Lancet*, II (1942), 59–63.

——— Heady, J. A., Raffle, P. A. B., Roberts, C. G., and Parks, J. W., 'Coronary Heart Disease and Physical Activity of Work', *Lancet*, II (1953), 1053–7, 1111–20.

Moss, L., *The Government Social Survey. A History* (London: HMSO, 1991).

Murard, L., 'Atlantic Crossings in the Measurement of Health; from U.S. Appraisal Forms to the League of Nations' Health Indices', in V. Berridge and K. Loughlin (eds.), *Medicine, the Market and the Mass Media. Producing Health in the Twentieth Century* (Abingdon: Routledge, 2005), 19–54.

Murphy, S., 'The Early Days of the MRC Social Medicine Research Unit', *Social History of Medicine*, 12(3) (1999), 389–406.

——— and Smith, G. Davey, 'The British Journal of Social Medicine: What Was in a Name?', *Journal of Epidemiology and Community Health*, 51 (1997), 2–8.

Nabarro, G., *Exploits of a Politician* (London: Arthur Barker, 1973).

Naidoo, J., and Wills, J., *Health Promotion. Foundations for Practice* (London: Bailliere Tindall, 1994).

Nathanson, C., 'Social Movements as Catalysts for Policy Change: The Case of Smoking and Guns', *Journal of Health Politics, Policy and Law*, 24(3) (1999), 421–88.

Ness, A. R., Reynolds, L. A., and Tansey, E. M. (eds.), *Population-Based Research in South Wales: The MRC Pneumoconiosis Research Unit and the MRC Epidemiology Unit*, Wellcome Witness seminars, vol. xiii (London: Wellcome Trust Centre for the History of Medicine at UCL, 2002).

Nicol, A., *The Social Sciences Arrive* (London: ESRC, 2001).

Oakley, A., 'Smoking in Pregnancy: Smokescreen or Risk Factor?', *Sociology of Health and Illness*, 11 (1989), 311–35.

——— 'Making Medicine Social: The Case of the Dog with Two Bent Legs', in D. Porter (ed.), *Social Medicine and Medical Sociology in the Twentieth Century* (Amsterdam: Rodopi, 1997), 81–96.

Obelkevich, J., 'Consumption', in J. Obelkevich and P. Catterall (eds.), *Understanding Post War British Society* (London: Routledge and Kegan Paul, 1994), 141–54.

Obelkevich, J., Review of A. Marwick, *The Sixties: Cultural Revolution in Britain, France, Italy, and the United States, c.1958–c.1974* (Oxford: Oxford University Press, 1998), *Twentieth Century British History*, 11 (2000), 333–6.

Owen, D., *Personally Speaking to Kenneth Harris* (London: Weidenfeld and Nicolson, 1987).

Packard, V., *The Hidden Persuaders*. (London: Longmans, Green, 1957).

——— *The Hidden Persuaders* (London: Penguin, 1960).

Palladino, P., 'Discourses of Smoking, Health, and the Just Society: Yesterday, Today, and the Return of the Same?', *Social History of Medicine*, 14 (2001), 313–35.

Parascandola, M., 'Cigarettes and the US Public Health Service in the 1950s', *American Journal of Public Health*, 91 (2001), 196–205.

——— 'Skepticism, Statistical Methods and the Cigarette', *Perspectives in Medicine and Biology*, 47 (2004), 246–61.

——— 'What Is an Epidemiologist? Biostatistics and Epidemiology at the National Cancer Institute', unpublished manuscript.

Parker, R., 'The Struggle for Clean Air', in P. Hall, H. Land, R. Parker, and A. Webb (eds.), *Change, Choice and Conflict in Social Policy* (London, 1975; repr. Aldershot: Gower, 1988), 371–409.

——— 'Comment and Oral History in the Transcript of the Witness Seminar on the Smog of 1952', in V. Berridge and S. Taylor (eds.), *The Big Smoke: Fifty Years after the 1952 London Smog* (London: Centre for History in Public Health, 2005), accessed at <http://www.lshtm.ac.uk/history>.

'Passive Smoking at Work', *British Medical Journal*, 297 (1988), 1565.

Pearson, G., *Hooligan. A History of Respectable Fears* (Basingstoke: Macmillan, 1983).

Peston, M. H., 'Economics of Cigarette Smoking', in R. G. Richardson (ed.), *The Second World Conference on Smoking and Health* (London: HEC/Pitman Medical, 1971), 100–10.

Peterson, A. R., and Lupton, D., *The New Public Health. Health and Self in the Age of Risk* (London: Sage, 1996).

Peto, J., 'Price and Consumption of Cigarettes; a Case for Intervention?', *British Journal of Social and Preventive Medicine*, 28 (1974), 241–5.

Phillips, M., ' "Curb smoking" Call Unheeded', *Guardian*, 6 May 1980.

Pollock, D., *Denial and Delay. The Political History of Smoking and Health, 1951–1964: Scientists, Government and Industry as Seen in the Papers at the Public Records* [sic] *Office* (London: ASH, 1999).

Porter, D., 'Changing Disciplines: John Ryle and the Making of Social Medicine in Britain in the 1940s', *History of Science*, 30 (1992), 137–64.

——— (ed.), *The History of Public Health and the Modern State* (Amsterdam: Rodopi, 1994).

——— (ed.), *Social Medicine and Medical Sociology in the Twentieth Century* (Amsterdam: Rodopi, 1997).

_____ *Health, Civilization and the State* (London: Routledge, 1999).

_____ 'From Social Structure to Social Behaviour in Britain after the Second World War', in. V. Berridge and S. Blume (eds.), *Poor Health. Social Inequality before and after the Black Report* (London: Frank Cass, 2003), 58–80.

Porter, R., 'The Drinking Man's Disease: The "Pre-history" of Alcoholism in Georgian Britain', *British Journal of Addiction*, 80 (1985), 383–96.

Pringle, P., *Dirty Business. Big Tobacco at the Bar of Justice* (London: Aurum Press, 1998).

Proctor, C., *Sometimes a Cigarette is Just a Cigarette* (London: Sinclair-Stevenson, 2003).

Proctor, R., *The Nazi War on Cancer* (Princeton, NJ: Princeton University Press, 1999).

Quirke, V., 'From Evidence to Market: Alfred Spinks's 1953 Survey of New Fields for Pharmacological Research, and the Origins of ICI's Cardio-vascular Programme', in V. Berridge and K. Loughlin (eds.), *Medicine, the Market and the Mass Media. Producing Health in the Twentieth Century* (Abingdon: Routledge, 2005), 146–71.

Raw, M., *Regulating Nicotine Delivery Systems: Harm Reduction and the Prevention of Smoking Related Disease* (London: Health Education Authority, 1997).

_____ Jarvis, M. J., Feyerabend, C., and Russell, M. A. H., 'Comparison of Nicotine Chewing Gum and Psychological Treatment for Dependent Smokers', *British Medical Journal*, 16 August 1980, 481–2.

_____ and Edwards, G., 'The Tobacco Habit as Drug Dependence', *British Journal of Addiction*, 86(5) (1991), 483–4.

_____ White, P., and McNeill, A., *Clearing the Air. A Guide for Action on Tobacco* (London: BMA/WHO, 1990).

Read, M., 'The Politics of Tobacco', PhD thesis, University of Essex, 1989.

_____ 'Policy Networks and Issue Networks. The Politics of Smoking', in D. Marsh and R. A. W. Rhodes (eds.), *Policy Networks in British Government* (Oxford: Oxford University Press, 1992).

_____ *The Politics of Tobacco. Policy Networks and the Cigarette Industry* (Aldershot: Ashgate, 1996).

Reisman, D., *Richard Titmuss: Welfare and Society* (London: Heinemann, 1977).

Reynolds, L. A., and Tansey, E. M. (eds.), *Cholesterol, Atherosclerosis and Coronary Disease in the UK, 1950–2000*, Wellcome Witnesses to Twentieth Century Medicine, vol. xxvii (London: Wellcome Trust Centre for the History of Medicine at UCL, 2006).

Richardson, R. G., *The Second World Conference on Smoking and Health. Conference Organized by the Health Education Council Held at Imperial College, 20–24 September 1971* (London: Pitman Medical HEC, 1971).

Riley, D., *War in the Nursery: Theories of the Child and Mother* (London: Virago, 1983).

Roberts, J., 'Economic Evaluation of Health Care : A Survey', *British Journal of Social and Preventive Medicine*, 28 (1974), 210–16.

Roemer, M. I., 'Henry Ernest Sigerist: Internationalist of Social Medicine', *Journal of the History of Medicine and Allied Sciences*, 13 (1958), 229–43.

Room, R., 'The World Health Organisation and Alcohol Control', *British Journal of Addiction*, 79 (1984), 85–92.

Rosenberg, C., *The Cholera Years: The United States in 1832, 1849, and 1866* (Chicago: University of Chicago Press, 1962).

Rosner, D., and Markowitz, G., *Are We Ready? Public Health since 9/11* (Berkeley: University of California Press, 2006).

Roth, D., 'The Scientific Basis of Epidemiology; An Historical and Philosophical Enquiry', PhD thesis, University of California at Berkeley, 1976.

Rothman, D. J., 'Serving Clio and Client: The Historian as Expert Witness', *Bulletin of the History of Medicine*, 77 (2003), 25–44.

Rothstein, W. G., *Public Health and the Risk Factor: A History of an Uneven Medical Revolution* (Rochester: University of Rochester Press, 2003).

Russell, M A. H., 'Cigarette Dependence: I, Nature and Classification', *British Medical Journal*, 21 (1971), 330–1.

——'Changes in Cigarette Price and Consumption by Men in Britain 1946–71: A Preliminary Analysis', *British Journal of Social and Preventive Medicine*, 27 (1973), 1–7.

——Reply to criticism by the epidemiologist Richard Peto, *British Medical Journal*, 285 (1982), 507.

——'Nicotine Use after the Year 2000', *Lancet*, 337 (1991), 1191–2.

——Cole, P. V., and Brown, E., 'Absorption by Non-smokers of Carbon Monoxide from Room Air Polluted by Tobacco Smoke', *Lancet*, 1 (1973), 576.

——Wilson, C., Patel, U. A., Feyerabend, C., and Cole P. V., 'Plasma Nicotine Levels after Smoking Cigarettes with High, Medium and Low Nicotine Levels', *British Medical Journal*, 2 (1975), 414–16.

—— ——Taylor, C., Baker, C. D., 'Effect of General Practitioners' Advice against Smoking', *British Medical Journal*, 2 (1979), 231–5.

Sellers, C., 'Worrying about the Water: Sprawl, Public Health and Environmentalism in Post World War Two Long Island', seminar paper at LSHTM 7 April 2006.

Sharpe, L. J., 'Government as Clients for Social Science Research', in M. Bulmer (ed.), *Social Policy Research* (Basingstoke: Macmillan, 1978).

Sheail, J., *An Environmental History of Twentieth Century Britain* (Basingstoke: Palgrave, 2002).

Sheard, S., and Donaldson, Sir L., *The Nation's Doctor. The Role of the Chief Medical Officer, 1855–1998* (Oxford: Radcliffe, 2005).

Shepherd, R., *Ian Macleod* (London: Hutchinson, 1994).

Simpson, D., 'ASH: Witness on Smoking', in S. Lock, L. Reynolds, and E. Tansey (eds.), *Ashes to Ashes: The History of Smoking and Health* (Amsterdam: Rodopi, 1998), 209.

Smee, C., *Effect of Tobacco Advertising on Tobacco Consumption: A Discussion Document Reviewing the Evidence* (Economic and Operational Research Division: Department of Health, 1992).

Smith, C., 'Networks of Influence: The Social Sciences in the UK since the War', in P. Wagner, C. Weiss, B. Wittrock, and H. Wollman (eds.), *Social Sciences and Modern States. National Experiences and Theoretical Cross Roads* (Cambridge: Cambridge University Press, 1991), 131–47.

Smith, D. F., 'The Social Construction of Dietary Standards: The British Medical Association–Ministry of Health Advisory Committee on Nutrition Report of 1934', in D. Maurer and J. Sobal (eds.), *Eating Agendas: Food and Nutrition as Social Problems* (New York: Aldine De Gruyter, 1995), 279–303.

Smith, G., 'The Rise of the "New Consumerism" in Health and Medicine in Britain, c.1948–1989', in J. Burr and P. Nicolson (eds.), *Researching Health Care Consumers* (Basingstoke: Palgrave/Macmillan, 2005), 13–38.

Smith, G. Davey, Strobele, S. A., Eggar, M., 'Smoking and Health Promotion in Nazi Germany', *Journal of Epidemiology and Community Health*, 48 (1994), 220–3.

Smith R., *Working Paper no 66. The National Politics of Alcohol Education: A Review* (Bristol: School of Advanced Urban Studies, 1987).

'Smoking, Pregnancy and Publicity', *Nature*, 245, (1973).

Stewart, J., *'The Battle for Health'. A Political History of the Socialist Medical Association, 1930–51* (Aldershot: Ashgate, 1999).

Stimson, G., 'Research on British Drug Policy', in V. Berridge (ed.), *Drugs Research and Policy in Britain. A Review of the 1980s* (Aldershot: Avebury, 1990), 260–81.

_____ and Lart, R., 'The Relationship between the State and Local Practice in the Development of National Policy on Drugs between 1920 and 1990', in J. Strang and M. Gossop (eds.), *Heroin Addiction and the British System. Treatment and Policy Responses. vol. ii* (Abingdon: Routledge, 2005), 177–86.

Stirling, H. F., Handley, J. E., Hobbs, A. W., 'Passive Smoking in Utero: Its Effect on Neonatal Appearance', *British Medical Journal*, 295 (1987), 627–8.

Swann, C., and Froggatt, Sir P., *The Tobacco Products Research Trust, 1982–1996* (London: RSM Press, 1996).

Szreter, S., 'The Importance of Social Intervention in Britain's Mortality Decline, c. 1850–1914: A Reinterpretation of the Role of Public Health', *Social History of Medicine*, 1(1) (1988), 1–37.

Talley, C., Kushner, H. I., and Sterk, C. E., 'Lung Cancer, Chronic Disease Epidemiology, and Medicine, 1948–1964', *Journal of the History of Medicine and Allied Sciences*, 59 (2004), 329–74.

Tansey, E. M., Catterall, P. P., Christie, D. A., Willhoft, S. V., and Reynolds, L. A. (eds.), *Technology Transfer in Britain: The Case of Monoclonal Antibodies;*

Self and Non-Self: A History of Autoimmunity; Endogenous Opiates; the Committee on Safety of Drugs, Wellcome Witnesses to Twentieth Century Medicine, vol. i (London: Wellcome Trust Centre for the History of Medicine at UCL, 1997).

Taylor, P., *Smoke Ring: The Politics of Tobacco* (London: Bodley Head, 1984).

Taylor, S., 'Remedicalising Cannabis; Science, Politics and Policy', upgrading document (LSHTM, 2006).

Teeling Smith, G., 'An Argument for Swingeing Taxation', in R. G. Richardson (ed.), *The Second World Conference on Smoking and Health. Conference Organized by the Health Education Council Held at Imperial College, 20–24 September 1971* (London: Pitman Medical HEC, 1971), 111–13.

Thom, B., *Dealing with Drink. Alcohol and Social Policy: From Treatment to Management* (London: Free Association Books, 1999).

Thomson, M., *Psychological Subjects. Identity, Culture and Health in Twentieth Century Britain* (Oxford: Oxford University Press, 2006).

Todd, G. F., *Statistics of Smoking in the United Kingdom. Tobacco Manufacturers Standing Committee, Research Paper Number 1* (London: TMSC, 1957).

——— *Reliability of Statements about Smoking Habits. Supplementary Report Tobacco Research Committee, 2A* (London: Tobacco Research Committee, 1966).

——— and Laws, J. T., *The Reliability of Statements about Smoking Habits Tobacco Manufacturers Standing Committee, Research Report Number 2* (London: TMSC, 1958).

Toon, E., 'Cancer Education in the 1950s', paper given at the NIH conference on cancer, November 2004, forthcoming in the *Bulletin of the History of Medicine*.

Townsend, J., 'Smoking and Class', *New Society*, 30 March 1978, 709–10.

Tulloch, J., 'Managing the Press in a Medium Sized European Power', in M. Bromley and H. Stephenson (eds.), *Sex, Lies and Democracy: The Press and the Public* (London: Longman, 1998), 63–83.

Tunstall, J., *The Media in Britain* (London: Constable, 1983).

Tweedale, G., *Magic Mineral to Killer Dust. Turner and Newall and the Asbestos Hazard* (Oxford: Oxford University Press, 2000).

Valverde, M., *Diseases of the Will. Alcohol and the Dilemmas of Freedom* (Cambridge: Cambridge University Press, 1998).

Walker, R. B., 'Medical Aspects of Tobacco Smoking and the Anti Tobacco Movement in Britain in the Nineteenth Century', *Medical History*, 24 (1980), 391–402.

Warren, M., *The Genesis of the Faculty of Community Medicine* (Canterbury: Centre for Health Service Studies, University of Kent, 1997).

Webb, M. Ogilvy, *The Government Explains: A Study of the Information Services* (London: Allen and Unwin, 1965).

Webster, C., 'Healthy or Hungry Thirties?', *History Workshop Journal*, 13 (1982), 110–29.

_____ 'Tobacco Smoking Addiction: A Challenge to the National Health Service', *British Journal of Addiction*, 79 (1984), 8–16.

_____ *The Health Services since the War, vol. ii: Government and Health Care. The British National Health Service 1958–1979* (London: HMSO, 1996).

_____ 'Investigating Inequalities in Health before Black,' in V. Berridge and S. Blume (eds.), *Poor Health. Social Inequality before and after the Black Report* (London: Frank Cass, 2003), 81–103.

_____ and French, J., 'The Cycle of Conflict: The History of Public Health and Health Promotion Movements', in L. Adams, M. Amos, and J. Munro (eds.), *Promoting Health. Politics and Practice* (London: Sage, 2002), 5–12.

Weeks, J., *Sex, Politics and Society. The Regulation of Sexuality since 1800* (London: Longman, 1981).

Weindling, P. (ed.), *International Health Organisations and Movements, 1918–39* (Cambridge: Cambridge University Press, 1995).

Welshman, J., 'Images of Youth: The Problem of Juvenile Smoking', *Addiction*, 91(9) (1996), 1379–86.

_____ *Municipal Medicine: Public Health in Twentieth Century Britain* (Oxford: Peter Lang, 2000).

_____ 'Ideology, Social Science and Public Policy: The Debate over Transmitted Deprivation', *Twentieth Century British History*, 16(3) (2005), 306–41.

Whelan, R., *Involuntary Action. How Voluntary is the 'Voluntary' Sector?* (London: Institute of Economic Affairs, Health and Welfare Unit, 1999).

Williams, K., *Get Me a Murder a Day!: History of Mass Communication in Britain* (London: Hodder Arnold, 1997).

Winston, B., 'The CBS Evening News, 7 April 1949: Creating an Ineffable Television Form', in J. Eldridge (ed.), *Getting the Message: News, Truth and Power* (London: Routledge, 1993), 181–208.

Worboys, M., *Spreading Germs. Disease Theories and Medical Practice in Britain, 1865–1900* (Cambridge: Cambridge University Press, 2000).

Yoshioka, A., 'Use of Randomization in the Medical Research Council's Clinical Trial of Streptomycin in Pulmonary Tuberculosis in the 1940s', *British Medical Journal*, 317 (1998), 1220–3.

Index

Tables are indicated in bold type.